D0895651

Clinical Anatomy
and Physiology

of the Visual
System

THIRD EDITION

Clinical Anatomy
and Physiology

of the Visual
System

THIRD EDITION

LEE ANN REMINGTON, OD, MS, FAAO
Professor of Optometry
Pacific University College of Optometry
Forest Grove, Oregon

ELSEVIER
BUTTERWORTH
HEINEMANN

3251 Riverport Lane
St. Louis, Missouri 63043

CLINICAL ANATOMY AND PHYSIOLOGY OF THE VISUAL SYSTEM, THIRD EDITION   ISBN: 978-1-4377-1926-0
Copyright © 2012, 2005, 1998 by Butterworth-Heinemann, an imprint of Elsevier Inc.

All rights reserved. No part of this publication may be reproduced or transmitted in any form or by any means, electronic or mechanical, including photocopy, recording, or any information storage and retrieval system, without permission in writing from the publisher.

No part of this publication may be reproduced or transmitted in any form or by any means, electronic or mechanical, including photocopying, recording, or any information storage and retrieval system, without permission in writing from the publisher. Details on how to seek permission, further information about the Publisher's permissions policies and our arrangements with organizations such as the Copyright Clearance Center and the Copyright Licensing Agency, can be found at our website: www.elsevier.com/permissions.

This book and the individual contributions contained in it are protected under copyright by the Publisher (other than as may be noted herein).

Notice

Knowledge and best practice in this field are constantly changing. As new research and experience broaden our understanding, changes in research methods, professional practices, or medical treatment may become necessary.

Practitioners and researchers must always rely on their own experience and knowledge in evaluating and using any information, methods, compounds, or experiments described herein. In using such information or methods they should be mindful of their own safety and the safety of others, including parties for whom they have a professional responsibility.

With respect to any drug or pharmaceutical products identified, readers are advised to check the most current information provided (i) on procedures featured or (ii) by the manufacturer of each product to be administered, to verify the recommended dose or formula, the method and duration of administration, and contraindications. It is the responsibility of practitioners, relying on their own experience and knowledge of their patients, to make diagnoses, to determine dosages and the best treatment for each individual patient, and to take all appropriate safety precautions.

To the fullest extent of the law, neither the Publisher nor the authors, contributors, or editors, assume any liability for any injury and/or damage to persons or property as a matter of products liability, negligence or otherwise, or from any use or operation of any methods, products, instructions, or ideas contained in the material herein.

978-1-4377-1926-0

Vice President and Publisher: Linda Duncan
Executive Editor: Kathryn Falk
Senior Developmental Editor: Christie M. Hart
Publishing Services Manager: Julie Eddy
Senior Project Manager: Andrea Campbell
Design Direction: Kim Denando

Printed in the United States of America

Last digit is the print number: 9 8 7 6 5 4

Working together to grow
libraries in developing countries

www.elsevier.com | www.bookaid.org | www.sabre.org

ELSEVIER   BOOK AID International   Sabre Foundation

QM511
R45
2012
c.4
OPTO

To Dan, Tracy, Ryan, Aaron, Angela, Isaiah, Shalane, Danielle, Taryn, Payton, and Taylor.

You bring joy to my life.

QM611
R45
2022

Preface

*C*linical Anatomy and Physiology of the Visual System was written to provide the optometry and ophthalmology student, as well as the clinician, with a single text that describes the embryology, anatomy, histology, physiology, blood supply, and innervation of the globe and ocular adnexa. The visual and pupillary pathways are covered as well. The text is fully referenced, and information gathered from historical and current literature is well documented. An overview of the visual system as well as a short review of histology and physiology is provided in the introductory chapter. Chapters 2 through 5 include the anatomy, the detailed histology, and the physiology of the structures constituting the globe. Each of the three coats of the eye—cornea-sclera, uvea, and retina—is covered in a separate chapter. Included in each is an emphasis on similarities and differences between regions within each coat and notations about layers that are continuous between structures and regions. The crystalline lens is covered in Chapter 5 and the globe is completed in Chapter 6, with descriptions of the chambers of the eye and the production and composition of the material that occupies those spaces.

In my experience, students can more easily grasp the intricacies of ocular development after gaining a comprehensive understanding of the composition of the structures; therefore, ocular embryology is covered in Chapter 7. The tissue and structures associated with and surrounding the globe are described in the next three chapters. First is a review of the bones and important foramen of the entire skull and then the detail regarding the orbital bones and connective tissue. This is followed by a chapter detailing eyelid structure and histology, including the roles that the muscles and glands have in tear film secretion and drainage. The chapter on the extraocular muscles describes movements that result from contraction of the muscles with the eye in various positions of gaze; an explanation of the clinical assessment of extraocular muscle function based on the anatomy is included.

The branches of the internal and the external carotid arteries that supply the globe and adnexa are identified in Chapter 11. The cranial nerve supply to orbital structures, including both sensory and motor pathways, is clarified in Chapter 12, with an emphasis on the clinical relevance and implications of interruptions along the pathways. Significant detail on the relationship between the structures of the visual pathway and neighboring structures and on the orientation of the fibers as they course through the cranium en route to the striate cortex is presented in Chapter 13. Examples are given of characteristic visual field defects associated with injury to various regions of the pathway. The final chapter presents the autonomic pathways to the smooth muscles of the orbit and to the lacrimal gland. The pupillary pathway is included in this chapter, as is a treatment of the more common pupillary abnormalities and the relation between the pathway and the clinical presentation. Some of the common pharmaceutical agents and their actions and pupillary effects are covered as well.

In the format used in the text, terms and names of structures are noted in bold print when they are first described or explained. The name for a structure that is more common in usage is presented first, followed by other terms by which that structure is also known. Current nomenclature tends to use the more descriptive name rather than proper nouns when identifying structures, but that is not always the case, especially when the proper name of an individual has been linked so closely historically (e.g., Schwalbe's line and Schlemm's canal).

Experienced clinicians know that the knowledge of structure and function provides a good foundation for recognizing and understanding clinical situations, conditions, diseases, and treatments. For this reason, "Clinical Comments" are included throughout the book to emphasize common clinical problems, disease processes, or abnormalities that have a basis in anatomy or physiology.

Lee Ann Remington

Acknowledgments

I have had the pleasure of interacting with many bright, engaging students during the past 25 years while teaching at Pacific University College of Optometry. Their questions, corrections, suggestions, and enthusiasm motivate me to continually improve and update my understanding of the process we call vision. I am grateful for their kindness; they make my days richer.

I am also fortunate to work with an extraordinary group of colleagues, the faculty at Pacific, who create an enjoyable environment conducive to academic growth. I am grateful to Dean Jennifer Smythe for the constant level of support she provides, and to the optometry faculty for their warm encouragement and help during this process.

I thank Seth Taylor for his diligence in assisting me in the search for pertinent literature sources. The histology photographs from the second edition were done by Neil VanderHorst, O.D., and the original line drawings included from the first edition were done by Tracey Asmus, O.D.

I am grateful to Dan, my husband and friend, for his patience, encouragement, and loving support during the months spent preparing this manuscript. I am indebted to my family for their love and support.

Christie Hart, my editor at Elsevier, has guided me with kindness and tact throughout the entire process, and for that I am grateful. Andrea Campbell, my project manager at Elsevier, competently combined the text and figures into a cohesive whole. I appreciated her thoughtful and gentle suggestions.

Contents

QM531
R45
2012

The visual system takes in information from the environment in the form of light and analyzes and interprets it. This process of sight and visual perception involves a complex system of structures, each of which is designed for a specific purpose. The organization of each structure enables it to perform its intended function.

The eye houses the elements that take in light rays and changes them to a neural signal; it is protected by its location within the bone and connective tissue framework of the orbit. The eyelids cover and protect the anterior surface of the eye and contain glands that produce the lubricating tear film. Muscles, attached to the outer coat of the eye, control and direct the globe's movement, and the muscles of both eyes are coordinated to provide binocular vision. A network of blood vessels supplies nutrients, and a complex system of nerves provides sensory and motor innervation to the eye and surrounding tissues and structures. The neural signal that carries visual information passes through a complex and intricately designed pathway within the central nervous system, enabling an accurate view of the surrounding environment. This information, evaluated by a process called visual perception, influences myriad decisions and activities.

This book examines the macroscopic and microscopic anatomy and physiology of the components in this complex system and the structures that support it.

THE EYE

ANATOMIC FEATURES

The eye is a special sense organ made up of three coats, or tunics, as follows:
1. The outer fibrous layer of connective tissue forms the cornea and sclera.
2. The middle vascular layer is composed of the iris, ciliary body, and choroid.
3. The inner neural layer is the retina.

Within this globe are three spaces: the anterior chamber, posterior chamber, and vitreous chamber. The crystalline lens is located in the region of the posterior chamber (Figure 1-1).

The outer dense connective tissue of the eye provides protection for the structures within and maintains the shape of the globe, providing resistance to the pressure of the fluids inside. The **sclera** is the opaque white of the eye and is covered by the transparent conjunctiva. The transparent **cornea** allows light rays to enter the globe and, by refraction, helps bring these light rays into focus on the retina. The region in which the transition from cornea to sclera and conjunctiva occurs is the **limbus.**

The vascular layer of the eye is the **uvea,** which is made up of three structures, each having a separate function but all are interconnected. Some of the histologic layers are continuous throughout all three structures and are derived from the same embryonic germ cell layer. The **iris** is the most anterior structure, acting as a diaphragm to regulate the amount of light entering the pupil. The two iris muscles control the shape and diameter of the pupil and are supplied by the autonomic nervous system. Continuous with the iris at its root is the **ciliary body,** which produces the components of the aqueous humor and contains the muscle that controls the shape of the lens. The posterior part of the uvea, the **choroid,** is an anastomosing network of blood vessels with a dense capillary network; it surrounds the retina and supplies nutrients to the outer retinal layers.

The neural tissue of the **retina,** by complex biochemical processes, changes light energy into a signal that can be transmitted along a neural pathway. The signal passes through the retina, exits the eye through the **optic nerve,** and is transmitted to various parts of the brain for processing.

The interior of the eye is made up of three chambers. The **anterior chamber** is bounded in front by the cornea and posteriorly by the iris and anterior surface of the lens. The **posterior chamber** lies behind the iris and surrounds the equator of the lens, separating it from the ciliary body. The anterior and posterior chambers are continuous with one another through the pupil, and both contain **aqueous humor** that is produced by the ciliary body. The aqueous humor provides nourishment for the surrounding structures, particularly the cornea and lens. The **vitreous chamber,** which is the largest space, lies adjacent to the inner retinal layer and is bounded in front by the lens. This chamber contains a gel-like substance, the **vitreous humor.**

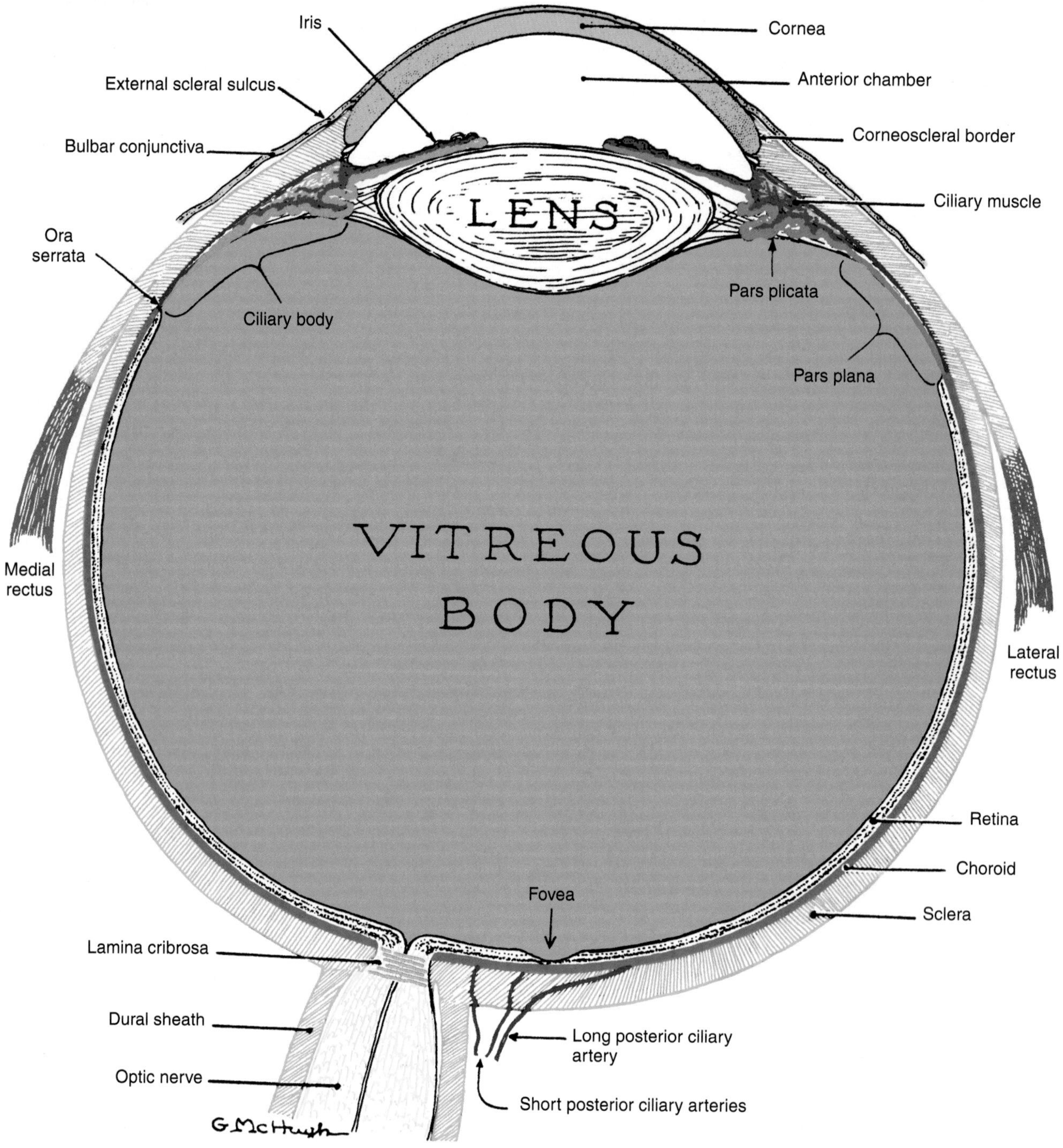

FIGURE 1-1
The visual system. (From Kronfeld PC: *The human eye*, Rochester, NY, 1943, Bausch & Lomb Press.)

The **crystalline lens** is located in the area of the posterior chamber and provides additional refractive power for accurately focusing images onto the retina. The lens must change shape to view an object that is close to the eye, through the mechanism of **accommodation.**

ANATOMIC DIRECTIONS AND PLANES

Anatomy is an exacting science, and specific terminology is basic to its discussion. The following anatomic directions should be familiar (Figure 1-2):

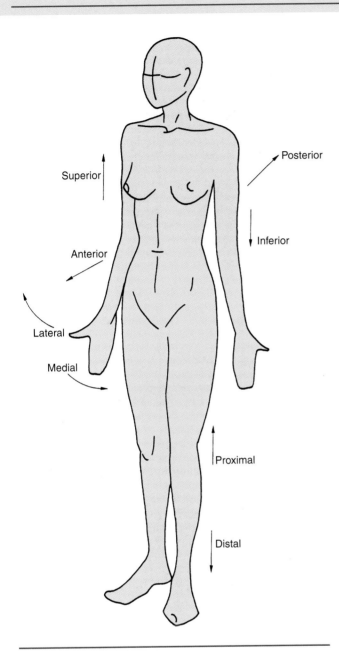

FIGURE 1-2
Anatomic directions. (From Palastanga N, Field D, Soames R: *Anatomy and human movement*, Oxford, UK, 1989, Butterworth-Heinemann.)

- Anterior, or ventral: toward the front
- Posterior, or dorsal: toward the back
- Superior, or cranial: toward the head
- Inferior, or caudal: away from the head
- Medial: toward the midline
- Lateral: away from the midline
- Proximal: near the point of origin
- Distal: away from the point of origin

The following planes are used in describing anatomic structures (Figure 1-3):

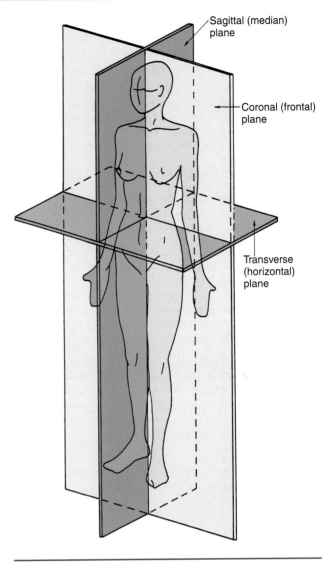

FIGURE 1-3
Anatomic planes. (From Palastanga N, Field D, Soames R: *Anatomy and human movement*, Oxford, UK, 1989, Butterworth-Heinemann.)

- Sagittal: vertical plane running from anterior to posterior locations, dividing the structure into right and left sides.
- Midsagittal: sagittal plane through the midline, dividing the structure into right and left halves.
- Coronal or frontal: vertical plane running from side to side, dividing the structure into anterior and posterior parts.
- Transverse: horizontal plane dividing the structure into superior and inferior parts.

Because the globe is a spherical structure, references to locations can sometimes be confusing. In references to **anterior** and **posterior** locations of the globe, the anterior pole (i.e., center of the cornea) is the reference point. For example, the pupil is anterior to the ciliary body (see Figure 1-1). When layers or structures are referred to as *inner* or *outer,* the reference is to the entire globe unless specified otherwise. The point of reference is the center of the globe, which would lie within the vitreous. For example, the retina is inner to the sclera (see Figure 1-1). In addition, the term *sclerad* is used to mean "toward the sclera," and *vitread* is used to mean "toward the vitreous."

REFRACTIVE CONDITIONS

If the refractive power of the optical components of the eye, primarily the cornea and lens, correlate with the distances between the cornea, lens, and retina so that incoming parallel light rays come into focus on the retina, a clear image will be seen. This condition is called **emmetropia** (Figure 1-4, *A*). No correction is necessary for clear distance vision. In **hyperopia** (farsightedness), the distance from the cornea to the retina is too short for the refractive power of the cornea and lens, thereby causing images that would come into focus behind the retina (Figure 1-4, *B*). Hyperopia can be corrected by placing a convex lens in front of the eye to increase the convergence of the incoming light rays. In **myopia** (nearsightedness), because the lens and cornea are too strong or, more likely, the eyeball is too long, parallel light rays are brought into focus in front of the retina (Figure 1-4, *C*). Myopia can be corrected by placing a concave lens in front of the eye, causing the incoming light rays to diverge.

OPHTHALMIC INSTRUMENTATION

Various instruments are used to assess the health and function of elements of the visual pathway and the supporting structures. This section briefly describes some of these instruments and the structures examined.

The curvature of the cornea is one of the factors that determine the corneal refractive power. A *keratometer* measures the curvature of the central 3 to 4 mm of the anterior corneal surface and provides information about the power and the difference in curvature between the principle meridians at that location. The smoothness of the corneal surface can also be assessed by the pattern reflected from the cornea during the measuring process. The *automated corneal topographer* maps the corneal surface and gives an indication of curvatures at selected points. This instrument is an important adjunct in the fitting of contact lenses in difficult cases.

The optometric physician can objectively determine the optical power of the eye with a set of lenses and a *retinoscope.* This instrument is beneficial also for assessing the accommodative function of the lens.

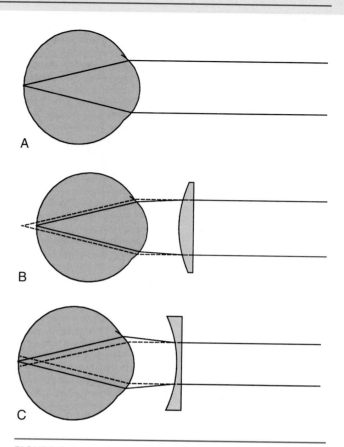

FIGURE 1-4
Refractive conditions. A, Emmetropia, in which parallel light comes to a focus on the retina. **B,** Hyperopia, in which parallel light comes to a focus behind the retina (*dotted lines*). A convex lens is used to correct the condition and bring the light rays into focus on the retina. **C,** Myopia, in which parallel light comes to a focus in front of retina (*dotted lines*). A concave lens is used to correct the condition and bring the light rays into focus on the retina. (Courtesy Karl Citek, OD, Pacific University College of Optometry, Forest Grove, Ore.)

The inside of the eye, called the **fundus**, is examined using an *ophthalmoscope,* which illuminates the interior with a bright light. The retina, optic nerve head, and blood vessels can be assessed and information about ocular and systemic health obtained. This is the only place in the body in which blood vessels can be viewed directly and noninvasively. Various systemic diseases, such as diabetes, hypertension, and arteriosclerosis, can alter ocular vessels. To obtain a more complete view of the inside of the eye, topical drugs are administered to influence the iris muscles, causing the pupil to become enlarged, or mydriatic. The *binocular indirect ophthalmoscope* allows stereoscopic viewing of the fundus.

The outside of the globe and the eyelids can be assessed with a *biomicroscope.* This combination of an illumination system and a binocular microscope allows stereoscopic views of various parts of the eye. Particularly beneficial is the view of the transparent structures, such as the cornea and lens. A number of auxiliary instruments can be used with the biomicroscope to measure intraocular pressure and to view the interior of the eye.

Technologic advances have produced instrumentation that can provide three-dimensional mapping of retinal and optic nerve head surfaces and measure the thickness of specific retinal layers. Additional instrumentation can allow visualization of corneal layers, cells, and nerves and can aid in the differentiation of bacterial, viral, parasitic, and fungal infection in corneal tissue.

The visual field is the area that a person sees when looking straight ahead, including those areas seen "out of the corner of the eye." A *perimeter* is used to test the extent, sensitivity, and completeness of this visual field. Computerized perimeters provide extremely detailed maps of the visual field, as well as statistical information on the reliability of the test and the probabilities of any defects.

BASIC HISTOLOGIC FEATURES

Because many of the anatomic structures are discussed in this book at the histologic level, this section briefly reviews basic human histology. Other details of tissues are addressed in the pertinent chapters.

All body structures are made up of one or more of the four basic tissues: epithelial, connective, muscle, and nervous tissue. A tissue is defined as a collection of similar cells that are specialized to perform a common function.

EPITHELIAL TISSUE

Epithelial tissue often takes the form of sheets of epithelial cells that either cover the external surface of a structure or that line a cavity. Epithelial cells lie on a basement membrane that attaches them to underlying connective tissue. The **basement membrane** can be divided into two parts: the **basal lamina,** secreted by the epithelial cell, and the **reticular lamina,** a product of the underlying connective tissue layer.[1] The free surface of the epithelial cell is the *apical surface,* whereas the surface that faces underlying tissue or rests on the basement membrane is the *basal surface.*

Epithelial cells are classified according to shape. Squamous cells are flat and platelike, cuboidal cells are of equal height and width, and columnar cells are higher than wide. Epithelium consisting of a single layer of cells is referred to as simple: simple squamous, simple cuboidal, or simple columnar. **Endothelium** is the special name given to the simple squamous layer that lines certain cavities. Epithelium consisting of several layers is referred to as *stratified* and is described by the shape of

the cells in the surface layer. Only the basal or deepest layer of cells is in contact with the basement membrane, and this layer usually consists of columnar cells.

Keratinized, stratified squamous epithelium has a surface layer of squamous cells with cytoplasm that has been transformed into a substance called *keratin,* a tough protective material relatively resistant to mechanical injury, bacterial invasion, and water loss. These keratinized surface cells constantly are sloughed off and are replaced from the layers below, where cell division takes place.

Glandular Epithelium

Many epithelial cells are adapted for secretion and, when gathered into groups, are referred to as *glands.* Glands can be classified according to the manner of secretion—*exocrine glands* secrete into a duct, whereas *endocrine glands* secrete directly into the bloodstream. Glands can also be classified according to the process of secretion production—*holocrine glands* secrete complete cells laden with the secretory material; *apocrine glands* secrete part of the cell cytoplasm in the secretion; and the secretion of *merocrine glands* is a product of the cell without loss of any cellular components. Glands can also be named according to the composition of their secretion: *mucous, serous,* or *sebaceous.*

CONNECTIVE TISSUE

Connective tissue provides structure and support and is a "space filler" for areas not occupied by other tissue. Connective tissue consists of cells, fibers, and ground substance. The ground substance consisting of glycoproteins and water, and the insoluble protein fibers collectively are called *matrix.* Connective tissue can be classified as *loose* or *dense.* Loose connective tissue has relatively fewer cells and fibers per area than dense connective tissue, in which the cells and fibers are tightly packed. Dense connective tissue can be characterized as *regular* or *irregular* on the basis of fiber arrangement.

Among the cells that may be found in connective tissue are *fibroblasts* (flattened cells that produce and maintain the fibers and ground substance), *macrophages* (phagocytic cells), *mast cells* (which contain heparin and histamine), and fat cells. Connective tissue composed primarily of fat cells is called *adipose tissue.*

The fibers found in connective tissue include flexible collagen fibers with high tensile strength, delicate reticular fibers, and elastic fibers, which can undergo extensive stretching. **Collagen fibers** are a major component of much of the eye's connective tissue. These fibers are composed of protein macromolecules of tropocollagen that have a coiled helix of three polypeptide chains. The individual polypeptide chains can differ in their amino acid sequences, and the tropocollagen has a banded pattern because of the sequence differences.[2] Collagen is separated into various types on the basis of such differences, and several types are components of ocular connective tissue structures.

The amorphous ground substance, in which the cells and fibers are embedded, consists of water bound to glycosaminoglycans and long-chain carbohydrates.

MUSCLE TISSUE

Muscle tissue is contractile tissue and can be classified as striated or smooth, *voluntary* or *involuntary*. **Striated muscle** has a regular pattern of light and dark bands and is subdivided into skeletal and cardiac muscle. Skeletal muscle is under voluntary control, whereas cardiac muscle is controlled involuntarily. The structure of skeletal muscle and the mechanism of its contraction are discussed in Chapter 10.

The **smooth muscle** fiber is an elongated, slender cell with a single centrally located nucleus. The tissue is under the involuntary control of the autonomic nervous system.

NERVE TISSUE

Nerve tissue contains two types of cells: **neurons,** which are specialized cells that react to a stimulus and conduct a nerve impulse, and **neuroglia,** which are cells that provide structure and metabolic support. The neuron cell body is the perikaryon, which has several cytoplasmic projections. The projections that conduct impulses *to* the cell body are **dendrites** (usually several), and the (usually single) projection that conducts impulses *away from* the cell body is an **axon. Schwann cells** encircle nerve fibers and can secrete a lipoprotein material, myelin, that then surrounds the Schwann cell covering the fiber. Nerve fibers thus are either *myelinated* or *unmyelinated;* myelinization improves impulse conduction speed.[3]

A nerve impulse passes between nerves at a specialized junction, the synapse. As the action potential reaches the presynaptic membrane of an axon, a neurotransmitter is released into the synaptic gap, triggering an excitatory or an inhibitory response in the postsynaptic membrane.

Neuroglial cells outnumber neurons by a ratio of 10 to 50:1, depending on the location.[3] Neuroglial cells include astrocytes, oligodendrocytes, and microglia. **Astrocytes** provide a framework that gives structural support and contributes to the nutrition of neurons. **Oligodendrocytes** produce myelin in the central nervous system, where there are no Schwann cells. **Microglia** possess phagocytic properties and increase in number in areas of damage or disease.[3]

BRIEF REVIEW OF HUMAN CELLULAR PHYSIOLOGY

The **cell membrane** surrounds each cell and is composed of a double layer of lipids; the hydrophobic lipid portion is in the center of the membrane and hydrophilic phosphate groups face aqueous solutions both inside and outside the cell. Cholesterol molecules found in the central fatty acid portion decrease the membrane's permeability to water soluble molecules. Protein molecules may be embedded in both surfaces of the lipid bilayer and membrane-spanning proteins have portions both inside and outside the cell.

The **cellular cytoplasm** (cytosol) contains various protein fibers: microtubules are the largest and are composed of the protein tubulin; other fibers may be tissue specific—keratin fibers in epithelium, microfilaments of actin and myosin fibers in sarcoplasm, and neurofilaments in neurons. The **cytoskeleton** is a three-dimensional scaffolding within the cytoplasm that gives the cell structure, support, and also provides intracellular transport. The **nucleus,** the control center for the cell, directs cellular function and contains most of the genetic material within its DNA, which is organized into **chromosomes.** The genes within the chromosomes are the **genome. Ribosomes,** granules of RNA within the cytoplasm, manufacture proteins as directed by the cellar DNA. The **endoplasmic reticulum (ER)** network, within the cytoplasm, provides sites for protein and lipid synthesis; smooth ER produces fatty acids, steroids, and lipids; rough ER produces proteins. **Golgi apparatus** modify and package proteins. **Mitochondria,** the power house of the cell, produce the cell's supply of energy in the form of adenosine triphosphate (ATP). The inner wall of the double-walled mitochondria is folded into cisternae, where biochemical processes produce the ATP. **Lysosomes,** intracellular digestive systems containing powerful enzymes, take up bacteria or old organelles and break them down into component molecules that are reused or reabsorbed into the cytoplasm to be transported to the cell membrane and out of the cell.

Fluid and solute transport across the cell membrane can occur passively by *diffusion* that occurs when molecules pass from a higher to a lower concentration down the concentration gradient; no energy is expended. *Channel proteins* within the cell membrane create water-filled passages linking the intracellular and extracellular spaces. A million ions per second may flow through such a channel and tens of millions of ions per second can enter or exit a cell.[4] These channels facilitate ion movement across the lipid bilayer and move ions, also without the expenditure of energy. Channels may be specific for ion type, molecule size, or charge (i.e., Na^+ channels, K^+ channels, cation channels). Channels can be gated, opening and closing in response to certain stimulants (i.e., *voltage-gated, chemical-gated, ligand-gated*). In *facilitated diffusion*, carrier proteins bind to substrates that they carry across the membrane (these are slower and selective but can carry larger molecules); they never form a direct connection between the intracellular and extracellular environments. Molecules such as glucose and amino acids are moved in this way. Active transport mechanisms use energy. *Transporters and co-transporters* move substance against the concentration gradient and need a steady supply of ATP. Transporting epithelia are polarized and the apical and basal membranes have differing properties; both often contain ion channels; however, the Na^+/K^+ *ATPase pumps* are generally located in the basolateral membranes. **Aquaporins** are bidirectional channels composed of major intrinsic proteins that specifically allow water passage but may not allow other materials to pass through the channel. Aquaporins are numerous in ocular tissues: cornea, lens, ciliary body epithelia, and retina. Membranes containing aquaporins have 100 times greater water permeability than membranes without them.[5] Aquaporins may have functions other than transport; some may regulate cell migration processes and some may have a role in neural signal transduction.[6]

Cellular metabolic functions are complex activities maintaining the viability of the cell. Amino acids, carbohydrates, and lipids are used as building blocks in the construction of cellular components or are broken down as a source of energy. Myriad biochemical pathways and processes function in cellular metabolism and are regulated by signals from either inside or outside the cell. Integrins are membrane-spanning proteins that can carry information from the extracellular matrix into the cell and activate intracellular enzymes that then influence cellular processes. Energy for metabolic processes is supplied by ATP molecules, produced either through aerobic or anaerobic metabolism; aerobic is more efficient, with 36 to 38 molecules of ATP produced per molecule of glucose; aerobic glycolysis yields 2 ATP per molecule.

INTERCELLULAR JUNCTIONS

Intercellular junctions join epithelial cells to one another and to adjacent tissue; some are named by their type and some by their shape. Protein components of intercellular junctions include cell adhesion molecules, transmembrane proteins (occludin, claudin), junctional adhesion molecules, and associated cytoplasmic proteins.[7] Junctions between cells or with connective tissue can have additional functions other than adhesion. Physical changes, such as pressure and biochemical or pharmaceutical factors, can modulate junctions and alter the junctional proteins. This allows information about changes in the extracellular environment to be relayed to the cell interior affecting intracellular processes.

In a **tight (occluding) junction**, the outer leaflet of the cell membrane of one cell comes into direct contact with its neighbor. Ridgelike elevations on the surface of the cell membrance fuse with complementary ridges on the surface of a neighboring cell.[8] As the paired strands meet, the neighboring cell membranes are fused.[9] The fibers of tight junctions are connected to the cytoskeleton within the cell.

A tight junction that forms a zone or belt around the entire cell, joining it with each of the adjacent cells is called a **zonula occludens (ZO)** (Figure 1-5). In these zones, row on row of interwining ridges effectively occlude the intercellular space. A substance cannot pass through a sheet of epithelium whose cells are joined by ZO by passing *between* the cells, but must pass *through* the cell. In stratified epithelia, whose surface layer is constantly being sloughed and replaced from below, ZO, if present, will be located in the surface layer. The components of the tight junction are found in increasing numbers as a cell moves from its origin in the basal layer until, finally when the cell reaches the surface, its occluding junction is complete.[10] The complex formed by the junctional proteins in the ZO can be affected in some diseases, causing in a breakdown in the barrier function, allowing a pathway to open through the network. Currently, researchers are developing pharmaceuticals that will cause a temporary disruption of the barrier, and that would allow other drugs or substances to pass through the intercellular route. In some instances, ridges in a tight junction are fewer and discontinuous, resulting in a "leaky epithelium."[8]

A **zonula adherens (ZA)**, an intermediate junction, is a similarly-shaped zone. However, the adjacent plasma membranes are separated, leaving a narrow intercellular space that contains a glycoporotein material causing cell adhesion but allowing intercellular passage.[12] ZA junctions produce relatively firm adhesions. Adjacent to the adhering junction are fine microfilaments that extend from a plaque just inside the membrane to filaments of the cytoskeleton, contributing to cell stability.[8] A terminal bar consists of a zonula occludens and a zonula adherens side by side, with the tight junction lying nearest the cell apex.[1,8]

Round, buttonlike intercellular junctions are either **macula occludens (MO)** or **macula adherens (MA)**, depending on the type of adhesion.

A **desmosome** is a strong, spotlike attachment between cells (see Figure 1-5). A dense disc or plaque is present within the cytoplasm adjacent to the plasma membrane at the site of the adherence. Hairpin loops of cytoplasmic filaments called tonofilaments extend from

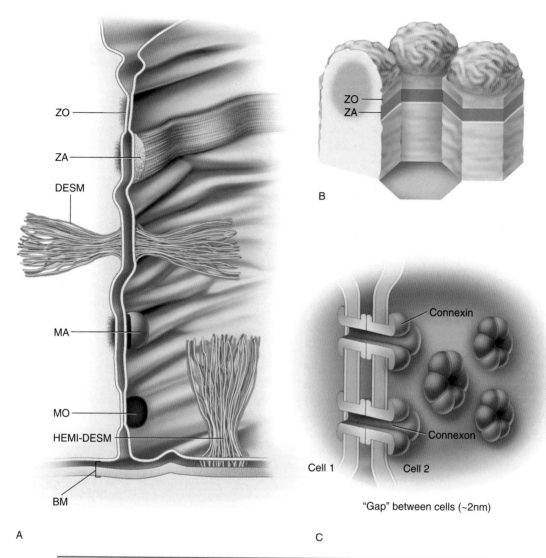

ZO

ZA

DESM

MA

MO

HEMI-DESM

BM

A

B

Connexin

Connexon

Cell 1

Cell 2

"Gap" between cells (~2nm)

C

FIGURE 1-5

Intercellular junctional complexes. A, Lateral cell membranes of adjacent cells. *ZO,* Zonula occludens, joins cells with no intercellular space present; *ZA,* zonula adherens, joins cells, membranes are not fused; *DESM,* desmosome, strong, circular junction, fibers extend into cytoplasm; *MA,* macula adherens; *MO,* macula occludens; *HEMI-DESM,* hemidesmosome, strong junction joining basal aspect of cell to its basement membrane. **B,** Adjacent ZO and ZA. **C,** Gap junctions joining two cells; six proteins (connexins) surround the central channel (connexon).

the disc into the cytoplasm and link to keratin filaments in the cytoskelton, contributing to cell stability. Other filaments, transmembrane linkers, cadherins, extend from the plaque across the intercellular space, holding the cell membranes together and forming a strong bond.[12] The intercellular space contains an acid-rich mucoprotein that acts as a strong adhesive.[8]

A **hemidesmosome** provides a strong connection between the cell and its basement membrane and underlying connective tissue. It contains similar intracellular components; the protein complex extends through the cell membrane to attach to keratin in the basement membrane. Bundles of filaments join the intracellular plaque to underlying connective tissue matrix, often attaching to a plaque embedded in the connective tissue.[10]

Gap junctions are formed by a group of (usually six) proteins, called *connexins,* that span the cell membrane and unite with connexins of a neighboring cell, forming a channel called a *connexon* (see Figure 5-1).[13] These narrow channels allow rapid cell-to-cell communication, i.e., passage of small molecules and ions from one cell to another. A group of cells with such connection act like a syncytium, that is, a single cell with multiple nuclei.

REFERENCES

1. Krause WJ, Cutts JH: Epithelium. In Krause WJ, Cutts JH, editors: *Concise text of histology*, Baltimore, 1981, Williams & Wilkins, p 27.
2. Copenhaver WM, Kelly DE, Wood RL: The connective tissues. In Copenhaver WM, Kelly DE, Wood RL, editors: *Bailey's textbook of histology*, ed 17, Baltimore, 1978, Williams & Wilkins, p 142.
3. Krause WJ, Cutts JH: Nervous tissue. In Krause WJ, Cutts JH, editors: *Concise text of histology*, Baltimore, 1981, Williams & Wilkins, p 137.
4. Mergler S, Pleyer U: The human corneal endothelium: new insights into electrophysiology and ion channels, *Prog Retin Eye Res* 26:359–378, 2007.
5. Agre P, Kozono D: Aquaporin water channels: molecular mechanisms for human diseases, *FEBS Lett* 555:72–78, 2003.
6. Verkman AS, Ruiz-Ederra J, Levin MH: Functions of aquaporins in the eye, *Prog Retin Eye Res* 27:420–433, 2008.
7. Teranishi S, Kimura K, Kawamoto K, et al: Protection of human corneal epithelial cells from hypoxia-induced disruption of barrier function by keratinocyte growth factor, *Invest Ophthalmol Vis Sci* 49:2432–2437, 2008.
8. Copenhaver WM, Kelly DE, Wood RL: Epithelium. In Copenhaver WM, Kelly DE, Wood RL, editors: *Bailey's textbook of histology*, ed 17, Baltimore, 1978, Williams & Wilkins, p 103.
9. Yoshida Y, Ban Y, Kinoshita S: Tight junction transmembrane protein claudin subtype expression and distribution in human corneal and conjunctival epithelium, *Invest Ophthalmol Vis Sci* 50:2103–2108, 2009.
10. Suzuki K, Tanaka T, Enoki M, et al: Coordinated reassembly of the basement membrane and junctional proteins during corneal epithelial wound healing, *Invest Ophthalmol Vis Sci* 41:2495–2500, 2000.
11. Delamere NA: Ciliary body and ciliary epithaliu. In Fischbarg J, editor: *The biology of the eye*, Amsterdam, The Netherlands, 2006, Elsevier, pp 127–148.
12. Fawcett DW, Jensh RP: *Bloom & Fawcett concise histology*, London, 1997, Chapman & Hall, p 19.
13. Shurman DL, Glazewski L, Gumpert A, Zieske JD, Richard G. In vivo and in vitro expression of connexins in the human corneal epithelium, *Invest Ophthalmol Vis Sci* 46:1957–1965, 2005.

CHAPTER 2

Cornea and Sclera

The outer connective tissue coat of the eye has the appearance of two joined spheres. The smaller, anterior transparent sphere is the cornea and has a radius of curvature of approximately 8 mm. The larger, posterior opaque sphere is the sclera, which has a radius of approximately 12 mm (Figure 2-1, A). The globe is not symmetric; its approximate diameters are 24 mm anteroposterior, 23 mm vertical, and 23.5 mm horizontal.[1]

CORNEA

CORNEAL DIMENSIONS

The transparent cornea appears from the front to be oval, as the sclera encroaches on the superior and inferior aspects. The anterior horizontal diameter is 12 mm, and the anterior vertical diameter is 11 mm.[1,2] If viewed from behind, the cornea appears circular, with horizontal and vertical diameters of 11.7 mm (Figure 2-1, B).[1]

In profile, the cornea has an elliptic rather than a spherical shape, the curvature being steeper in the center and flatter near the periphery. The radius of curvature of the central cornea at the anterior surface is 7.8 mm and at the posterior surface is 6.5 mm.[1,3] The central corneal thickness is 0.53 mm, whereas the corneal periphery is 0.71 mm thick (Figure 2-1, C).[1,3-5] (All values given are approximations.)

Clinical Comment: Astigmatism

ASTIGMATISM is a condition in which light rays coming from a point source are not imaged as a point. This results from the unequal refraction of light by different meridians of the refracting elements. Because it is usually elliptic in profile, the cornea contributes to astigmatism in the eye because it refracts light and helps to focus the rays onto the retina. The curvature of the surface of the cornea (central 3 to 4 mm) can be determined by keratometric measurement to give a clinical assessment of the corneal contribution to astigmatism.

Regular astigmatism occurs when the longest radius of curvature and shortest radius of curvature lie 90 degrees apart. The usual presentation occurs when the radius of curvature of the vertical meridian differs from that of the horizontal meridian. The most common situation, called **with-the-rule astigmatism** *(Figure 2-2, A), occurs when*

the steepest curvature lies in the vertical meridian. Thus the vertical meridian has the shortest radius of curvature. **Against-the-rule astigmatism** *(Figure 2-2, B) is not as common and occurs when the horizontal meridian is the steepest; the greatest refractive power is found in the horizontal meridian. If the meridians that contain the greatest differences are not along the 180- and 90-degree axes (± 30 degrees) but lie along the 45- and 135-degree axes (± 15 degrees), the astigmatism is called* **oblique.** **Irregular astigmatism** *is an uncommon finding in which the meridians corresponding to the greatest differences are not 90 degrees apart.*

In addition to the cornea, the lens is a refractive element that focuses light rays and might contribute to astigmatism. In fact, when considering the refractive condition, the tendency of with-the-rule astigmatism to convert to against-the-rule astigmatism with aging is attributable primarily to the lens, which continues to grow throughout life.

CORNEAL HISTOLOGIC FEATURES

The **cornea** is the principal refracting component of the eye. Its transparency and avascularity provide optimal light transmittance. The anterior surface of the cornea is covered by the tear film, and the posterior surface borders the aqueous-filled anterior chamber. At its periphery, the cornea is continuous with the conjunctiva and the sclera. From anterior to posterior, the five layers that compose the cornea are epithelium, Bowman's layer, stroma, Descemet's membrane, and endothelium (Figure 2-3).

Epithelium

The outermost layer of **stratified corneal epithelium** is five to seven cells thick and measures approximately 50 μm.[1,6] The epithelium thickens in the periphery and is continuous with the conjunctival epithelium at the limbus.

The surface layer of corneal epithelium is two cells thick and displays a very smooth anterior surface. It consists of *nonkeratinized* squamous cells, each of which contains a flattened nucleus and fewer cellular organelles than deeper cells. Cell size varies but a superficial cell can be 50 μm in diameter and 5 μm

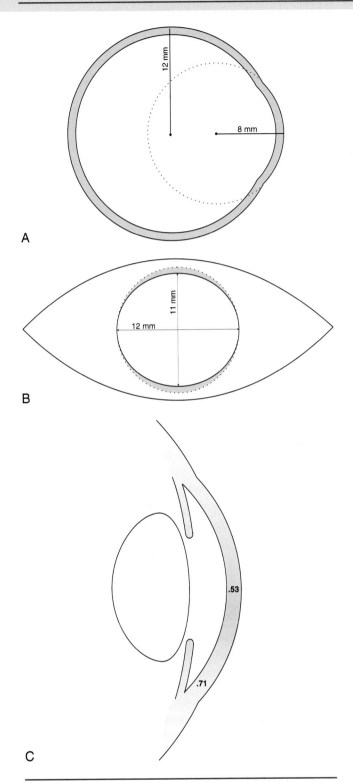

A

B

C

FIGURE 2-1
Corneal dimensions. A, Radius of curvature of cornea and sclera. **B,** View from in front of the eye. The sclera encroaches on the corneal periphery inferiorly and superiorly. Dotted lines show the extent of the cornea in the vertical dimension posteriorly. **C,** Sagittal section of cornea showing central and peripheral thickness (0.53 to 0.71 mm).

in height.[7] The plasma membrane of the surface epithelial cells secretes a **glycocalyx** component that adjoins the mucin layer of the tear film.[8-10] Many projections located on the apical surface of the outermost cells increase the surface area, thus enhancing the stability of the tear film. The fingerlike projections are *microvilli*, and the ridgelike projections are *microplicae* (Figure 2-4).

Tight junctions **(zonula occludens)** join the surface cells along their lateral walls, near the apical surface. These junctures provide a barrier to intercellular movement of substances from the tear layer and prevent the uptake of excess fluid from the tear film. A highly effective, semipermeable membrane is produced, allowing passage of fluid and molecules *through* the cells but not *between* them. Additional adhesion between the cells is provided by numerous desmosomes.

As the surface cells age, they degenerate. The cytoskeleton disassembles and the cytoplasm condenses. The cells lose their attachments and are sloughed off, being constantly replaced from the layers below. On scanning electron microscopy, the corneal surface consists of variously sized cells, ranging from small to large. The lighter cells are newer replacement cells, whereas the darker cells are those that are degenerating and will soon be sloughed.[11]

The middle layer of the corneal epithelium is made up of two to three layers of **wing cells.** These cells have winglike lateral processes, are polyhedral, and have convex anterior surfaces and concave posterior surfaces that fit over the basal cells (Figure 2-5). The diameter of a wing cell is approximately 20 μm.[7] Desmosomes and gap junctions join wing cells to each other, and desmosomes join wing cells to surface and basal cells.[12]

The innermost **basal cell layer** of the corneal epithelium is a single layer of columnar cells, with diameters ranging from 8 to 10 μm (Figure 2-6).[7] These cells contain oval-shaped nuclei displaced toward the apex and oriented at right angles to the surface. The rounded, apical surface of each cell lies adjacent to the wing cells, and the basal surface attaches to the underlying basement membrane (basal lamina). The basal cells secrete this basement membrane, which attaches the cells to the underlying tissue through hemidesmosomes. Anchoring fibrils pass from these junctions through Bowman's layer into the stroma.[13] Although less numerous here than in the wing cell layer, desmosomes and gap junctions join the columnar cells; interdigitations and desmosomes connect the basal cells with the adjacent layer of wing cells. The basal layer is the germinal layer where mitosis occurs.

The basal cells are joined to keratin filaments in the basement membrane by **hemidesmosomes.** Opposite

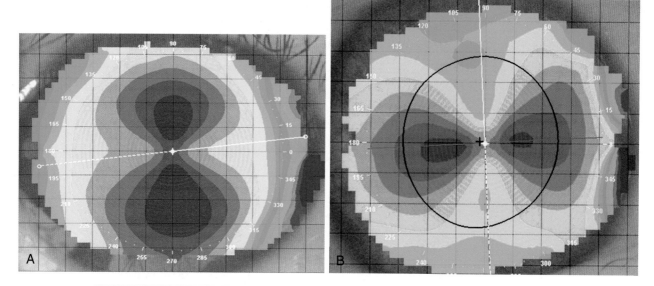

FIGURE 2-2

Corneal topography provides a map of the corneal surface curvature. A, Corneal topography demonstrating with-the-rule corneal astigmatism. **B,** Corneal topography demonstrating against-the-rule corneal astigmatism. (Courtesy Patrick Caroline, C.O.T., Pacific University College of Optometry, Forest Grove, Ore.)

the plaque, fine anchoring collagen fibrils form a complex branching and anastomosing network that runs from the basement membrane through Bowman's layer and penetrates 1.5 to 2 μm into the stroma.[13-18] The linkage between the hemidesmosome and the anchoring network is likely composed of basement membrane components.[5] The anchoring fibrils attach to anchoring laminin-containing plaques of extracellular matrix within the stroma.[16,19]

Clinical Comment: Evaluation of Corneal Surface

Fluorescein dye can be used to evaluate the barrier function of the surface layer. When instilled in the tear film, it will not penetrate the epithelial tissue as long as the zonula occludens are intact. If the tight junctions are disrupted, the dye can pass easily through Bowman's layer and into the anterior stroma. An epithelial defect will usually appear a vivid green fluorescence when viewed with the cobalt blue filter of the slit lamp.

Epithelial Replacement

Maintenance of the smooth corneal surface depends on replacement of the surface cells that are continually being shed into the tear film. This renewal of the stratified epithelium involves cell division, migration, differentiation, and senescence. Cell proliferation occurs in the basal layer. Basal cells move up to become wing cells, and wing cells move up to become surface cells. Only the cells in contact with the basement membrane have the ability to divide; the cells that are displaced into the wing cell layers lose this ability.[20] Stem cells located in a 0.5- to 1-mm-wide band around the corneal periphery are the source for renewal of the corneal basal cell layer. A slow migration of basal cells occurs from the periphery toward the center of the cornea.[21,22] Turnover time for the entire corneal epithelium is approximately 7 days, which is more rapid than for other epithelial tissues.[23,24] Repair to corneal epithelial tissue proceeds quickly; minor abrasions heal within hours, and larger ones often heal overnight. If the basement membrane is damaged, however, complete healing with replacement basement membrane and hemidesmosomes can take months.[14,15]

Despite cells constantly being sloughed, the barrier function is maintained as the cell below moves into position to replace the one that has been shed. Tight junctions are present exclusively between the squamous cells that occupy the superficial position. The protein components necessary to form these junctions are not present in the basal cells but are increasingly present as the cells move up to the surface where the zonula occludens junctions become complete.[25]

The basal cell layer is continually losing and reestablishing the hemidesmosome junctions as cells divide and move up into the wing cell layers. The plaque sites remain present in the stroma for reattachment.[15]

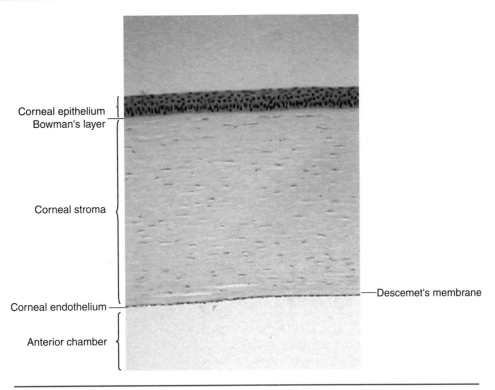

FIGURE 2-3
Light micrograph of corneal layers.

Corneal epithelium
Bowman's layer

Corneal stroma

Descemet's membrane

Corneal endothelium

Anterior chamber

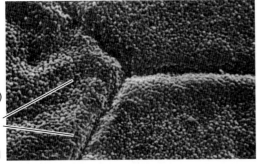

Fine ridges
(microplicae)
and
processes
(microvilli)
of corneal
surface cell

FIGURE 2-4
Scanning electron micrograph of junction of three superficial cells in cornea. (×5000.) (From Krause WJ, Cutts JH: *Concise text of histology*, Baltimore, 1981, Williams & Wilkins.)

Clinical Comment: Recurrent Corneal Erosion

RECURRENT CORNEAL EROSION is a condition in which the corneal epithelium sloughs off either continually or periodically. This condition may occur because of either poor attachment between the epithelium and its basement membrane or poor attachment between the basement membrane and the underlying tissue. Recurrent corneal erosion can occur after incomplete healing of an abrasion in which the hemidesmosomes are malformed, or it may be caused by an epithelial basement membrane dystrophy stemming from defective nutrition or metabolism.[5]

Age-related changes also can play a role in recurrent corneal erosion. Epithelium continues to secrete basement membrane throughout life; in the corneal epithelium, the thickness of the basement membrane doubles by 60 years of age. In addition, areas of reduplication of the membrane can occur with aging.[26] As the basement membrane thickens or as reduplication occurs, the thickness of the membrane can exceed the length of the anchoring fibrils, allowing sloughing of epithelial layers.

Corneal erosions are very painful because the dense network of sensory nerve endings in the epithelium is disrupted. A number of treatments may be used. Acute cases may be patched and antibiotic ointment applied to allow healing of the surface without the shearing effect of opening and closing the eyelids. Bandage soft contact lenses or collagen shields often are applied in chronic situations to alleviate pain.[26-29] For cases in which the suspected cause is a faulty basement membrane, treatment might include corneal puncture in which multiple perforations are made through the epithelial layers to induce new basement membrane formation and adhesion[30-32] (Figure 2-7). If reduplication is the cause of corneal erosion, the doubled membrane can be removed.[32]

Bowman's Layer

The second layer of the cornea is approximately 8 to 14 μm thick.[1,6,33] **Bowman's layer** is a dense, fibrous sheet of interwoven collagen fibrils randomly arranged in a mucoprotein ground substance. The fibrils have a

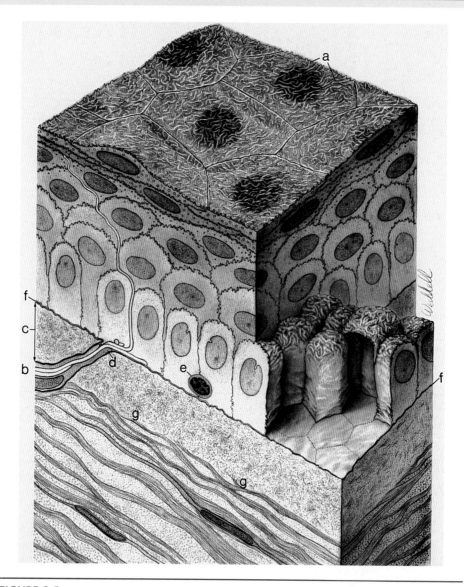

FIGURE 2-5

Three-dimensional drawing of corneal epithelium showing five layers of cells. Polygonal shape of basal and surface cells and their relative size are apparent. Wing cell processes fill spaces formed by dome-shaped apical surface of basal cells. Turnover time for these cells is 7 days, and during this time the columnar basal cell gradually is transformed into a wing cell and then into a thin, flat surface cell. During this transition, cytoplasm changes and Golgi apparatus becomes more prominent. Numerous vesicles develop in the superficial wing and surface layers, and glycogen appears in surface cells. Intercellular space separating the outermost surface cells is closed by a zonula occludens, forming a barrier that prevents passage of precorneal tear film into corneal stroma. Cell surface shows extensive net of microplicae (*a*) and microvilli that might be involved in retention of the precorneal film. Corneal nerve (*b*) passes through Bowman's layer (*c*); the nerve loses its Schwann cell sheath near basement membrane (*d*) of basal epithelium. It then passes as a naked nerve between the epithelial cells toward the superficial layers. Lymphocyte (*e*) is seen between two basal epithelial cells. Basement membrane is seen at (*f*). Some of the most superficial corneal stromal lamellae (*g*) are seen curving forward to merge with Bowman's layer. The regular arrangement of the corneal stromal collagen differs from the random disposition in Bowman's layer. (From Hogan MJ, Alvarado JA, Weddell JE: *Histology of the human eye*, Philadelphia, 1971, Saunders.)

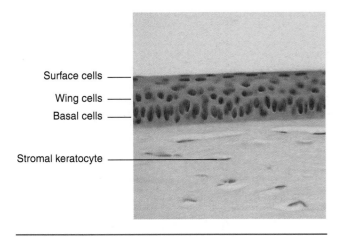

Surface cells ——
Wing cells ——
Basal cells ——

Stromal keratocyte ——

FIGURE 2-6
Light micrograph of corneal epithelium showing columnar basal cells, wing cells, and squamous surface cells of cornea; Bowman's layer and anterior stroma are also evident.

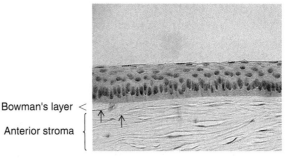

Bowman's layer <
Anterior stroma {

FIGURE 2-8
Light micrograph of corneal epithelium, Bowman's layer, and anterior stroma. There is a change in the direction of the superficial lamellae as they curve forward to merge with Bowman's layer (*arrows*).

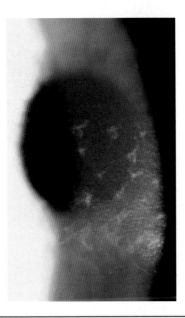

FIGURE 2-7
Corneal puncture. In recurrent corneal erosion, defective adhesion of the epithelium and basement membrane complex to underlying stroma exists. A hypodermic needle is passed through epithelium and anterior stroma to create focal areas of scarring that help to cause "spot welds." (From Krachmer JH, Palay DA: *Cornea color atlas*, St Louis, 1995, Mosby.)

diameter. Bowman's layer might provide biomechanical rigidity and shape to the cornea. The pattern of the anterior surface is irregular and reflects the contour of the bases of the basal cells of the epithelium. Posteriorly, as the layer transitions into stroma, the fibrils gradually adopt a more orderly arrangement and begin to merge into bundles that intermingle with those of the stroma (Figure 2-8). The posterior surface is not clearly defined.[33]

Bowman's layer is produced prenatally by the epithelium and is not believed to regenerate. Therefore, if injured, the layer usually is replaced by epithelial cells or stromal scar tissue. However, Bowman's layer is very resistant to damage by shearing, penetration, or infection. Speculation continues regarding the function of Bowman's layer and whether it is necessary to maintain corneal function. No long-term effects have been documented in patients with Bowman's layer removed by photorefractive keratoplasty, a procedure performed since the late 1980s.[34]

Corneal nerves passing through Bowman's layer typically lose their Schwann cell covering and pass into the epithelium as naked nerves (see Figure 2-5). The layer tapers and ends at the corneal periphery and does not have a counterpart in either the conjunctiva or the sclera.

Stroma or Substantia Propria

The middle layer of the cornea is approximately 500 μm thick, or about 90% of the total corneal thickness[7] (see Figure 2-3). The **stroma** (*substantia propria*) is composed of collagen fibrils, keratocytes, and extracellular ground substance.

The **collagen fibrils** have a uniform 25- to 35-nm diameter and run parallel to one another, forming flat

diameter of 20 to 25 nm, run in various directions, and are not ordered into bundles. Bowman's layer sometimes is referred to as a "membrane," but it is more correctly a *transition layer* to the stroma rather than a true membrane. It differs from the stroma in that it is acellular and contains collagen fibrils of a smaller bundles called **lamellae.**[33] The 200 to 300 lamellae are distributed throughout the stroma and lie parallel to the corneal surface. Each contains uniformly straight collagen fibrils arranged with regular spacing, sometimes described as a "latticework." The fibrils are also oriented parallel to the corneal surface. Adjacent lamellae lie at angles to one another, but all fibrils within a lamella run in the same direction (Figure 2-9). Each lamella extends across the entire cornea, and each fibril runs from limbus to limbus. Interweaving occurs between the lamellae.[35,36]

The arrangement of the lamellae varies slightly within the stroma. In the anterior one third of the stroma, the lamellae are thin (0.5 to 30 µm wide and 0.2 to 1.2 µm thick), and they branch and interweave more than in the deeper layers.[33,37] In the posterior two thirds of the stroma, the arrangement is more regular, and the lamellae become larger (100 to 200 µm wide and 1 to 2.5 µm thick).[33] Anterior cornea has a higher incidence of cross-linking and is more rigid, helping to maintain corneal curvature.[38]

In the innermost layer, adjacent to Descemet's membrane, the fibrils interlace to form a thin collagenous sheet that contributes to the binding between stroma and Descemet's membrane.[33]

Keratocytes (corneal fibroblasts) are flattened cells that lie between and occasionally within the lamellae[39] (Figure 2-10). The cells are not distributed randomly; a corkscrew pattern is recognizable from anterior to posterior, with the density higher in anterior stroma.[40] Keratocytes have extensive branching processes joined by gap junctions along the lateral extensions, as well as the anteroposterior branches.[41,42] These are active cells that maintain the stroma by synthesizing collagen and extracellular matrix components. Other cells may be found between lamellae, including white blood cells, lymphocytes, macrophages, and polymorphonuclear leukocytes, which can increase in number in pathologic conditions.

Ground substance fills the areas between fibrils, lamellae, and cells. It contains *proteoglycans* (PG), macromolecules consisting of a core protein with one or more attached glycosaminoglycan (GAG) side chains. The corneal proteoglycans were once classified by their side chains: keratan sulphate (KS) and chondroitin/dermatan sulphate (CS/DS).[43] They are now named for their core proteins, decorin is a CS/DS proteoglycan, and lumican, keratocan, and mimican are KS proteoglycans. Decorin is more abundant in anterior stroma; lumican, keratocan, and mimican are more abundant in posterior stroma.[44] Lumican controls collagen fibril diameter keeping it within a very limited range.[45] PGs have a significant role in maintaining corneal tensile strength and the GAGs contribute to the relatively high stromal hydration.[44] **Glycosaminoglycans** are hydrophilic, negatively charged carbohydrate molecules located at specific sites around each collagen fibril. They

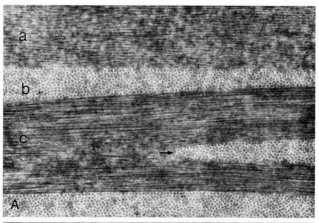

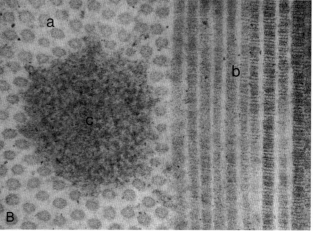

FIGURE 2-9

Corneal stroma. A, View of lamellae cut in three planes. The upper lamella (a) is cut obliquely, the next (b) is cut in cross section, and the third (c) is cut longitudinally. This lamella splits into two lamellae (*arrow*) (×28,000). **B,** Cross-sectional (a) and longitudinal (b) views of the two lamellae. The fibrils measure 340 to 400 Å in diameter and are separated from each other by a space measuring 200 to 500 Å. Large, round granular mass (c) is observed within the lamella cut in cross section. Such masses are seen in most of the collagenous tissues of the eye and may represent a stage in formation of the mature fiber (×104,000). (From Hogan MJ, Alvarado JA, Weddell JE: *Histology of the human eye*, Philadelphia, 1971, Saunders.)

attract and bind with water, maintaining the precise spatial relationship between individual fibrils.[45]

The very regular arrangement of the stromal components, as well as the small diameter of the fibrils, contributes to stromal transparency.[46] The index of refraction of the fibrils is 1.411 and that of the extracellular matrix is 1.365. Studies have shown that the distance between areas of different refractive indices can affect transparency. If the change in the index of refraction occurs across a distance that is less than one half the wavelength of visible light (400 to 700 nm), *destructive interference* occurs, and *light scattering* is reduced significantly.[40,47,48] In the stroma the very specific spacing between the fibrils allows destructive interference

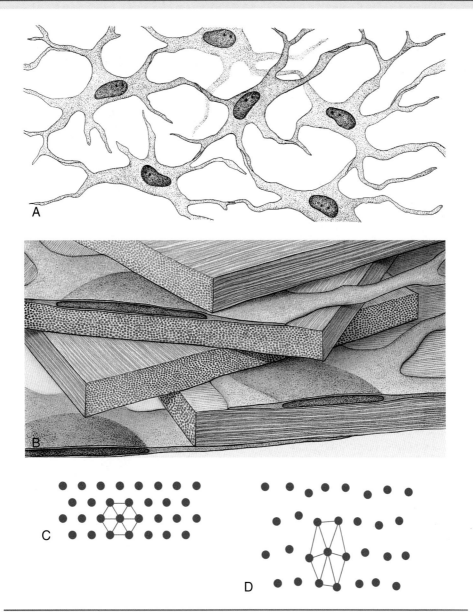

FIGURE 2-10

Summary diagram of corneal stroma. A, Fibroblasts. Diagram shows six fibroblasts lying between stromal lamellae. Cells are thin and flat with long processes that contact fibroblast processes of other cells lying in same plane. These cells once were believed to form a true syncytium, but electron microscopy has disproved this theory. There is almost always a 200-Å-wide intercellular space that separates the cells. Unlike fibroblasts elsewhere, these cells occasionally join one another at a macula occludens. **B,** Lamellae. Cornea is composed of orderly, dense, fibrous connective tissue. Its collagen, which is a stable protein with an estimated half-life of 100 days, forms many lamellae. Collagen fibrils within a lamella are parallel to one another and run the full length of cornea. Successive lamellae run across cornea at an angle to one another. Three fibroblasts are seen between the lamellae. **C,** Theoretic orientation of corneal collagen fibrils. Each of the fibrils is separated from the others by an equal distance. Maurice[46] has explained the transparency of cornea on the basis of this equidistant separation. As a result of this arrangement, stromal lamellae form a three-dimensional array of diffraction gratings. Scattered rays of light passing through such a system interact with one another in an organized way, resulting in elimination of scattered light by destructive interference. Mucoproteins, glycoproteins, and other components of ground substance are responsible for maintaining proper position of fibrils. **D,** Orientation of collagen fibrils in an opaque cornea. Diagram shows that orderly position of fibrils has been disturbed. Because of this disarrangement, scattered light is not eliminated by destructive interference, and cornea becomes hazy. Edematous fluid in ground substance also produces clouding of cornea by disturbing interfibrillar distance. (From Hogan MJ, Alvarado JA, Weddell JE: *Histology of the human eye,* Philadelphia, 1971, Saunders.)

of rays reflecting from adjacent fibrils. Although the components of the epithelium, Bowman's layer, and Descemet's membrane are arranged irregularly, the scattering particles are separated by such small distances that light scattering is minimal in these layers.[37] The cornea scatters less than 1% of the light that enters it.[6,49]

Clinical Comment: Keratoconus

KERATOCONUS is a corneal dystrophy that first presents with focal disruptions of basement membrane and Bowman's layer. Metabolic and nutritional disturbances are among the possible causes. Normal corneal shape and strength are maintained by the arrangement and density of the collagen fibrils that lie parallel to each other and the surface. Two mechanisms likely play some role in keratoconus: tissue loss caused by enzymatic degradation and the loss of adhesive forces between collagen fibrils that can cause slippage and displacement of lamellae.[50] The process usually begins in central cornea; the stroma eventually degenerates and thins, and the affected area projects outward in a cone shape because of the force exerted on the weakened area by intraocular pressure (Figure 2-11, A). The cone shape is most evident in downgaze when the lower lid conforms to the cone shape; this is known as Munson's sign (Figure 2-11, B). Folds occur in the posterior stroma and Descemet's membrane.[51,52]

Spectacles may be used for a time for correction of refractive error, but with increasing irregular astigmatism, rigid gas-permeable contact lenses usually are necessary to achieve best corrected vision.[53] When contact lenses no longer correct vision, penetrating keratoplasty may be performed to replace the defective cornea with a donor cornea.

Currently clinical trials are being conducted to evaluate a procedure called collagen cross-linking. In this treatment, after removing the epithelium, the stroma is saturated with topical riboflavin; it is then exposed to ultraviolet radiation that interacts with the riboflavin creating chemical bonds between and within the collagen fibrils. The corneal collagen stiffens, decreasing the progression of keratoconus.[54] Initial results are promising.[55,56]

Descemet's Membrane

Descemet's membrane is considered the basement membrane of the endothelium. It is produced continually and therefore thickens throughout life, such that it has doubled by age 40 years.[26] In children it is 5 μm thick and will increase to approximately 15 μm over a lifetime (Figure 2-12).

Descemet's membrane consists of two laminae. The *anterior lamina*, approximately 3 μm thick, exhibits a banded appearance and is a latticework of collagen fibrils secreted during embryonic development. The *posterior lamina* is nonbanded and homogeneous; it is the portion secreted by the endothelium throughout life.[57]

Although no elastic fibers are present, the collagen fibrils are arranged in such a way that Descemet's

membrane exhibits an elastic property; if torn, the membrane will curl into the anterior chamber. Descemet's membrane is very resistant to trauma, proteolytic enzymes, and some pathologic conditions but can be regenerated if damaged. A thickened area of collagenous connective tissue may be seen at the membrane's termination in the limbus; this circular structure is called **Schwalbe's line** (or ring).

The method of attachment between Descemet's membrane and the neighboring layers is poorly understood. Attachment sites between the stroma and Descemet's membrane are relatively weak; the membrane can be detached easily from the posterior stroma.[19] The anchoring fibrils characteristic of the connective tissue component of the hemidesmosome are not seen in Descemet's[58] and so the adhesions between Descemet's membrane and the endothelium are not the typical hemidesmosomes.[59]

Endothelium

The innermost layer of the cornea, the **endothelium,** lies adjacent to the anterior chamber and is composed of a single layer of flattened cells. It normally is 5 μm thick.[6] The basal part of each cell rests on Descemet's membrane, and the apical surface, from which microvilli extend, lines the anterior chamber (Figure 2-13). Endothelial cells are polyhedral: five-sided and seven-sided cells can be found in normal cornea, but 70% to 80% are hexagonal. The hexagon is considered the most efficacious shape to provide area coverage without gaps.[5,60] The very regular arrangement of these cells is described as the *endothelial mosaic* (Figure 2-14).

Although Descemet's membrane is considered a basement membrane, the nature of the junctions joining it to the endothelium are undefined.[61] Extensive interdigitations join the lateral walls of the cells, and gap junctions provide intercellular communication.[12] Tight junctional complexes joining the endothelial cells are located near the cell apex; these are a series of macula occludens rather than zonula occludens.[62,63]

The barrier formed by these adhesions is slightly leaky; in experiments, large molecules have penetrated the intercellular spaces.[64] This incomplete barrier allows the entrance of nutrients, including glucose and amino acids, from the aqueous humor. Excess water that accompanies these nutrients must be moved out of the cornea if proper hydration is to be maintained. Metabolic pump mechanisms are active throughout the cells of the endothelium and function continually to move ions across the cell membranes; lateral infoldings increase the surface area providing space necessary for the number of ionic pumps needed. With changes in solute concentration, water flows down the concentration gradient, thus maintaining a balance of fluid movement across the endothelium. The endothelial cell is rich in cellular

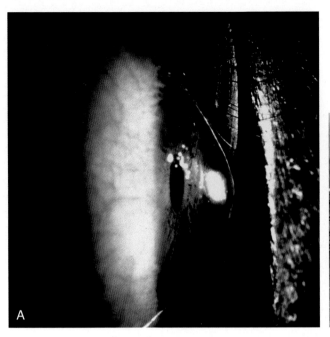
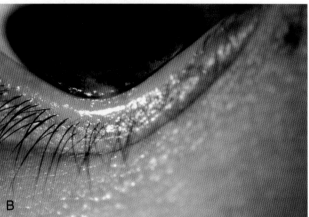

FIGURE 2-11
A, Keratoconus. (Courtesy Patrick Caroline, C.O.T., Pacific University College of Optometry, Forest Grove, Ore.) **B,** Munson's sign; the lower lid conforms to the shape of the keratoconic cornea in downgaze. (Courtesy Edward B. Mallett, O.D., Pacific University, Family Vision Center, Forest Grove, Ore.)

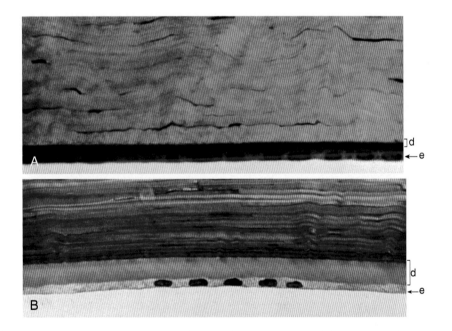

FIGURE 2-12
Thickness of Descemet's membrane changes with increasing age. A, Eye of 1½-year-old child. Light micrograph showing the endothelium (e) and Descemet's membrane (d), which are approximately the same thickness (×500). **B,** Eye of 50-year-old adult. Descemet's membrane (d) is a little more than double the thickness of the endothelium (e) (×800). (From Hogan MJ, Alvarado JA, Weddell JE: *Histology of the human eye*, Philadelphia, 1971, Saunders, p 94.)

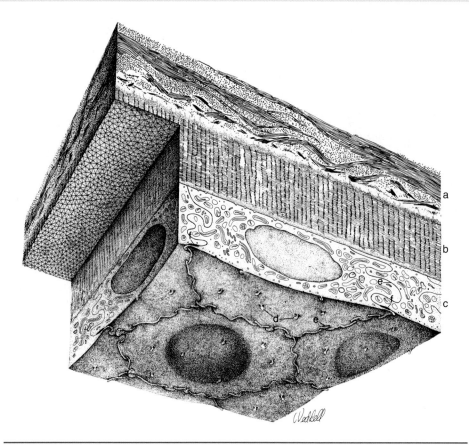

FIGURE 2-13
Three-dimensional drawing of deep cornea showing deepest corneal lamellae (*a*), Descemet's membrane (*b*), and endothelium (*c*). The deeper stromal lamellae split, and some branches curve posteriorly to merge with Descemet's membrane. Descemet's membrane is seen in meridional and tangential planes. Collagenous lattice of this membrane has intersecting filaments that form nodes. These nodes are separated from one another by 100 Å and are exactly superimposed on one another to form a linear pattern in meridional sections. Endothelial cells are polygonal, measuring approximately 3.5 mm in thickness and 7 to 10 mm in length. Microvilli (*d*) protrude into anterior chamber from posterior cell, and marginal folds (*e*) at intercellular junctions project into anterior chamber. Intercellular space near anterior chamber is closed by a tight junction (*f*). Cytoplasm contains an abundance of rod-shaped mitochondria. Nucleus is round and flattened in anteroposterior axis. (From Hogan MJ, Alvarado JA, Weddell JE: *Histology of the human eye*, Philadelphia, 1971, Saunders.)

organelles; mitochondria reflect high metabolic activity and are more numerous in these cells than in any other cells of the eye, except the retinal photoreceptor cells.[6]

Endothelial cells do not divide and replicate. Studies now suggest that endothelial cells in the adult possess proliferative capacity but are in an arrested phase in the cell cycle. The cell-to-cell contact may be one factor that maintains this layer in the nonproliferative state.[59,61,65] The lack of proliferation may be necessary for the layer to maintain its barrier and pump functions.[59] Even in children, cells migrate and spread out to cover a defect, with resultant cell thinning. The cell density (cells per unit area) of the endothelium decreases normally with aging because of cell disintegration; density ranges from 3000 to 4000 cells/mm^2 in children to 1000 to 2000 cells/mm^2 at age 80 years.[5,62,66,67] The minimum cell density necessary for adequate function is in the range of 400 to 700 cells/mm^2.[68] Disruptions to the endothelial mosaic can include endothelial cell loss or an increase in the variability of cell shape (*pleomorphism*) or size (*polymegathism*) (Figure 2-15). The active pump function can be detrimentally affected by polymegathism or morphologic changes, although the endothelial barrier function is not compromised by a moderate loss of cells.[69] An excessive loss of cells can disrupt the intercellular junctions and allow excess aqueous to flow into the stroma, and the endothelial pumps may be unable to compensate for this loss of barrier function.

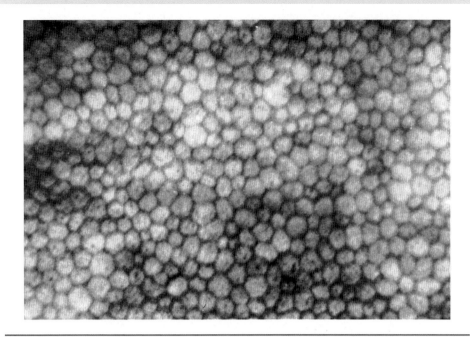

FIGURE 2-14
View with specular reflection through biomicroscope showing the endothelial mosaic.
(Courtesy Patrick Caroline, C.O.T., Pacific University College of Optometry, Forest Grove, Ore.)

Clinical Comment: Hassall-Henle Bodies and Guttata

*The endothelium can produce mounds of basement membrane material, which are seen as periodic thickenings in Descemet's membrane that bulge into the anterior chamber. Those located near the corneal periphery are called **Hassall-Henle bodies**. These bodies are a common finding, and their incidence increases with age. Such deposits of basement membrane in the central cornea are called **corneal guttata** and are indicative of endothelial dysfunction. The endothelium that covers these mounds is thinned and altered, and the endothelial barrier may be compromised. Both Hassall-Henle bodies and guttata are visible as dark areas when viewed with specular reflection with the biomicroscope. These may be interpreted as holes in the endothelium, but the endothelium is merely displaced posteriorly from the plane of reflection (Figure 2-16).*

Clinical Comment: Effects of Contact Lenses

Clinical studies indicate that epithelial thinning, stromal thinning, and a decreased number of keratocytes are associated with long-term extended wear of contact lenses.[70,71] Numerous studies show that contact lens wear can induce changes in the regularity of the endothelial mosaic.[72-76] Pleomorphism and polymegathism have been documented after only six years of either rigid gas-permeable or soft contact lens wear, although cell density remained normal.[77,78] Endothelial stress resulting from contact lens wear, disease, surgery, or age can lead to endothelial remodeling, including change in size and shape or both.

CORNEAL FUNCTION

The cornea has two primary functions: to refract light and to transmit light. Factors that affect the amount of corneal refraction include (1) the curvature of the anterior corneal surface, (2) the change in refractive index from air to cornea (actually the tear film), (3) corneal thickness, (4) the curvature of the posterior corneal surface, and (5) the change in refractive index from cornea to aqueous humor. The total refractive power of the eye focused at infinity is between 60 and 65 diopters (D), with 43 to 48 D attributable to the cornea.[5]

In the transmission of light through the cornea, it is important that minimal scattering and distortion occur. Scattering of incident light is minimized by the smooth optical surface formed by the corneal epithelium and its tear film covering. The regular arrangement of the surface epithelial cells provides a relatively smooth surface, and the tear film fills in slight irregularities between cells producing negligible scatter of incident light. The absence of blood vessels and the maintenance of the correct spatial arrangement of components account for minimal scattering and distortion as light rays pass through the tissue. The cornea scatters less than 1% of the visible incident light[6,49] and the majority of that scatter as determined by examination with the confocal microscope occurs due to the epithelium and endothelium.[48] The epithelial and endothelial cell cytoplasm contain large amounts of water-soluble proteins, which enable the cytoplasm to appear homogenous and help to diminish light scattering. These proteins are now

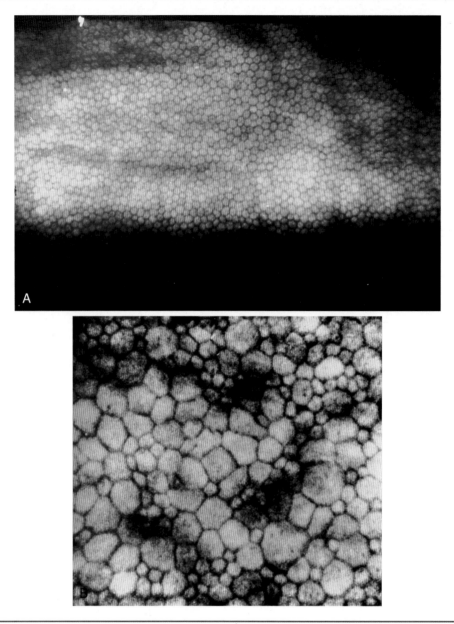

FIGURE 2-15
Endothelial integrity can be evaluated by determining the coefficient of variation (CV) of cell size. Normal endothelium has a CV of 0.25. **A,** Endothelium of healthy 25-year-old non-contact lens wearer. Endothelial cell density is 2000 cells/mm^2, hexagonality is 69%, and CV is 0.25. **B,** Endothelium of 40-year-old patient who has worn polymethyl methacrylate contact lenses for 23 years. Endothelial cell density is 1676 cells/mm^2, hexagonality is 24%, and CV is 0.66. (**A** courtesy Scott MacRae, M.D., Oregon Health Sciences University, Portland, Ore.; **B** from MacRae SM, Matsuda M, Shellans S et al: The effects of hard and soft contact lenses on the corneal endothelium, *Am J Ophthalmol* 102:50, 1986.)

called corneal crystallins, and they share many of the attributes of the long recognized lens crystallins, important in maintaining the transparency of the lens.[77]

Because the stroma makes up 90% of the cornea, the regularity of spacing between the collagen fibrils is important in maintaining corneal transparency. The negatively charged molecules located around each collagen fibril maintain this precise arrangement by their bonds with water molecules, and corneal transparency is optimal when the stroma is 75% to 80% water.[4,78]

Corneal Hydration

This relative *corneal deturgescence* (78% water content) requires precise control of stromal extracellular water content and is dependent upon: (1) the barrier

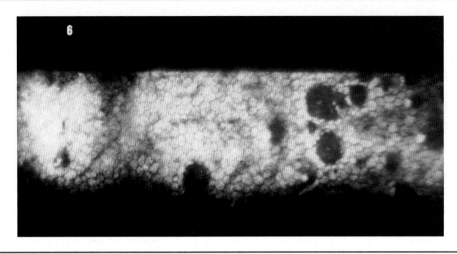

FIGURE 2-16
Guttata. Endothelium of a patient with Fuchs endothelial dystrophy. Numerous guttata are evident by the dark areas; endothelial cell density is 1600 cells/mm^2. (Courtesy Scott MacRae, M.D., Oregon Health Sciences University, Portland, Ore.)

functions of the epithelium and endothelium, (2) the anionic characteristics of molecules within the stromal matrix that account for the tendency of the stroma to imbibe water, and (3) water and ion transport through the epithelial and endothelial cell membranes (including ion channels, ion cotransporters, and energy-utilizing ion pumps). Fluid is continually entering the cornea through the leaky barrier formed by the junctions joining the endothelial cells. Ion transporters in both the epithelium and the endothelium help to maintain the concentration gradient change that can facilitate water movement from the stroma into the tear film through the epithelium and into the anterior chamber through the endothelium. Net transport of solute into the anterior chamber exceeds that into the tears and corneal deturgescence is primarily reliant on endothelium and minimally on epithelium.[79]

The movement of water out of the cornea from the stroma through the endothelium and into the aqueous or through the epithelium into tears is mediated by ion flow and osmotic gradients. As ions are exchanged and the concentration is altered, water passage follows, moving down its concentration gradient. Cl$^-$ extrusion and Na$^+$ absorption are the major driving forces for water transport across the epithelium and endothelium.[80] However, an additional avenue of water movement occurs through water transport channels called aquaporins, identified in human corneal epithelial and endothelial cell membranes.

Aquaporins

Aquaporins (AQPs) are small integral membrane proteins residing in the plasma membrane; some are water-selective and others also transport glycerol.[81] They form bidirectional osmotic water transport channels across the plasma membrane. The most constricted portion of the channel might allow only single file water molecule flow.[82] AQP1, AQP2, AQP4, AQP5, and AQP8 are water selective and AQP3, AQP7, and AQP9 transport glycerol and perhaps other small solutes.[81] AQP1 is found in corneal epithelium, endothelium, and keratocytes; AQP3 is found in cornea and conjunctival epithelium; and AQP5 is found in corneal epithelium.[81] AQP5 is a significant pathway for water movement into the hypertonic tear film and water moves from the stroma into the aqueous through AQP1.[81] Aquaporins function not only as channels but have some role in cellular processes, particularly in cell migration.[81]

The contributions to corneal hydration by the epithelium, the stroma, and the endothelium will be discussed next.

Epithelium. The barrier produced by the tight junctions **(zonula occludens)** joining the surface cells of the corneal epithelium prevents water influx from the tear film. All molecules (water included) entering the cornea from the tear film must pass through the cell. Aquaporins in both apical and basal membranes provide channels for water passage.

The cations, Na$^+$ and K$^+$, and the anion Cl$^-$ move across the epithelial cell membrane by various mechanisms (Figure 2-17). Channels in the apical membrane allow Na$^+$ to move into the epithelium from the tear film; Na$^+$ is extruded from the cell via Na$^+$/K$^+$ ATPase pumps in the basolateral membrane. Na$^+$, K$^+$, and Cl$^-$ are transported from stroma into the cell via the Na$^+$/K$^+$/2Cl$^-$ cotransporter in the basolateral membrane.[83] Cl$^-$ moves out of the cell through channels in the apical surface. K$^+$ movement out of the cell down its concentration gradient through channels in the basal membrane is opposed by the cotransporter and the

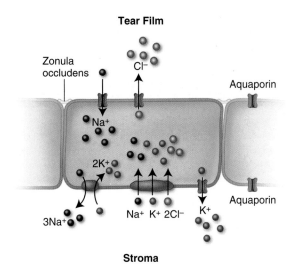

Tear Film

Zonula
occludens

Cl⁻

Aquaporin

Na⁺

2K⁺

Aquaporin

3Na⁺

Na⁺ K⁺ 2Cl⁻

K⁺

Stroma

FIGURE 2-17

Diagram depicting ion and water movement through corneal epithelial cells. Although the corneal epithelium is several cell layers think, it is represented as a single layer because of the gap junctions joining cells, they act as a syncytium.

Na⁺/K⁺ ATPase pump resulting in intracellular accumulation of K⁺. The net K⁺ transport creates the electrical force for Cl⁻ diffusion across the apical side of the cell.[83] This Cl⁻ movement in turn has been identified as the driving force for osmotic water transport out of the epithelial cell into the tear film.[82]

Stroma. The stroma imbibes water because of the large anionic proteoglycans within the extracellular matrix that produce a swelling pressure that "pulls water in." It is the sulfonation of the glycosaminoglycan side chains that accounts for the water-binding properties of these molecules, thus ensuring the hydrophilic environment in the stroma responsible for maintaining the regular spacing contributing to transparency.

Endothelium. The endothelial layer allows a slow leak of fluids and solutes from the aqueous into the cornea due to the "leaky" occluding type of tight junction that joins them. Discontinuity and focal disruptions have been observed between the adhesion molecules forming these tight junctions.[84] The rate of leakage into the cornea is dependent upon the swelling pressure of the stroma and must be balanced by water exit through the endothelium to maintain homeostasis and prevent edema.[85]

Water movement through the endothelium into the anterior chamber follows the concentration gradient as ions accumulate in the anterior chamber. In addition there are aquaporins throughout the endothelial

cell membrane.[86] Several types of processes transport ions across the membrane. The Na⁺/K⁺ ATPase pump located in the basolateral membrane of the endothelial cell is the most thoroughly understood; other methods of ion movement include channels, cotransporters, and exchangers. Figure 2-18 depicts some of the established methods, however there is still uncertainty about the control of many of these processes. The Na⁺/K⁺/2Cl⁻ cotransporter and the Na⁺/2HCO₃⁻ cotransporter (although there is some question whether these two ions are directly coupled[87]) move ions into the cell from the stroma. Ion channels transport K⁺ and Cl⁻ out of the cell into the intracellular space; however, the gating mechanism governing these channels is uncertain.[85] Cl⁻ and HCO₃⁻ also exit the apical membrane via ion channels, some of which are permeable to both ions.[87] H⁺ and HCO₃⁻, (both generated intracellularly as by-products of metabolism,) are moved out of the endothelial cell via Cl⁻/HCO₃⁻ and Na⁺/H⁺ exchangers. Water movement out of the endothelium and into the anterior chamber is believed to be driven by the anions Cl⁻ and HCO₃⁻.[86]

Clinical Comment: Fuchs' Dystrophy

FUCHS' DYSTROPHY (see Figure 2-16) is a bilateral, noninflammatory loss of endothelial function. It is inherited and progressive and may be caused by mutation of the gene that codes for collagen VII. The changes start in central cornea and gradually extend to the periphery. Guttata first form and endothelial cells lose Na⁺K⁺ ATPase pumps, although the barrier function remains. As guttata increase in number, some will fuse and the disruption of the endothelial mosaic, visible with specular reflection, is described as having the appearance of beaten metal. Stromal edema occurs with the reduction of ion movement. If the edema moves into the epithelium, it can cause a painful microcystic epithelial edema and recurrent corneal erosion can follow.[85] Fuchs' dystrophia was given as the reason for 15% of penetrating keratoplasty procedures performed in the United States in 2000.[88]

Corneal Metabolism

The metabolically active cornea depends on a stable supply of oxygen and glucose. Oxygen is derived primarily from atmospheric oxygen dissolved in the tear film, with small amounts obtained from the aqueous humor and limbal capillaries. In closed eye conditions, approximately two thirds of the oxygen is supplied by palpebral capillaries with the rest from the aqueous.[89] Most nutrients, including glucose, amino acids, and vitamins, readily enter the cornea from the aqueous humor through the leaky endothelium; a lesser amount is obtained from limbal capillaries.[90,91]

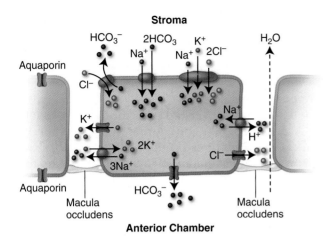

Stroma

Anterior Chamber

FIGURE 2-18
Diagram depicting ion and water movement through corneal endothelial cells.

Glucose is metabolized by aerobic glycolysis via the tricarboxylic acid cycle (TCA or Krebs cycle), anaerobic glycolysis, and the hexose monophosphate shunt. About 85% of the glucose utilized by the cornea is metabolized anaerobically.[92,93] Because the basal cells of the corneal epithelium are in a constant state of replication, they have significant stores of glycogen, and 35% of the glucose processed within the epithelium is via the hexose monophosphate shunt.[79] The hexose monophosphate shunt provides NADP, a reducing agent (part of the defense against free radicals) and nucleotides for the synthesis of cellular components necessary for the constant replacement of epithelial cells.

The endothelium requires significant stores of energy to maintain its metabolic function; each cell contains a large number of mitochondria and each cell is estimated to have 1.5×10^6 Na+/K+ ATPase pumps.[49] In certain diseases, in which there is an increase in the permeability of the endothelial layer, the body can increase the number of pumps per cell, thus expanding pump function and compensating for the increased membrane permeability.[94]

When the oxygen supply is reduced in the hypoxic cornea, the rate of anaerobic glycolysis increases causing an increase in the concentration of lactate. As lactate accumulates, only a small amount can move into tears; the rest must move through the stroma and then through the endothelium into the anterior chamber facilitated by an H+/lactate cotransporter. This is a slow process and lactate builds up, shifting the osmotic balance, pulling water into the corneal stroma, and inducing edema. A poorly fit contact lens that does not allow adequate tear exchange and diminishes the amount of oxygen present at the tear/cornea interface can produce an hypoxic condition.

Hydrogen ions (also a by-product of glycolysis) can also build up, causing a decrease in intracellular pH. Acidification can prompt a change in K+ channels, resulting in a rapid and massive loss of intracellular K+, which causes cell shrinkage and apoptosis.[95] If acidification involves keratocytes, cellular damage can cause a dysfunction in collagen production, resulting in scar formation.

Clinical Comment: Overnight Corneal Swelling

During sleep the cornea swells because of the limited oxygen available to the endothelium.[96] The cornea is thickest upon awakening but returns to baseline within the first two hours of waking.[97] With stromal hydration increase, there is a decrease in swelling pressure and for a short time, the endothelial pumps exceed the water leak, decreasing the edema and reattaining normal hydration.[87]

Clinical Comment: Corneal Edema

CORNEAL EDEMA is manifested by a change in corneal thickness; the swelling is directed posteriorly and the anterior surface curvature remains the same (due to the fixed nature of Bowman's layer).[98] The more closely packed lamellae in the anterior cornea may make the anterior stroma more resistant to edema than the posterior stroma, with the larger spaces between lamellae in the posterior stroma allowing more fluid collection.[40] The reduction in the curvature of the posterior surface can cause buckling of Descemet's membrane and the appearance of vertical folds (striae). Corneal diameter remains the same. An increase in corneal hydration is positively and linearly correlated with corneal thickness. Normally the cornea scatters 1% of incident light, but with fluid retention light scattering increases.

A minor abrasion of the corneal epithelium causing a loss of the zonular occludens barrier results in a localized area of edema and haziness. Epithelial edema can decrease visual acuity when it separates cells causing surface irregularities; it is uncomfortable and can be painful. More extensive epithelial abrasions also allow fluid entrance into the stroma.

Corneal edema caused by the loss of endothelial function is generally of a magnitude greater than that caused by the loss of the epithelial barrier and causes generalized stromal edema.[85] Fluid accumulates in the stromal matrix around the collagen fibrils. Moderate stromal edema is usually symptom-free. Mild to moderate corneal edema can temporarily be cleared with instillation of a hypertonic solution of glycerin.

Age, disease, surgery, or injury can all result in a reduction of endothelial cell number, causing cells to spread out to cover the loss with resultant endothelial cell thinning. As the cell architecture changes to cover more area, cellular function can be reduced and endothelial cell function can be adversely affected by either a change in the size or the shape of the cell. The loss of cells can result in increased permeability of the layer, and damage at the cellular level can also result in a loss of pump function.

Clinical Comment: High Intraocular Pressure

VERY HIGH INTRAOCULAR PRESSURE (IOP) on the order of 50 mm Hg or higher can move excessive water into the corneal stroma from the anterior chamber and overwhelm the endothelial transport system. This is an ocular emergency and must be treated quickly to prevent permanent corneal damage.

Corneal Repair: Wound Healing

Corneal injury initiates a cascade of mechanisms designed to repair damaged tissue. These processes are directed by various biomolecules such as integrins, cytokines, and growth factors Corneal *integrins* are integral membrane glycoproteins that have multiple roles in maintaining corneal function. Some facilitate interactions between cells and extracellular matrix; some have a role in matrix assembly; some impact cell adhesion and the formation of intercellular junctions; and others sense change in the extracellular environment and communicate to the cell nucleus by an alteration in the cytoskeleton.[99] *Cytokines* are signaling molecules that facilitate cellular communication between cells and with surrounding tissues. Cellular proliferation and differentiation are mediated by *growth factors.*[100-108]

Epithelium

Because of the high rate of cell turnover, mitosis is constantly occurring in the basal layer of corneal epithelium. With corneal injury mitosis stops, and growth factors and cytokines are released from damaged epithelial and stromal cells. These molecules play key roles in initiating and continuing the processes necessary for corneal repair.[99,109] Hemidesmosomes in the basal layer are dissembled along the leading edge of the wound.[110] Changes in the cytoskeleton occur allowing for a rapid change in cell shape as those cells at the wound edges develop membrane extensions (filopodia) enabling the cell to migrate and cover the wound.[99,111,112] Cell migration requires precise control of the hemidesmosomes, the cytoskeleton structure, and cell-to-matrix adhesion, which preserves the structural integrity of the epithelial sheet.[109]

Adhesion molecules allow the leading edge of the epithelial sheet to adhere to the basement membrane, in the absence of hemidesmosomes, and also to "pull cells forward" as the sheet moves to cover the injury. Growth factors stimulate the production of matrix components that enhance this cell-to-substrate adhesion; fibronectin is likely a key factor in the substrate that establishes adhesion during cell migration.[113] Proliferation is suppressed until migration occurs, but then proliferation is enhanced in the region behind the advancing front.[109]

Once the defect is covered by a single layer of cells, cell-to-cell junctions are constructed between neighboring cells. Mitosis resumes and glycogen utilization and protein synthesis increases.[80] Cell proliferation continues until normal cell density is reached and the stratified nature of the tissue is reestablished; apoptosis prevents epithelial hyperplasia.[114] Biochemical bonds hold the basal cell to its substrate before hemidesmosomes are formed.[14,15] A small lesion in the epithelium can heal in 24 to 48 hours with hemidesmosomes reformed, but if the basement membrane is damaged, normal adhesion may take months to complete.[17,110] Basal cells are replenished by proliferation in the limbus. Epithelial healing generally is scar-free.

Bowman's

Bowman's layer will not regenerate if damaged but will be replaced either by stromalike fibrous tissue or by epithelium.

Stroma

When corneal injury extends into the stroma, keratocytes increase in number and some are stimulated to become *myofibroblasts.* These cells cause the wound bed to contract, allowing for more rapid wound coverage by the epithelium.[99] The characteristics of the newly formed connective tissue components of the stroma differ slightly from those of the original tissue. The diameter of regenerated corneal stromal collagen is larger than the original fibrils, comparable to that found in the sclera, and the alignment and organization of the replacement fibrils are not as precise. These factors increase the probability that a scar will result.[115] The tensile strength of the collagen fibrils in repaired cornea is diminished and may take months to approach the typical strength.[116] Once healing is complete, the myofibroblasts undergo apoptosis or revert back to keratocytes.[99]

Descemet's

Descemet's membrane is a strong, resistant membrane but, if damaged, can be secreted and re-formed by stromal keratocytes and the endothelium.

Endothelium

Very little mitosis occurs in the endothelium; with cell loss, the neighboring cells generally enlarge and flatten to cover the area of loss; a decrease in endothelial cell density results. The cells remodel into the hexagonal shape, and pump and barrier functions are reestablished. In certain conditions, the number of ion pumps in an endothelial cell can increase dramatically to compensate for the loss of pumps that occur when cells are lost.[94] There may be endothelial cells with proliferative ability that are inhibited and quiescent because of some as yet unknown factor.[59,117]

Absorption of Ultraviolet Radiation (UVR)

The cornea transmits light with wavelengths between 310 and 2500 nm.[49,118] Wave lengths below 300 nm are absorbed by the epithelium and Bowman's layer and do not penetrate deeper; those between 300 to 320 nm are absorbed by corneal stroma.[119-121] The ability of the cornea to absorb the shorter wavelengths of ultraviolet radiation is *protective* to deeper structures (lens and retina), but the cornea is vulnerable to damage from this constant exposure.[119] UVR induces oxidative stress by generating reactive oxygen species (ROS). These free radicals are highly reactive because of an unpaired electron and can damage cellular structures. The corneal epithelium has some protection against the damage caused by UVR absorption. Its cells have high concentrations of ascorbate (vitamin C) and glutathione. Ascorbate can absorb UVR, and is also a cellular antioxidant that can reduce free radicals and neutralize their activity.[119] Glutathione is both a reducing agent and a free radical scavenger.[77] Crystallins, present in cellular cytoplasm, also absorb UVR and are free radical scavengers.[77] The epithelial cell also has a cellular repair system to minimize or reverse UVR damage to DNA.[77]

Clinical Comment: UVR Overexposure or Photokeratitis

Because the epithelium and Bowman's layer are the primary sites for UVR absorbance, acute overexposure to UVR can result in a painful photokeratitis. This can occur with exposure to sunlamps, tanning beds, a welder's arc, or the highly reflective rays from snow. Cellular defense mechanisms are overcome causing disruption of the epithelial tight junctions, inducing edema. Hyperactivation of the K+ channels in cell membranes results in a massive loss of intracellular K+, which causes cell shrinkage and apoptosis.[95] Chronic exposure can result in keratopathies affecting the epithelium and anterior stroma or can cause endothelial pleomorphism.[122]

CORNEAL INNERVATION

The cornea is densely innervated with sensory fibers. Seventy to 80 large nerves, branches of the long and short ciliary nerves, enter the peripheral stroma. Approximately 2 to 3 mm after they pass into the cornea, the nerves lose their myelin sheath, but the covering from the Schwann cell remains.[123,124] Considerable branching occurs, and three nerve networks are formed. One network is located in midstroma, and a subepithelial network is located in the region of Bowman's layer and anterior stroma. Branches from this second network enter the epithelium, where the final nerve network is located (see Figure 12-2).

As the sensory nerves pass through Bowman's layer, the Schwann cell covering is lost, and the fibers terminate as free nerve endings between the tightly packed epithelial cells.[6,124] With surface cell turnover, the nerve endings retract and shift position. As they reinsert between the new surface cells, the nerve ending pattern changes slightly. No nerve endings are located in Descemet's membrane or the endothelium. Any abrasion of the cornea, even a superficial one, is quite painful because of the density of this sensory innervation. The density of sensory nerve endings in the epithelium is approximately 400 times that of the epidermis of the skin, with approximately 7000 nociceptors per square millimeter in the cornea.[44]

Stimulation of the cornea, even just touch, is recognized as pain because of the density of nociceptors. The cornea also recognizes changes in temperature. Contact lens wear over time and aging cause a decrease in sensitivity. The corneal sensory nerves have a neurotrophic effect (i.e., they influence corneal metabolism and aid in tissue maintenance).[125] Individuals with corneal anesthesia and a loss of nerve endings may have increased epithelial permeability, reduced mitosis, decreased cell adhesion, and impaired wound healing.[49,126,127]

In addition to the rich sensory innervation, the cornea contains sympathetic nerve fibers that may have some regulatory effect on Cl⁻ channels.[49] Acetylcholine is found in significant quantities in the corneal epithelium where it functions, not as a neurotransmitter, but as a cellular signaling molecule helping to maintain transparency and cellular homeostasis. It is believed to have a role in pain recognition, cellular proliferation, ion transport, and wound healing.[121,128]

When corneal nerves are damaged in central cornea, the normal nerve pattern is present by week 4, but reinnervation of peripheral branches can take longer than 60 days, resulting in a less dense nerve network than is found in the normal cornea. Repair of the subepithelial plexus can occur by two methods: new nerve fibers can arise from already existing but damaged superficial nerves or new fibers might sprout from deeper stromal nerves that have not been damaged.

Clinical Comment: Assessing Corneal Sensitivity

CORNEAL SENSITIVITY can be "measured" clinically by touching the cornea gently with a wisp of cotton from a swab and initiating a blink response. It can be measured quantitatively by using a measuring device, an esthesiometer. A small, fine filament is introduced from the side to just touch the cornea. Because rigidity depends on the length of the filament, the longer the filament (the more flexible the filament) that initiates a blink, the more sensitive the cornea.

Clinical Comment: Neurotrophic Keratitis

NEUROTROPHIC KERATITIS is a rare degenerative disease caused by the loss of corneal sensory innervation. It confirms the role of nerve endings in maintaining corneal function. Causes include viral herpetic infection, chemical burn, corneal injury or surgery, or intracranial involvement that compromises the trigeminal innervation to the cornea. The clinical presentation can include punctate keratopathy, epithelial thinning, increased epithelial permeability, neovascularization, persistent epithelial defect, and corneal ulceration that can lead to perforation.[126] Treatment can be challenging.

CORNEAL BLOOD SUPPLY

The cornea is avascular and obtains its nourishment by diffusion from the aqueous humor and from the conjunctival and episcleral capillary networks located in the limbus. Absence of blood vessels is an important factor in corneal transparency and although it is surrounded by conjunctival capillary loops a balance between angiogenic and antiangiogenic factors maintains its avascular state.[129,130] The healthy limbus also forms a physical barrier to blood vessels, preventing encroachment of conjunctival tissue into the cornea. The compact composition of the stroma impedes vessel growth.[129-131] Corneal avascularity helps to establish "immune privilege" that gives some protection against immune rejection of grafts.[96] The cornea is normally devoid of antigen processing but under certain conditions, such as inflammatory disease, or with mechanical irritation (such as contact lens wear) immunologically active macrophages, Langerhans cells, can migrate from the limbal periphery.[132,133]

Clinical Comment: Corneal Neovascularization

*In response to oxygen deprivation, the body may produce new blood vessels in an attempt to supply the oxygen-depleted area. This growth of abnormal blood vessels is termed **neovascularization**. In a contact lens wearer, neovascularization is usually an indication that the cornea is not receiving enough oxygen. It can be a sign of a poorly fitting or poorly moving lens or a thick edge. The incidence of neovascularization is higher in soft contact lens wearers than in those wearing rigid gas-permeable lenses and increases in those who wear their lenses for extended periods.*

New vessels sprout from the perilimbal capillaries; first enzymes degrade the basement membrane of the capillary, then the endothelial cells migrate, and finally endothelial cells proliferate to form new vessels that enter the cornea (Figure 2-19, A and B). Careful monitoring of patients with neovascularization and elimination of the causative factor may prevent extensive neovascularization. When the oxygen supply to the cornea resumes, the vessels will no longer carry blood, but the structures will remain and atrophy. These are known as ghost vessels and appear as fine white lines on biomicroscopy (see Figure 2-19, C).

Corneal infections and inflammations also may induce neovascularization in the body's attempt to increase blood supply and some diseases can release vascular endothelial growth factor (VEGF), a protein that stimulates the multiplication of vascular endothelial cells.[127]

Clinical Comment: Keratoplasty

In conditions where the cornea thins and perforation is a danger, or when central corneal scarring (perhaps from injury or infection) causes loss of visual acuity, or when the endothelium is compromised and function is lost, the cornea can be replaced by a donor cornea. The cornea is normally devoid of antigen processing because of the lack of blood vessels and so the rate of graft rejection is usually quite low.

*Full thickness **penetrating keratoplasty** (PK) has been the traditional method for replacing diseased and compromised corneas. PK has significant complications such as irregular cornea and irregular astigmatism (sutures run the entire circumference of the corneal donor button, and are often left in place for years), infection, wound rupture, and sometimes graft rejection or failure. It can take months to years to heal and reestablish tensile strength.[134]*

New surgical methods, which may replace some penetrating keratoplasty procedures, involve replacement of only the posterior cornea in those patients in whom corneal decompensation is due to endothelial dysfunction. One of these procedures is Descemet's stripping automated endothelial keratoplasty (DSAEK). In DSAEK, Descemet's membrane and the endothelium are removed and replaced with donor membrane and endothelium. This method offers a more stable postoperative refraction, reduced corneal surface irregularity, decreased infection risk and wound rupture, and a quicker visual recovery.[134] It requires a skilled and experienced surgeon.

Clinical Comment: Corneal Reshaping

Reducing myopic refractive error can be accomplished by remodeling the corneal curvature either by a method of contact lens fitting (orthokeratology) or by procedures that remove corneal tissue.

*In **orthokeratology**, a rigid, gas-permeable contact lens is fit that gradually changes corneal shape. This lens is worn for a certain period, often overnight, and with time causes the center of the cornea to flatten. Wearing time is gradually reduced, and a minimal wearing time may be established that maintains the corrected corneal shape.*

*The earliest surgical procedure for modifying corneal curvature, **radial keratotomy (RK)**, involved radial incisions from the corneal periphery to a point just outside the pupillary zone. This weakened the corneal periphery and the normal pressure within the eye, pushed the periphery out, thus flattening central cornea, shortening the optical length of the eye, and reducing myopia. Numerous complications resulted, the most serious of which was endothelial compromise when the incision extended to the endothelium.*

*Greatly improved procedures have enhanced the methods for corneal restructuring and in these procedures corneal stroma is removed. The amount of stroma to be removed is determined by the target refractive correction desired. In **photorefractive keratoplasty** (PRK), the epithelium is removed first, usually by mechanical means; then Bowman's layer and anterior stroma are ablated by laser. Bowman's layer does not regenerate, and the basement membrane of the epithelium must be laid down on the remaining stromal surface. In **laser-assisted in situ keratomileusis (LASIK)**, an incision is made to produce a flap consisting of epithelium and Bowman's layer. This flap is folded back, and stroma is removed by laser. The flap is laid back down, and the edges seal as the epithelium heals. In both procedures anterior stroma is removed. Some endothelial cell loss is reported but has not been found to be clinically significant.[135-139] Speculation continues about long-term effects resulting from loss of Bowman's layer, although none has yet been determined. The role of Bowman's layer in UVR absorption may be one of the considerations when deciding between PRK and LASIK.*

The reduction of corneal thickness may have other clinical effects, considering that removal of anterior stroma eliminates an area having significant rigidity and stability.[40] Studies have shown a correlation between corneal thickness and the measurement of intraocular pressure (IOP), and between corneal thickness and the incidence of glaucoma.[140,141] The clinician must be aware of the increased risk of inaccurate IOP readings, as well as any implications for glaucoma risk, in patients who have had removal of stromal tissue.[142,143] Pachometry (measurement of corneal thickness) may be a relevant addition to the diagnosis of glaucoma, especially in those who have had refractive surgery.

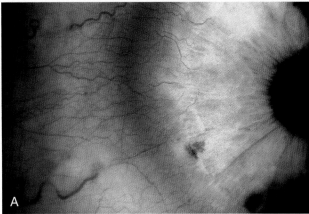
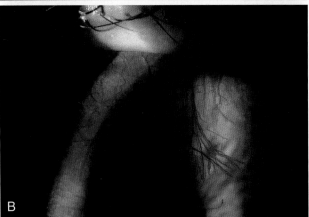
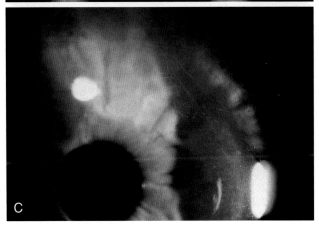

FIGURE 2-19
A, Early neovascularization from conjunctival loops. **B,** Several large vessels have invaded the corneal stroma. **C,** Corneal ghost vessels remain after vessels empty. (**A** Courtesy Family Vision Center, Pacific University, Forest Grove, Ore. **B, C** Courtesy Christina Schnider, O.D.)

SCLERA

The **sclera** forms the posterior five-sixths of the connective tissue coat of the globe. The sclera maintains the shape of the globe, offering resistance to internal and external forces, and provides an attachment for the extraocular muscle insertions. The thickness of the sclera varies from 1 mm at the posterior pole to 0.3 mm just behind the rectus muscle insertions.[151]

SCLERAL HISTOLOGIC FEATURES

Episclera

The **episclera** is a loose, vascularized, connective tissue layer that lies just outer to the sclera. The larger episcleral vessels are visible through the conjunctiva. Branches of the anterior ciliary arteries form a capillary network in the episclera just anterior to the rectus muscle insertions and surrounding peripheral cornea. The episclera, which is joined to Tenon's capsule by strands of connective tissue, becomes thinner towards the back of the eye.

Clinical Comment: Ciliary Injection

The episcleral network becomes congested in **ciliary injection**, *giving the limbus a light-purple or rose coloration in serious corneal inflammation or diseases of the iris or ciliary body.*

Sclera

The **sclera** is a thick, dense connective tissue layer that is continuous with the corneal stroma at the limbus. The diameter of the collagen fibrils in this tissue varies from 25 to 230 nm. These fibrils are arranged in irregular bundles that branch and interlace.[33,144] The fibril size, orientation, and arrangement are influenced by proteoglycans in the extracellular matrix.[145] Bundle widths and thicknesses vary, with the external bundles narrower and thinner than the deeper bundles. The orientation of these scleral lamellae is very irregular compared with corneal lamellae organization. The lamella in the outer regions of the sclera run approximately parallel to the surface, with interweaving between them, whereas in the inner regions the lamellae run in all directions.[33] This random arrangement and the amount of interweaving contributes to the strength and flexibility of the eye. Generally, the fibrils parallel the limbus anteriorly; the pattern becomes meridional near the rectus muscle insertions and circular around the optic nerve exit. The collagen of the extraocular muscle tendon at its insertion merges and interweaves with the fibrils of the sclera.[146]

Elastic fibers have a low incidence in the sclera between and sometimes within bundles.[33,145,147,148] Fibroblasts are also present, although they are less numerous than in the cornea. The stromal ground substance is similar to the corneal ground substance but contains fewer GAGs.[78] The innermost aspect of the sclera merges with the choroidal tissue in the suprachoroid layer.

PHYSIOLOGY OF SCLERAL CHANGES IN MYOPIA

Early childhood growth of the eye requires coordinated changes in refractive components and in eye size for the eye to become emmetropic. When these factors are not coordinated, refractive error develops. A myopic eye generally is larger than emmetropic or hyperopic eyes, and changes in scleral tissue may be a factor when emmetropization does not occur. Most myopia develops between ages 8 to 14 and is caused by the elongation of the vitreal chamber.[145] The sclera is a dynamic tissue; the connective tissue components can change in response to changes in the visual environment.[145] Animal studies have shown that poor image quality on the retina can elicit a signal to scleral tissue components to strengthen or weaken in an attempt to move the retina to the best location for a clear image.

Scleral remodeling causes the axial lengthening that occurs in myopia; the scleral tissue is weakened and thins. In progressive myopia existing collagen is degraded, the production of new collagen is reduced, and matrix proteoglycans are lost.[149,150] Studies attribute these alterations during myopia development to changes in the extracellular matrix but an additional piece of the puzzle may be the role played by scleral fibroblasts; if stimulated to become myofibroblasts, they can provide biochemical signals leading to changes in collagen production and degradation of tissue.[149,150]

Clinical Comment: Scleral Ectasia

The progression of myopia caused by axial elongation in a highly myopic eye often causes scleral thinning, particularly at the posterior pole where the collagen fibril diameter and the bundle size are reduced.[145] As the sclera thins, the tissue can bulge outward causing **scleral ectasia.**

SCLERAL SPUR

The **scleral spur** is a region of circularly oriented collagen bundles that extends from the inner aspect of the sclera. In its entirety, the scleral spur is actually a ring, although on cross section it appears wedge shaped, resembling a spur (Figure 2-20). At the spur's posterior edge, its fibers blend with the more obliquely arranged scleral fibers. The posterior scleral spur is the origin of the longitudinal ciliary muscle fibers and most of the trabecular meshwork sheets attach to its anterior aspect, such that the collagen of the spur is continuous with that of the trabeculae.

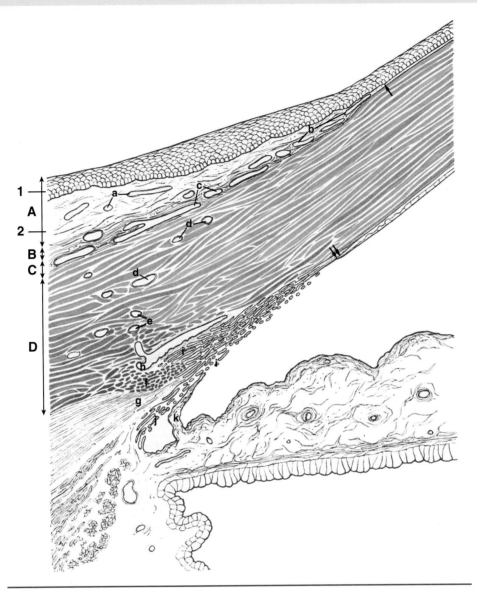

FIGURE 2-20

Limbus. Limbal conjunctiva (*A*) is formed by an epithelium (*1*) and a loose connective tissue stroma (*2*). Tenon capsule (*B*) forms a thin, poorly defined connective tissue layer over episclera (*C*). Limbal stroma occupies the area (*D*) and is composed of scleral and corneal tissues that merge in this region. Conjunctival stromal vessels are also seen (*a*). They form peripheral corneal arcades (*b*), which extend anteriorly to termination of Bowman's layer (*arrow*). Episcleral vessels (*c*) are cut in different planes. Vessels forming intrascleral (*d*) and deep scleral plexus (*e*) are shown within limbal stroma. Scleral spur has coarse and dense collagen fibers (*f*). Anterior part of longitudinal portion of ciliary muscle (*g*) merges with scleral spur and trabecular meshwork. Lumen of Schlemm canal (*h*) and loose tissues of its wall are seen clearly. Sheets of the trabecular meshwork (*i*) are outer to cords of uveal meshwork (*j*). An iris process (*k*) is seen to arise from iris surface and join trabecular meshwork at level of anterior portion of scleral spur. Descemet's membrane terminates (*double arrows*) within anterior portion of the triangle, outlining aqueous outflow system. (From Hogan MJ, Alvarado JA, Weddell JE: *Histology of the human eye*, Philadelphia, 1971, Saunders.)

SCLERAL OPACITY

The opacity of the sclera depends on a number of factors, including the number of GAGs, the amount of water, and the size and distribution of the collagen fibrils. The sclera contains one-fourth the number of GAGs that are present in the cornea, and as a probable consequence, the sclera is relatively dehydrated (68%) compared with the cornea.[151] The greater variation in fibril size and the irregular spacing between scleral components induce light scattering, which renders the sclera opaque.[33,145]

SCLERAL COLOR

The anterior sclera is visible through the conjunctiva and, if healthy, is white but may appear colored as a result of age or disease. In the newborn, the sclera has a bluish tint because it is almost transparent and the underlying vascular uvea shows through. The sclera also may appear blue in connective tissue diseases that cause scleral thinning. The sclera might appear yellow in the presence of fatty deposits, which can occur with age. Likewise, the sclera may appear yellow in liver disease because of the buildup of metabolic wastes.

SCLERAL FORAMINA AND CANALS

The sclera contains a number of foramina and canals. The *anterior scleral foramen* is the area occupied by the cornea. The optic nerve passes through the *posterior scleral foramen*, which is bridged by a network of scleral tissue called the **lamina cribrosa.** It is similar to a sieve, with interwoven collagen fibrils forming canals through which the optic nerve bundles pass.[146,152] The lamina cribrosa is the weakest area of the outer connective tissue tunic.[1]

Clinical Comment: Optic Nerve Cupping

Because it is the weakest area of the outer connective tissue layer, the lamina cribrosa is the area that will most likely be affected by increased pressure inside the eye. A cupping out or ectasia of the center area of the surface of the optic nerve may be evident in patients with elevated intraocular pressure and is one of the clinical signs sometimes noted in glaucoma. This cupping can also be attributable to the loss of nerve fiber tissue of the optic nerve head.

The canals that pass through the sclera carry nerves and vessels, and are possible routes by which disease can exit or enter the eye. The canals are designated by their location. The *posterior apertures* are located around the posterior scleral foramen and are the passages for the posterior ciliary arteries and nerves. The *middle apertures* lie approximately 4 mm posterior to the equator and carry the vortex veins (Figure 2-21). The *anterior apertures* are near the limbus at the muscle insertions and are the passages for the anterior ciliary vessels, which are branches from the muscular arteries.

SCLERAL BLOOD SUPPLY

Because it is relatively inactive metabolically, the sclera has a minimal blood supply. A number of vessels pass through the sclera to other tissues, but the sclera is considered avascular because it contains no capillary beds. Nourishment is furnished by small branches from the episcleral and choroidal vessels, and branches of the long posterior ciliary arteries.[151]

SCLERAL INNERVATION

Sensory innervation is supplied to the posterior sclera by branches of the short ciliary nerves; the remainder of the sclera is served by branches of the long ciliary nerves.[151]

LIMBUS

The **limbus,** located at the corneoscleral junction, is a band approximately 1.5 to 2 mm wide that encircles the periphery of the cornea. The radius of curvature abruptly changes at this junction of cornea and sclera, creating a narrow furrow, the *external scleral sulcus*. Internally at this juncture, there is a larger furrow, the *internal scleral sulcus*, which has a scooped-out appearance and contains the trabecular meshwork and the canal of Schlemm, the major route for drainage of the aqueous humor. These structures are discussed in Chapter 6.

Histologically, the *anterior boundary* of the limbus consists of a plane connecting the termination of Bowman's layer and the termination of Descemet's membrane (see Figure 2-20). The *posterior boundary* is a plane perpendicular to the surface of the globe and passing through the posterior edge of the scleral spur.[153] These boundaries are used in this discussion, although clinically the boundaries are not as definitive.

The limbus is the transitional zone between cornea and conjunctiva, and between cornea and sclera. Some layers of the cornea continue into the limbal area and others terminate (see Figure 2-20). In the limbus, (1) the very regular squamous corneal epithelium becomes the thicker columnar conjunctival epithelium, (2) the very regular corneal stroma becomes the irregularly arranged scleral stroma, (3) the corneal endothelial

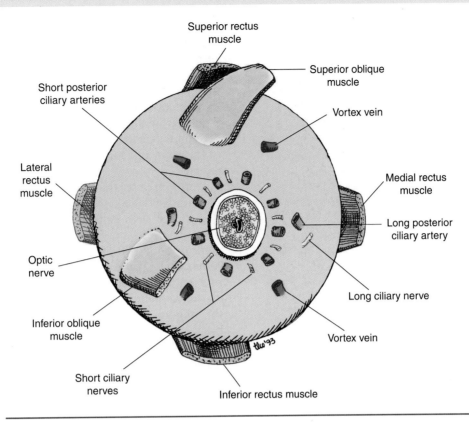

FIGURE 2-21
Posterior sclera. Optic nerve passes through the posterior scleral foramen; long and short ciliary arteries and nerves pass through the posterior apertures; and vortex veins pass through the middle apertures.

sheet becomes discontinuous to wrap around the strands of the trabecular meshwork, (4) Bowman's layer and Descemet's membrane terminate at the anterior border, and (5) the conjunctival stroma, episclera, and Tenon's capsule begin within the limbal area.

LIMBAL HISTOLOGIC FEATURES

The epithelium increases at the limbus from a layer five cells thick to a layer 10 to 15 cells thick (Figure 2-22).[1,153,154] Melanocytes may be present in the basal layer, and pigmentation may be evident in the limbus and conjunctiva, especially in darker-skinned individuals. Bowman's layer tapers and terminates.

The limbus contains the transition from the very regular corneal lamellae to the irregular and random organization of collagen bundles in the sclera. This change is gradual such that, as the transparent cornea merges into the opaque sclera, no line of demarcation can be identified. The scleral fibrils extend further anteriorly on the external than on the internal side of the limbus.[2] Within the limbal stroma at the corneal periphery, a distinct group of collagen fibrils has been identified that lies circumferentially, forming an annulus. This ring

structure is postulated to help maintain the correct corneal curvature.[50,155]

Descemet's membrane tapers at the anterior limbal boundary, and the posterior nonbanded portion becomes interlaced with the connective tissue of the anterior sheets of the trabecular meshwork. The corneal endothelium continues into the anterior chamber angle as the endothelial covering of the sheets of the trabecular meshwork.[19,62]

The conjunctival stroma (*submucosa*) begins in the limbus and has no counterpart in the cornea. This stromal tissue forms mounds that project toward the surface epithelium at the limbus, giving an undulating appearance to the anterior surface of the stroma. The basal layer of the epithelium follows these ridges, called papillae, which are also found near the eyelid margin. Papillae give the inner aspect of the epithelium a wavy appearance, although the surface remains smooth.

Tenon's capsule lies just inner to the conjunctival submucosa, and the episclera is inner to Tenon's capsule. Both begin in the limbus but do not continue into the cornea. Tenon's capsule, the episclera, and the conjunctival stroma fuse in the anterior limbal area.[2]

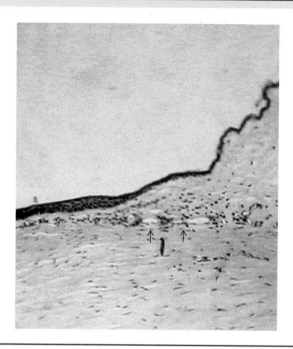

FIGURE 2-22
Light micrograph showing limbal area, cornea to left, conjunctiva and sclera to right. The loose connective tissue of the conjunctival stroma appears inner to the thickened epithelium. Episcleral vessels (*arrows*), cut in cross section, are outer to dense connective tissue of sclera.

LIMBAL BLOOD VESSELS AND LYMPHATICS

Capillary loops from conjunctival and episcleral vessels form networks in the limbus, which surround the cornea and provide nourishment to the avascular corneal tissue. Limbal veins collect blood from the anterior conjunctival veins and drain into the radial episcleral veins, which then empty into the anterior ciliary veins.[156] Lymphatic channels located in the limbal area do not enter the cornea.

PALISADES OF VOGT

The **palisades of Vogt** are radial projections of fibrovascular tissue in spokelike fashion around the corneal periphery.[16] They are concentrated in the superior and inferior limbus and contain nerves, blood vessels, and lymphatics. On biomicroscopy these projections appear as thin, gray pegs approximately 0.04 mm wide and 0.36 mm long.[157] The surface of the limbal area where the palisades of Vogt arise remains flat. The interpalisade region contains thickened conjunctival epithelium and is the likely site for limbal stem cells.[156,158-166]

A population of cells residing in the basal epithelial layer in this area has been identified as possessing the characteristics of stem cells; that is, (1) a cell with self-renewal properties (i.e., after cell division one of the daughter cells remains a stem cell); (2) the cell is undifferentiated but has differentiation ability; and (3) the cell is in an arrested state most of the time, but can be stimulated to divide.[117,129] The low mitotic ability of the stem cell helps to decrease possibility of DNA damage.[117]

Cords of cells that run from the palisade periphery into limbal stroma are the likely anatomical location of the stem cells and are called *limbal epithelial crypts*.[167] They serve as a reserve for corneal cell proliferation; upon cell division a cell migrates toward the center of the cornea and then differentiates into a corneal epithelial cell in the basal layer.[168] This centripetal movement from the limbal area is responsible for the migration and replacement of corneal epithelial basal cells in both normal cell replacement and wound healing.[15] Stem cells are a source for corneal repair in disease.

Stem cells are generally located in a "niche," a specific environment that provides the factors necessary to maintain the cell in its "stemness."[167] The palisades of Vogt are the "niche" for limbal stem cells. The undulations of the epithelium between the palisades provides increased surface area for a large number of cells. The limbal epithelial crypts are located mainly superiorly and inferiorly and thus are protected by the eyelids. The palisades contain melanocytes safeguarding against UVR damage and contain conjunctival blood vessel loops, a source of nutrition.[117,129,157] The stem cells have contact with limbal stroma with no intervening Bowman's layer and it is speculated that the contact with stroma facilitates the distribution of growth factors and cytokines and maintains the cell in its stemness.[131]

Clinical Comment: Limbal Stem Cell Deficiency

IN LIMBAL STEM CELL DEFICIENCY the limbus is nonfunctioning, stem cell loss occurs, and conjunctival tissue can invade the cornea, leading to neovascularization and corneal opacity. Because a key feature of limbal stem cell deficiency is corneal neovascularization, the stem cells may have a role in maintaining the antiangiogenic state of normal cornea, and when stem cells are lost neovascularization ensues. In a novel approach to treating limbal stem cell deficiency, a sheet of epithelial cells fabricated from the patient's own oral mucosal epithelium is transplanted into the limbal area. Initial studies are promising.[169]

PHYSIOLOGICAL AGING CHANGES IN CORNEA

Alterations to cellular integrins in the corneal epithelium can occur with age and result in a reduction in the adhesion molecules necessary for intercellular junction construction. This causes a breakdown in the barrier function of the corneal epithelium.[170] Decreased keratocyte density can adversely affect wound healing and collagen fibril degradation produces spaces that can disrupt transparency and create opacities.[170] Descemet's membrane increases in thickness, Hassall-Henle bodies increase in the periphery, and endothelial cell density decreases with cell loss.

Clinical Comment: Clinical Aging Changes

*AGING produces changes in corneal appearance, but most are not detrimental to vision. Iron deposits in epithelial cell cytoplasm, more concentrated in the basal cells,[171] produce a horizontal pigmented line, the **Hudson-Stähli line**, often evident at the level of the lower lid margin. Degeneration of Bowman's layer produces the **limbal girdle of Vogt**. This yellowish white opacity is located at the 3 and 9 o'clock positions, interpalpebrally, but does not encircle the cornea. A clear interval separating the opacity from the limbus may or may not be seen. The area may include degeneration of the anterior stroma, calcium deposits, and hypertrophy of the overlying epithelium.*

***Corneal arcus** is the most common corneal aging change. An annular yellow-white deposit located within peripheral stroma is evident (Figure 2-23). This ring is separated from the limbus by a zone of clear cornea. The deposits are cholesterol and cholesterol esters and can result from age or elevated blood cholesterol levels. With time the arcus can extend anteriorly to Bowman's layer or into central cornea. There is no clinical significance in elderly persons, but in those under age 40, hyperlipidemia should be suspected.*

Hassall-Henle bodies, located in peripheral Descemet's membrane and described earlier, are of no clinical significance.

*Aging changes in the corneal endothelium include a decrease in cell density, polymegathism, and pleomorphism.[66,67,172] Pigment deposits on the posterior cornea that have a vertical orientation are called **Krukenberg's spindle**, and their incidence increases with age.*

There is no evident change in the wavelengths transmitted by the aging cornea.[173]

A decrease in corneal sensitivity corresponds to a loss of corneal nerves with age.[174]

Fatty deposits may cause the sclera to appear yellow. Scleral collagen and elastic fibers degenerate, the concentration of certain proteoglycans is decreased, causing scleral thinning and loss of elasticity.[145] The fibers of the lamina cribrosa become stiffer and less resilient with age. Changes in the laminar pores in the aged lamina cribrosa may make the nerve fibers passing through the openings more susceptible to injury, contributing to an increased susceptibility to glaucomatous damage.[175-178]

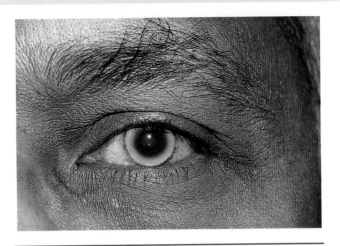

FIGURE 2-23
The white limbal band of corneal arcus. (From Kanski JJ, Nischal JJ: *Ophthalmology: clinical signs and differential diagnosis,* St Louis, 1998, Mosby.)

REFERENCES

1. Warwick R: *Eugene Wolff's anatomy of the eye and orbit,* ed 7, Philadelphia, 1976, Saunders, p 30.
2. Van Buskirk EM: The anatomy of the limbus, *Eye* 3:101, 1989.
3. Martola EL, Baun JL: A clinical study on central and peripheral corneal thickness, *Arch Ophthalmol* 79:28, 1968.
4. Pepose JS, Ubels JL: The cornea. In Hart WM Jr, editor: *Adler's physiology of the eye: clinical application,* ed 9, St Louis, 1992, Mosby, p 29.
5. Siu A, Herse P: The effect of age on human corneal thickness. Statistical implications of power analysis, *Acta Ophthalmol (Copenh)* 71(1):51, 1993.
6. Hogan MJ, Alvarado JA: The cornea. In Hogan MJ, Alvarado JA, Weddell JE, editors: *Histology of the human eye,* Philadelphia, 1971, Saunders, p 55.
7. Guthoff RF, Zhivov A, Stachs O: *In vivo* confocal microscopy, an inner vision of the cornea—a major review, *Clin Exp Ophthalmol* 37:100–117, 2009.
8. Gipson IK, Yankauckas M, Spurr-Michaud SJ, et al: Characteristics of a glycoprotein in the ocular surface glycocalyx, *Invest Ophthalmol Vis Sci* 33:218, 1992.
9. Nichols B, Dawson CR, Togni B: Surface features of the conjunctiva and cornea, *Invest Ophthalmol Vis Sci* 24:570, 1983.
10. Watanabe H, Fabricant M, Tisdale AS, et al: Human corneal and conjunctival epithelia produce a mucin-like glycoprotein for the apical surface, *Invest Ophthalmol Vis Sci* 36(2):337, 1995.
11. Pfister RR: The normal surface of corneal epithelium: a scanning electron microscopic study, *Invest Ophthalmol* 12:654, 1973.
12. Williams KK, Watsky MA: Dye spread through gap junctions in the corneal epithelium of the rabbit, *Curr Eye Res* 16:445, 1997.
13. Gipson IK, Spurr-Michaud SJ, Tisdale AS: Anchoring fibrils form a complex network in human and rabbit cornea, *Invest Ophthalmol Vis Sci* 28(2):212, 1987.
14. Gipson IK, Spurr-Michaud S, Tisdale A, et al: Reassembly of the anchoring structures of the corneal epithelium during wound repair in the rabbit, *Invest Ophthalmol Vis Sci* 30:425, 1989.
15. Gipson IK, Spurr-Michaud SJ, Tisdale AS: Hemidesmosome and anchoring fibril collagen appears synchronously during development and wound healing, *Dev Biol* 126:253, 1988.

16. Gipson IK: The epithelial basement membrane zone of the limbus, *Eye* 3:132, 1989.

17. Khodadoust AA, Silverstein AM, Kenyon DR, et al: Adhesion of regenerating epithelium. The role of basement membrane, *Am J Ophthalmol* 65(3):339, 1968.

18. Tisdale AS, Spurr-Michaud SJ, Rodrigues M, et al: Development of the anchoring structures of the epithelium in rabbit and human fetal corneas, *Invest Ophthalmol Vis Sci* 29(5):727, 1988.

19. Binder PS, Rock ME, Schmidt KC, et al: High-voltage electron microscopy of normal human cornea, *Invest Ophthalmol Vis Sci* 32:2234, 1991.

20. Kruse FE: Stem cells and corneal epithelial regeneration, *Eye* 8:170, 1994.

21. Thoft R, Friend J: The X, Y, Z hypothesis of corneal epithelial maintenance, *Invest Ophthalmol Vis Sci* 24(10):1442, 1983.

22. Tseng SC: Concept and application of limbal stem cells, *Eye* 3:141, 1989.

23. Hanna C, O'Brien JE: Cell production and migration in the epithelial layer of the cornea, *Arch Ophthalmol* 64:536, 1960.

24. Hanna C, Bicknell DS, O'Brien JE: Cell turnover in the adult human eye, *Arch Ophthalmol* 65:695, 1961.

25. McCartney ND, Cantu-Crouch D: Rabbit corneal epithelial wound repair: tight junction reformation, *Curr Eye Res* 11:15, 1992.

26. Alvarado J, Murphy C, Juster R: Age-related changes in the basement membrane of the human corneal epithelium, *Invest Ophthalmol Vis Sci* 24(8):1015, 1983.

27. Bartlett JD, Jaanus SD: *Clinical ocular pharmacology*, ed 2, Boston, 1989, Butterworth, p 379.

28. Susický P: Use of soft contact lenses in the treatment of recurrent corneal erosions, *Cesk Oftalmol* 46(5):381, 1990:(abstract).

29. Robin JB, Keys CL, Kaminski LA, et al: The effect of collagen shields on rabbit corneal reepithelialization after chemical debridement, *Invest Ophthalmol Vis Sci* 31(7):1294, 1990.

30. Geggel HS: Successful treatment of recurrent corneal erosion with Nd:YAG anterior stromal puncture, *Am J Ophthalmol* 110(4):404, 1990.

31. Katsev DA, Kincaid MC, Fouraker BD, et al: Recurrent corneal erosion: pathology of corneal puncture, *Cornea* 10(5):418, 1991.

32. Pfister RR: Clinical measures to promote corneal epithelial healing, *Acta Ophthalmol Suppl* 202:73, 1992.

33. Komai Y, Ushiki T: The three-dimensional organization of collagen fibrils in the human cornea and sclera, *Invest Ophthalmol Vis Sci* 32:2244, 1991.

34. Wilson SE, Hong JW: Bowman's layer structure and function: critical or dispensable to corneal function? A hypothesis, *Cornea* 19(4):417, 2000.

35. Radner W, Zehetmayer M, Aufreiter R, et al: Interlacing and cross-angle distribution of collagen lamellae in the human cornea, *Cornea* 17(5):537, 1998.

36. Radner W, Mallinger R: Interlacing of collagen lamellae in the midstroma of the human cornea, *Cornea* 21(6):598, 2002.

37. Goldman J, Benedek G, Dohlman C, et al: Structural alterations affecting transparency in swollen human corneas, *Invest Ophthalmol* 7(5):501, 1968.

38. Müller LJ, Pels E, Vrensen GF: The specific architecture of the anterior stroma accounts for maintenance of corneal curvature, *Br J Ophthalmol* 85:437–443, 2001.

39. Poole CA, Brookes NH, Clover GM: Keratocyte networks visualized in the living cornea using vital dyes, *J Cell Sci* 106:685, 1993.

40. Müller LJ, Pels E, Vrensen GF: The specific architecture of the anterior stroma accounts for maintenance of corneal curvature, *Br J Ophthalmol* 85:437, 2001.

41. Müller LJ, Pels L, Vrensen GF: Novel aspects of the ultrastructural organization of human corneal keratocytes, *Invest Ophthalmol Vis Sci* 36(13):2557, 1995.

42. Snyder MC, Bergmanson JP, Doughty MJ: Keratocytes: no more the quiet cells, *J Am Optom Assoc* 69:180, 1998.

43. Davies Y, Lewis D, Fullwood NJ, et al: Proteoglycans on normal and migrating human corneal endothelium, *Exp Eye Res* 68:303–311, 1999.

44. Ehlers N, Hjortdal J: The Cornea. In Fischbarg J, editor: *The biology of the eye, vol. 10*, 2006, Elsevier, pp 83–111.

45. Scott JE, Haigh M: "Small" proteoglycan: collagen interactions: Keratin sulfate proteoglycan associates with rabbit corneal collagen fibrils at the "a" and "c" bands, *Biosci Rep* 5:765, 1985.

46. Maurice DM: The structure and transparency of the cornea, *J Physiol* 136:263, 1957.

47. Farrell RA, McCally RL, Tatham PE: Wave-length dependencies of light scattering in normal and cold swollen rabbit corneas and their structural implications, *J Physiol* 233:589, 1973.

48. Jester JV: Corneal crystallins and the development of cellular transparency, *Semin Cell Dev Biol* 19:82–93, 2008.

49. Edelhauser HF, Ubels JL: The cornea and the sclera. In Kaufman PL, Alm A, editors: *Adler's physiology of the eye: clinical application*, ed 10, St Louis, 2003, Elsevier Science, p 47.

50. Meek KM, Tuft SJ, Huang Y, et al: Changes in collagen orientation and distribution in keratoconus corneas, *Invest Ophthalmol Vis Sci* 46:1948–1956, 2005.

51. Bron AJ: Keratoconus, *Cornea* 7(3):163, 1988.

52. Chi HH, Katzin HM, Teng CC: Histopathology of keratoconus, *Am J Ophthalmol* 42:847, 1956.

53. Astin C: Contact lens fitting after anterior segment disease, *Contact Lens J* 20(5):11, 1992.

54. http://www.nkcf.org/treatment-options/corneal-crosslinking/70-corneal-collagen-crosslinking.html. Accessed April 10, 2011.

55. Whikehart DR, Parikh CH, Vaughn AV, et al: Evidence suggesting the existence of stem cells for the human corneal endothelium, *Mol Vis* 11:816–824, 2005.

56. Raiskup-Wolf F, Hoyer A, Spoerl E, et al: Collagen crosslinking with riboflavin and ultraviolet-A light in keratoconus: long-term results, *J Cataract Refract Surg* 34(5):796–801, 2008.

57. Johnson DH, Bourne WM, Campbell RJ: The ultrastructure of Descemet's membrane: I. Changes with age in normal corneas, *Arch Ophthalmol* 100:1942, 1982.

58. Gipson IK, Grill SM, Spurr SJ, et al: Hemidesmosomes formation in vitro, *J Cell Biol* 9(97):849–857, 1983.

59. Joyce NC: Proliferative capacity of the corneal endothelium, *Prog Retin Eye Res* 22:359, 2003.

60. Doughty MJ: Toward a quantitative analysis of corneal endothelial cell morphology: a review of techniques and their application, *Optom Vis Sci* 66:626, 1989.

61. Joyce NC, Harris DL, Mello DM: Mechanisms of miotic inhibition in corneal endothelium: contact inhibition and TGF-beta2, *Invest Ophthalmol Vis Sci* 43:2152, 2002:(abstract).

62. Waring GO 3rd, Bourne WM, Edelhauser HF, et al: The corneal endothelium. Normal and pathologic structure and function, *Ophthalmology* 89(6):531, 1982.

63. Barry PA, Petroll WM, Andrews PM, et al: The spatial organization of corneal endothelial cytoskeletal proteins and their relationship to the apical junctional complex, *Invest Ophthalmol Vis Sci* 36(6):1115, 1995.

64. Kaye GI, Sibley RC, Hoefle FB: Recent studies on the nature and function of the corneal endothelial layer, *Exp Eye Res* 15:585, 1973.

65. Senoo T, Joyce NC: Cell cycle kinetics in corneal endothelium from old and young donors, *Invest Ophthalmol Vis Sci* 41:660, 2000.

66. Mustonen RK, McDonald MB, Srivannaboon S, et al: Normal human corneal cell populations evaluated by in vivo scanning slit confocal microscopy, *Cornea* 17(5):485, 1998.

67. Abib FC, Barreto J Jr: Behavior of corneal endothelial density over a lifetime, *J Cataract Refract Surg* 27:1574, 2001.

68. Bourne WM, Kaufman HE: Specular microscopy of the human corneal endothelium in vivo, *Am J Ophthalmol* 81:319, 1976.

69. Bergmanson JP: Histopathological analysis of corneal endothelial polymegathism, *Cornea* 11:133, 1992.

70. Efron N, Perez-Gomez I, Morgan PB: Confocal microscopic observations of stromal keratocytes during extended contact lens wear, *Clin Exp Optom* 85(3):156, 2002.

71. Lui ZG, Pflugfelder SC: The effects of long-term contact lens wear on corneal thickness, curvature, and surface regularity, *Ophthalmology* 107:105, 2000.

72. Connor CG, Zagrod ME: Contact lens-induced corneal endothelial polymegathism: functional significance and possible mechanisms, *Am J Optom Physiol Opt* 63:539, 1986.

73. Holden BA, Sweeney DF, Vannas A, et al: Effects of long-term extended contact lens wear on the human cornea, *Invest Ophthalmol Vis Sci* 26:1489, 1985.

74. Holden BA, Vannas A, Nilsson L, et al: Epithelial and endothelial effects from the extended wear of contact lenses, *Curr Eye Res* 4:739, 1985.

75. Matsuda M, Inaba M, Suda T, et al: Corneal endothelial changes associated with aphakic extended contact lens wear, *Arch Ophthalmol* 106:70, 1988.

76. MacRae SM, Matsuda M, Shellans S, et al: The effects of hard and soft contact lenses on the corneal endothelium, *Am J Ophthalmol* 102:50, 1986.

77. Lassen N, Black WJ, Estey T, et al: The role of corneal crystallins in the cellular defense mechanisms against oxidative stress, *Semin Cell Dev Biol* 19:100–112, 2008.

78. McCulley JP: The circulation of fluid at the limbus (flow and diffusion at the limbus), *Eye* 3:114, 1989.

79. Mishima S, Hedbys BO: Physiology of the cornea, *Int Ophthalmol Clin* 8:527–560, 1968.

80. Levin MH, Verkman AS: Aquaporin-3-dependent cell migration and proliferation during corneal re-epithelialization, *Invest Ophthalmol Vis Sci* 47:4365–4372, 2006.

81. Verkman AS: Aquaporins and water transport in the cornea. In Tombran-Tink J, Barnstable CJ, editors: *Ophthtlamology research: ocular transporters in ophthalmic diseases and drug delivery*, Totowa NJ, 2008, Hamana Press.

82. Candia OA: Electrolyte and fluid transport across corneal, conjunctival and lens epithelia, *Exp Eye Res* 78:527–535, 2004.

83. Reinach PS, Capó-Aponte JE, Mergler S, et al: Roles of corneal epithelial ion transport mechanisms in mediating responses to cytokines and osmotic stress. In Tombran-Tink J, Barnstable CJ, editors: *Ophthalmology research: ocular transporters in ophthalmic diseases and drug delivery*, Totowa NJ, 2008, Hamana Press.

84. Mandell KJ, Berglin L, Severson EA, et al: Expression of JAM-A in the human corneal endothelium and retinal pigment epithelium: localization and evidence for role in barrier function, *Invest Ophthalmol Vis Sci* 48:3928–3936, 2007.

85. Mergler S, Pleyer U: The human corneal endothelium: new insights into electrophysiology and ion channels, *Prog Retin Eye Res* 26:359–378, 2007.

86. Fischbarg J: The corneal endothelium. In Fischbarg J, editor: *The biology of the eye*, vol 10, 2006, Elsevier, pp 113–125.

87. Bonanno JA: Identity and regulation of ion transport mechanism in the corneal epithelium, *Prog Retin Eye Res* 22:69–94, 2003.

88. McDermott ML, Atluri HKS: Corneal endothelium. In Yanoff M, Duker JS, editors: *Ophthalmology*, ed 2, 2004, Mosby, pp 422–430.

89. Fatt I, Bieber MT, Pye SD: Steady state distribution of oxygen and carbon dioxide in the in vivo cornea of an eye covered by a gas-permeable contact lens, *Am J Optom Arch Am Acad Optom* 46:3–14, 1969.

90. Hill RM, Fatt I: How dependent is the cornea on the atmosphere? *J Am Optom Assoc* 5:873, 1964.

91. Smelser GK, Ozanics V: Importance of atmospheric oxygen for maintenance of the optical properties of the human cornea, *Science* 115:140, 1952.

92. Baum JP, Maurice DM, McCarey BE: The active and passive transport of water across the corneal endothelium, *Exp Eye Res* 39:335, 1984.

93. Larrea X, Büchler P: A transient diffusion model of the cornea for the assessment of oxygen diffusivity and consumption, *Invest Ophthalmol Vis Sci* 50:1076–1080, 2009.

94. Geroski DH, Matsuda M, Yee RW, et al: Pump function of the human corneal endothelium. Effects of age and cornea guttata, *Ophthalmology* 92:759–763, 1985.

95. Lu L: Stress-induced corneal epithelial apoptosis mediated by K+ channel activation, *Prog Retin Eye Res* 25:515–538, 2006.

96. Beebe DC: Maintaining transparency: a review of the developmental physiology and pathophysiology of two avascular tissues, *Semin Cell Dev Biol* 19:125–133, 2008.

97. Mertz GW: Overnight swelling of the living human cornea, *J Am Optom Assoc* 51:211–214, 1980.

98. Rom ME, Keller WB, Meyer CJ, et al: Relationship between corneal edema and topography, *CLAO J* 21(3):191, 1995.

99. Stepp MA: Corneal integrins and their functions, *Exp Eye Res* 83:3–15, 2006.

100. Brazzell RK, Stern ME, Aquavella JV, et al: Human recombinant epidermal growth factor in experimental corneal wound healing, *Invest Ophthalmol Vis Sci* 32(2):336, 1991.

101. Hoppenreijs VP, Pels E, Vrensen GF, et al: Effects of human growth factor on endothelial wound healing of human corneas, *Invest Ophthalmol Vis Sci* 33(6):1946, 1992.

102. Hoppenreijs VP, Pels E, Vrensen GF, et al: Platelet-derived growth factor: receptor expression in corneas and effects on corneal cells, *Invest Ophthalmol Vis Sci* 34(3):637, 1993.

103. Kim KS, Oh JS, Kim IS, et al: Clinical efficacy of topical homologous fibronectin in persistent corneal epithelial disorders, *Korean J Ophthalmol* 6(1):12, 1992.

104. Mooradian DL, McCarthy JB, Skubitz AP, et al: Characterization of FM-C/H-V, a novel synthetic peptide from fibronectin that promotes rabbit corneal epithelial cell adhesion, spreading, and motility, *Invest Ophthalmol Vis Sci* 34(1):153, 1993.

105. Pastor JC, Calonge M: Epidermal growth factor and corneal wound healing. A multicenter study, *Cornea* 11(4):311, 1992.

106. Rieck P, Hartmann C, Jacob C, et al: Human recombinant bFGF stimulates corneal endothelial wound healing in rabbits, *Curr Eye Res* 11(12):1161, 1992.

107. Schultz G, Chegini N, Grant M, et al: Effects of growth factors on corneal wound healing, *Acta Ophthalmol Suppl* 202:60, 1992.

108. Fullwood NJ, Davies Y, Nieduszynski IA, et al: Cell surface-associated keratan sulfate on normal and migrating corneal endothelium, *Invest Ophthalmol Vis Sci* 37(7):1256, 1996.

109. Zelenka PS, Arpitha P: Coordinating cell proliferation and migration in the lens and cornea, *Semin Cell Dev Biol* 19:113–124, 2008.

110. Suzuki K, Tanaka T, Enoki M, et al: Coordinated reassembly of the basement membrane and junctional proteins during corneal epithelial wound healing, *Invest Ophthalmol Vis Sci* 41:2495–2500, 2000.

111. Crosson CE, Klyce SD, Beuerman RW: Corneal epithelial wound closure, *Invest Ophthalmol Vis Sci* 27(4):464, 1986.

112. Tervo T, van Setten GB, Päällysaho T, et al: Wound healing of the ocular surface, *Ann Med* 24:19, 1992.

113. Nishida T, Nakagawa S, Awata T, et al: Fibronectin promotes epithelial migration of cultured rabbit cornea in situ, *J Cell Biol* 97:1653–1657, 1983.

114. Stapleton F, Kim JM, Kasses J, et al: Mechanisms of apoptosis in human corneal epithelial cells, *Adv Exp Med Biol* 506:827–834, 2002.

115. Karamichos D, Lakshman N, Petroll WM: Regulation of corneal fibroblast morphology and collagen reorganization by extracellular matrix mechanical properties, *Invest Ophthalmol Vis Sci* 48:5030–5037, 2007.

116. Davison PF, Galbary EJ: Connective tissue remodeling in corneal and scleral wounds, *Invest Ophthalmol Vis Sci* 27(10):1478, 1986.

117. Takács L, Tóth E, Berta A, et al: Stem cells of the adult cornea: from cytometric markers to therapeutic applications, (Cytometry Part A: The Journal of the International Society for Analytical Cytology) *Cytometry A* 75:54–66, 2009.

118. Boettner EA, Wolter JR: Transmission of the ocular media, *Invest Ophthalmol Vis Sci* 1:776, 1962.

119. Podskochy A: Protective role of corneal epithelium against ultraviolet radiation damage, *Acta Ophthalmol Scand* 82:714–717, 2004.

120. Kolozsvári L, Nógrádi A, Hopp B, et al: UV absorbance of the human cornea in the 240- to 400-nm range, *Invest Ophthalmol Vis Sci* 43(7):2165, 2002.

121. Ringvold A: Corneal epithelium and UV-protection of the eye, *Acta Ophthalmol Scand* 76:149, 1998.

122. Karai I, Matsumura S, Takise S, et al: Morphological change in the corneal endothelium due to ultraviolet radiation in welders, *Br J Ophthalmol* 68:544, 1984.

123. Lawrenson JG, Ruskell GL: The structure of corpuscular nerve endings in the limbal conjunctiva of the human eye, *J Anat* 177:75, 1991.

124. Müller LJ, Pels E, Vrensen GF: Ultrastructural organization of human corneal nerves, *Invest Ophthalmol Vis Sci* 37(4):476, 1996.

125. Müller LJ, Marfurt CF, Kruse F, et al: Corneal nerves: structure, contents and function, *Exp Eye Res* 76(5):521–542, 2003.

126. Bonini S, Rama P, Olzi D, et al: Neurotrophic keratitis: A review, *Eye* (17):989–995, 2003.

127. Yu CQ, Zhang M, Matis KI, et al: Vascular endothelial growth factor mediates corneal nerve repair, *Invest Ophthalmol Vis Sci* 49:3870–3878, 2008.

128. Liu S, Li J, Tan DT, et al: Expression and function of muscarinic receptor subtypes on human cornea and conjunctiva, *Invest Ophthalmol Vis Sci* 48:2987–2996, 2007.

129. Lim P, Fuchsluger TA, Jurkunas UV: Limbal stem cell deficiency and corneal neovascularization, *Semin Ophthalmol* 24:139–148, 2009.

130. Klintworth GK, Burger PC: Neovascularization of the cornea: current concepts of its pathogenesis, *Int Ophthalmol Clin* 23(1):27, 1983.

131. Secker GA, Daniels JT: Corneal epithelial stem cells: Deficiency and regulation, *Stem Cell Rev* 4:159–168, 2008.

132. Efron N, Al-Dossari M, Pritchard N: Confocal microscopy of the bulbar conjunctiva in contact lens wear, *Cornea* 29(1):43–52, 2010.

133. Chen W, Lin H, Dong N, et al: Cauterization of central cornea induces recruitment of major histocompatibility complex class II+ Langerhans cells from limbal basal epithelium, *Cornea* 29(1):73–79, 2010.

134. Chih A, Lugo M, Kowing D: Descemet stripping and automated endothelial keratoplasty: an alternative to penetrating keratoplasty, *Optom Vis Sci* 85:152–157, 2008.

135. Pallikaris JG, Siganos DS: Laser in situ keratomileusis to treat myopia: early experience, *J Cataract Refract Surg* 23:39, 1997.

136. Collins MJ, Carr JD, Stulting RD, et al: Effects of laser in situ keratomileusis (LASIK) on the corneal endothelium 3 years postoperatively, *Am J Ophthalmol* 131:1, 2001.

137. Jabbur NS: Endothelial cell studies in patients after photorefractive keratectomy for hyperopia, *J Refract Surg* 19:142, 2003.

138. Fagerholm P: Phototherapeutic keratectomy: 12 years of experience, *Acta Ophthalmol Scand* 81(1):19, 2003.

139. Simaroj P, Kosalprapai K, Chuckpaiwong V: Effect of laser in situ keratomileusis on the corneal endothelium, *J Refract Surg* 19:S237, 2003.

140. Brandt JD, Beiser JA, Kass MA, et al: Central corneal thickness in the Ocular Hypertension Treatment Study (OHTS), *Ophthalmology* 108(10):1779, 2001.

141. Bhan A, Browning AC, Shah S, et al: Effect of corneal thickness on intraocular pressure measurements with the pneumotonometer, Goldmann applanation tonometer, and Tono-Pen, *Invest Ophthalmol Vis Sci* 43(5):1389, 2002.

142. Rashad KM, Bahnassy AA: Changes in intraocular pressure after laser in situ keratomileusis, *J Refract Surg* 17(4):420, 2001.

143. Arimoto A, Shimizu K, Shoji N, et al: Underestimation of intraocular pressure in eyes after laser in situ keratomileusis, *Jpn J Ophthalmol* 46(6):645, 2002.

144. Quantock AJ, Meek KM: Axial electron density of human scleral collagen, Location of proteoglycans by x-ray diffraction, *Biophys J* 54:159, 1988.

145. Rada JA, Shelton S, Norton TT: The sclera and myopia, *Exp Eye Res* 82(2):185–200, 2006.

146. Thale A, Tillmann B: The collagen architecture of the sclera—SEM and immunohistochemical studies, *Ann Anat* 175:215, 1993.

147. Marshall GE: Human scleral elastic system: an immunoelectron microscopic study, *Br J Ophthalmol* 79:57, 1995.

148. Alexander RA, Garner A: Elastic and precursor fibres in the normal human eye, *Exp Eye Res* 36:305, 1983.

149. McBrien NA, Cornell LM, Gentle A: Structural and ultrastructural changes to the sclera in a mammalian model of high myopia, *Invest Ophthalmol Vis Sci* 42:2179, 2001:(abstract).

150. McBrien NA, Gentle A: The role of visual information in the control of scleral matrix biology in myopia, *Curr Eye Res* 23(5):313, 2001.

151. Hogan MJ, Alvarado JA: The sclera. In Hogan MJ, Alvarado JA, Weddell JE, editors: *Histology of the human eye*, Philadelphia, 1971, Saunders, p 183.

152. Elkington AR, Inman CB, Steart PV, et al: The structure of the lamina cribrosa of the human eye: an immunocytochemical and electron microscopical study, *Eye* 4:42, 1990.

153. Hogan MJ, Alvarado JA: The limbus. In Hogan MJ, Alvarado JA, Weddell JE, editors: *Histology of the human eye*, Philadelphia, 1971, Saunders, p 112.

154. Kikkawa DO, Lucarelli MJ, Shovlin JP, et al: Ophthalmic facial anatomy and physiology. In Kaufman PL, Alm A, editors: *Adler's physiology of the eye: clinical application*, ed 10, St Louis, 2003, Elsevier Science, p 16.

155. Newton RH, Meek KM: Circumcorneal annulus of collagen fibrils in the human limbus, *Invest Ophthalmol Vis Sci* 39(7):1125, 1998.

156. Meyer PA: The circulation of the human limbus, *Eye* 3:121, 1989.

157. Goldberg MF, Bron AJ: Limbal palisades of Vogt, *Trans Am Ophthalmol Soc* 80:155–171, 1982.

158. Davanger M, Evensen A: Role of the pericorneal papillary structure in renewal of corneal epithelium, *Nature* 229:560, 1971.

159. Dua HS, Azuara-Blanco A: Limbal stem cells of the corneal epithelium, *Surv Ophthalmol* 44(5):415, 2000.

160. Kinoshita S, Adachi W, Sotozono C, et al: Characteristics of the human ocular surface epithelium, *Prog Retin Eye Res* 20(5):639, 2001.

161. Cotsarelis G, Cheng SZ, Dong GE, et al: Existence of slow-cycling limbal epithelial basal cells that can be preferentially stimulated to proliferate: implications on epithelial stem cells, *Cell* 57:201, 1989.

162. Ebato B, Friend J, Throft RA: Comparison of central and peripheral human corneal epithelium in tissue culture, *Invest Ophthalmol Vis Sci* 28:1450, 1987.

163. Lauweryns B, van den Oord JJ, De Vos R, et al: A new epithelial cell type in the human cornea, *Invest Ophthalmol Vis Sci* 34(6):1983, 1993.

164. Thoft RA, Wiley LA, Sundarraj N: The multipotential cells of the limbus, *Eye* 3:109, 1989.

165. Zieske JD, Bukusoglu G, Yankauckas MA: Characterization of a potential marker of corneal epithelial stem cells, *Invest Ophthalmol Vis Sci* 33(1):143, 1992.

166. Wolosin JM, Xiong X, Schütte M, et al: Stem cells and differentiation stages in the limbo-corneal epithelium, *Prog Retin Eye Res* 19(2):223, 2000.

167. Shanmuganathan VA, Foster T, Kulkarni BB, et al: Morphological characteristics of the limbal epithelial crypt, *Br J Ophthalmol* 91:514–519, 2007.

168. Chang CY, Green CR, McGhee CN, et al: Acute wound healing in the human central corneal epithelium appears to be independent of limbal stem influence, *Invest Ophthalmol Vis Sci* 49:5279–5286, 2008.

169. Nishida K, Yamato M, Hayashida Y, et al: Corneal reconstruction with tissue-engineered cell sheets composed of autologous oral mucosal epithelium, *N Engl J Med* 351:1187–1196, 2004.

170. Faragher RG, Mulholland B, Tuft SJ, et al: Aging and the cornea, *Br J Ophthalmol* 81:814–817, 1997.

171. Barraquer-Somers E, Chan CC, Green WR: Corneal epithelial iron deposition, *Ophthalmology* 90:729, 1983.

172. Bourne WM, Nelson LR, Hodge DO: Central corneal endothelial cell changes over a ten-year period, *Invest Ophthalmol Vis Sci* 38(3):779, 1997.

173. van den Berg TJ, Tan KE: Light transmittance of the human cornea from 320 to 700 nm for different ages, *Vision Res* 34(11):1453, 1994.

174. Hollingsworth J, Perez-Gomez I, Mutalib HA, et al: A population study of the normal cornea using an in vivo, slit-scanning confocal microscope, *Optom Vis Sci* 78(10):706, 2001.

175. Albon J, Karwatowski WS, Easty DL, et al: Age related changes in the non-collagenous components of the extracellular matrix of the human lamina cribrosa, *Br J Ophthalmol* 84:311, 2000.

176. Sawaguchi S, Yue BY, Fukuchi T, et al: Collagen fibrillar network in the optic nerve head of normal monkey eyes and monkey eyes with laser-induced glaucoma—a scanning electron microscopic study, *Curr Eye Res* 18(2):143, 1999.

177. Albon J, Purslow PP, Karwatowski WS, et al: Age related compliance of the lamina cribrosa in human eyes, *Br J Ophthalmol* 84:318, 2000.

178. Albon J, Karwatowski WS, Avery N, et al: Changes in the collagenous matrix of the aging human lamina cribrosa, *Br J Ophthalmol* 79:368, 1995.

The middle layer of the eye, the uvea (uveal tract), is composed of three regions (from front to back): the iris, ciliary body, and choroid. The uvea sometimes is called the vascular layer because its largest structure, the choroid, is composed mainly of blood vessels, which supply the outer retinal layers.

IRIS

The **iris** is a thin, circular structure located anterior to the lens, often compared with a diaphragm of an optical system. The center aperture, the **pupil,** actually is located slightly nasal and inferior to the iris center.[1] Pupil size regulates retinal illumination. The diameter can vary from 1 mm to 9 mm depending on lighting conditions. The pupil is very small **(miotic)** in brightly lit conditions and fairly large **(mydriatic)** in dim illumination. The average diameter of the iris is 12 mm, and its thickness varies. It is thickest in the region of the **collarette,** a circular ridge approximately 1.5 mm from the pupillary margin. This slightly raised jagged ridge was the attachment site for the fetal pupillary membrane during embryologic development.[1,2] The collarette divides the iris into the **pupillary zone,** which encircles the pupil, and the **ciliary zone,** which extends from the collarette to the iris root (Figure 3-1). The color of these two zones often differs.

The pupillary margin of the iris rests on the anterior surface of the lens and, in profile, the iris has a truncated cone shape such that the pupillary margin lies anterior to its peripheral termination, the **iris root** (Figure 3-2). The root, approximately 0.5 mm thick, is the thinnest part of the iris and joins the iris to the anterior aspect of the ciliary body (Figure 3-3).[1] The iris divides the anterior segment of the globe into anterior and posterior chambers, and the pupil allows the aqueous humor to flow from the posterior into the anterior chamber with no resistance.

Clinical Comment: Blunt Trauma

*With blunt trauma to the eye or head, the thin root may tear away from the ciliary body, creating a condition called **iridodialysis,** which can result in damaged blood vessels and nerves. Blood may hemorrhage into either the anterior or the posterior chamber, or both, and nerve damage may cause sector paralysis of the iris muscles.*

HISTOLOGIC FEATURES OF IRIS

The iris can be divided into four layers: (1) the anterior border layer, (2) stroma and sphincter muscle, (3) anterior epithelium and dilator muscle, and (4) posterior epithelium.

Anterior Border Layer

The surface layer of the iris, the **anterior border layer,** is a thin condensation of the stroma. In fact, some do not consider this to be a separate layer. It is composed of fibroblasts and pigmented melanocytes. The highly branching processes of the cells interweave to form a meshwork in which the fibroblasts are on the surface and the melanocytes are located below[1,2] (Figure 3-4). The thickness of the melanocyte layer may vary throughout the iris, with accumulations of melanocytes forming elevated frecklelike masses, evident in the anterior border layer. The density and arrangement of the meshwork differ among irises and are contributing factors in iris color.

The anterior border layer is absent at the oval-shaped **iris crypts.** Near the root, extensions of this layer form finger-shaped iris processes that can attach to the trabecular meshwork. The number of these processes varies, but they usually do not impede aqueous outflow. The anterior border layer ends at the root.

Iris Stroma and Sphincter Muscle

The connective tissue **stroma** is composed of pigmented and nonpigmented cells, collagen fibrils, and extensive ground substance. The pigmented cells include melanocytes and clump cells, whereas the nonpigmented cells are fibroblasts, lymphocytes, macrophages, and mast cells.[1] Although melanocytes and fibroblasts have many branching processes, the cells are widely spaced in the stroma, so their branches do not form a meshwork. *Clump cells* are large, round, darkly pigmented cells and are likely "altered macrophages" and are scavengers of free pigment within the iris.[1,3] Clump cells usually are located in the pupillary portion of the stroma, often near the sphincter muscle (Figure 3-5). The collagen fibrils are arranged in radial columns (trabeculae) that are seen easily as white fibers in light-colored irises.[3]

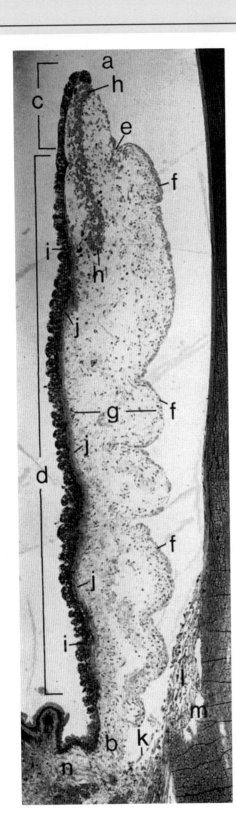

FIGURE 3-1
Light micrograph of the iris and anterior chamber. The cornea, anterior chamber angle, trabecular meshwork, canal of Schlemm, and part of the ciliary body are included. Anterior and posterior iris contraction furrows are accentuated by slight dilation of pupil. Pupil and pupillary ruff are at *a,* and iris root (*b*), pupillary portion of iris (*c*), and ciliary portion (*d*). Collarette (*e*) and minor arterial circle of the iris lie at the junction of these two portions. Cellular anterior border layer (*f*) is distinct from loosely arranged stromal tissue (*g*). Sphincter muscle lies in the stroma (*h*). Posterior iris shows posterior (*i*) and anterior (*j*) epithelium; the latter forms the dilator muscle. Anterior chamber angle shows part of a uveal band (*k*). Trabecular meshwork (*l*) and canal of Schlemm (*m*) lie external to chamber angle. Ciliary body and its muscle are posterior to iris (*n*). (×60.) (From Hogan MJ, Alvarado JA, Weddell JE: *Histology of the human eye,* Philadelphia, 1971, Saunders.)

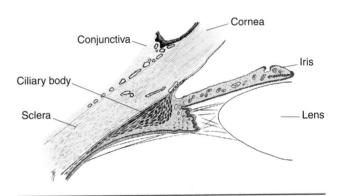

FIGURE 3-2
Periphery of anterior segment of the globe.

The iris arteries are branches of a circular vessel, the **major circle of the iris,** located in the ciliary body near the iris root. The iris vessels usually follow a radial course from the iris root to the pupil margin. These vessels were historically thought to have an especially thick tunica adventitia and have been called "thick-walled blood vessels."[1-3] Improved histologic staining has shown, however, that the bundles of collagen fibrils encircling the vessels are continuous with the collagen network of the stroma and not part of the actual vessel wall. This fibril network anchors the vessels in place and protects them from kinking and compression during the extensive iris movement that occurs with miosis and mydriasis.[4] An incomplete circular vessel, the **minor circle of the iris,** is located in the iris stroma inferior to the collarette and is a remnant of embryologic development. The iris capillaries are not fenestrated and form part of the *blood-aqueous barrier.*[1] The iris stroma is continuous with the stroma of the ciliary body.

The **sphincter muscle** lies within the stroma (see Figure 3-5) and is composed of smooth-muscle cells joined by tight junctions.[1] As its name implies, the sphincter is a circular muscle 0.75 to 1 mm wide, encircling the pupil and located in the pupillary zone of the

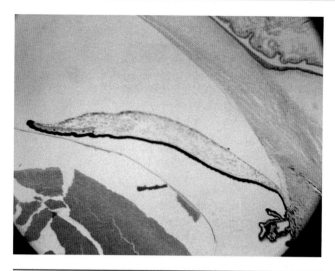

FIGURE 3-3
Light micrograph of anterior segment section. The pupillary zone of the iris rests on lens, lens fibers are fragmented, the iris root is evident at its attachment to the ciliary body; remnants of the zonular fibers are seen betweens lens equator and ciliary process.

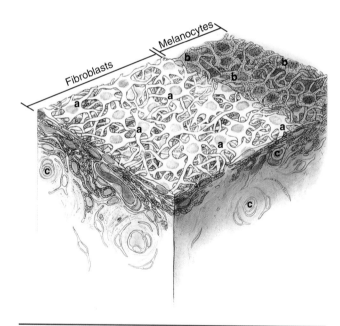

FIGURE 3-4
Anterior layers of the iris. Anterior border layer is covered by a single layer of fibroblasts (*a*), the long, branching processes of which interconnect. Branching processes of fibroblasts form variably sized openings on iris surface. Beneath the layer of fibroblasts is a fairly dense aggregation of melanocytes and a few fibroblasts. The superficial layer of fibroblasts has been removed (*b*) to show these cells. Number of cells in anterior border layer is greater than that in underlying stroma. Iris stroma contains a number of capillaries (*c*), which may be quite close to the surface. (From Hogan MJ, Alvarado JA, Weddell JE: *Histology of the human eye*, Philadelphia, 1971, Saunders.)

stroma[1,2] (Figure 3-6). The sphincter muscle is anchored firmly to adjacent stroma and retains its function even if severed radially.[1] Contraction of the sphincter causes the pupil to constrict in *miosis*. The muscle is innervated by the parasympathetic system.

Clinical Comment: Iridectomy

> In some cases of glaucoma, an **iridectomy** is performed to facilitate the movement of aqueous from the posterior chamber to the anterior chamber. In this surgical procedure a wedge-shaped, full-thickness section of tissue is removed from the iris. If the sphincter muscle is cut during this procedure, the ability of the muscle to contract is not lost. **Iridotomy**, a similar procedure in which an opening is made in the iris without excising tissue, often is accomplished using a laser. The muscle is usually not involved.

Anterior Epithelium and Dilator Muscle

Posterior to the stroma are two layers of epithelium. The first of these, the epithelial layer lying nearest to the stroma, is the **anterior iris epithelium,** which is composed of the unique *myoepithelial cell*. The apical portion is pigmented cuboidal epithelium joined by tight junctions and desmosomes, whereas the basal portion is composed of elongated, contractile, smooth muscle processes (Figure 3-7). The muscle fibers extend into the stroma, forming three to five layers of **dilator muscle** fibers joined by tight junctions (Figure 3-8).

The dilator muscle is present from the iris root to a point in the stroma below the midpoint of the sphincter.[1] The stroma separating the sphincter and dilator muscles is a particularly dense band of connective tissue. Near the termination of the dilator muscle, small projections insert into the stroma or, more accurately, into the sphincter[1,2] (see Figure 3-6). Because the fibers are arranged radially, contraction of the dilator muscle pulls the pupillary portion toward the root, thereby enlarging the pupil in *mydriasis*. The dilator is sympathetically innervated.

The anterior iris epithelium continues to the pupillary margin as cuboidal epithelial cells, and the anterior iris epithelium continues posteriorly as the pigmented epithelium of the ciliary body.

Posterior Epithelium

The second epithelial layer posterior to the stroma is the **posterior iris epithelium,** a single layer of heavily pigmented, approximately columnar cells joined by tight junctions and desmosomes.[2,3] In the periphery, the posterior iris epithelium begins to lose its pigment as it continues into the ciliary body as the nonpigmented

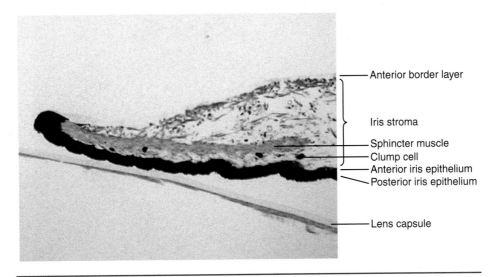

— Anterior border layer

Iris stroma

— Sphincter muscle
— Clump cell
— Anterior iris epithelium
— Posterior iris epithelium

— Lens capsule

FIGURE 3-5
Light micrograph of transverse section of pupillary portion of the iris showing the sphincter muscle. Clump cells are evident between the muscle and the anterior epithelium.

epithelium. A thin basement membrane covers the basal aspect of this cellular layer, which lines the posterior chamber.

The anterior and posterior iris epithelial layers are positioned *apex to apex*, a result of events during embryologic development. Apical microvilli extend from both surfaces, and desmosomes join the two apical surfaces. The epithelial cells curl around from the posterior iris to the anterior surface at the pupillary margin, forming the pigmented **pupillary ruff** (or frill), which encircles the pupil; this normally has a serrated appearance (see Figure 3-6).

Clinical Comment: Iris Synechiae

*IRIS SYNECHIA is an abnormal attachment between the iris surface and another structure. In a **posterior synechia**, the posterior iris surface is adherent to the anterior lens surface. In an **anterior synechia**, the anterior iris surface is adherent to the corneal endothelium or the trabecular meshwork. Synechiae can occur as a result of a sharp blow to the head or a whiplash-type movement that brings the two structures forcefully together. Alternatively, cells and debris from a uveal infection that are circulating in the aqueous humor can make the surfaces "sticky" and so cause synechiae.[5]*

If a posterior synechia involves a large portion of the pupillary margin, aqueous will accumulate in the posterior chamber. Continual production of aqueous causes the pressure in the posterior chamber to increase, which in turn causes the iris to bow forward in a configuration called iris bombé. This can push the peripheral iris against the trabecular meshwork, setting the stage for a dramatic increase of intraocular pressure (IOP). A drug-induced

dilation usually will break a posterior synechia. The break usually occurs between the epithelial layers, leaving remnants of the posterior epithelium on the anterior surface of the lens.

An anterior synechia usually occurs at the iris periphery and involves the meshwork. It is called a peripheral anterior synechia (PAS). Aqueous outflow is impeded by a PAS, causing an increase in IOP if the adhesion occupies a considerable amount of the trabecular meshwork.

ANTERIOR IRIS SURFACE

Thin, radial, collagenous columns or trabeculae are evident in lightly pigmented irises. Thicker, radially oriented, branching trabeculae encircle depressions or openings in the surface called crypts.[3] Crypts are located on both sides of the collarette **(Fuchs' crypts)** and near the root (peripheral crypts). They allow the aqueous quick exit and entrance into spaces in the iris stroma as the volume of the iris changes with iris dilation and contraction.

Circular contraction folds, evident on the anterior surface of the ciliary zone, result from tissue moving toward the iris root during pupillary dilation. Figure 3-9 shows the topography of the anterior and posterior iris surfaces.

POSTERIOR IRIS SURFACE

The posterior surface of the iris is fairly smooth, but when viewed with magnification, small circular furrows are evident near the pupil. **Radial contraction furrows (of Schwalbe)** are located in the pupillary zone, and the deeper **structural furrows (of Schwalbe)** run

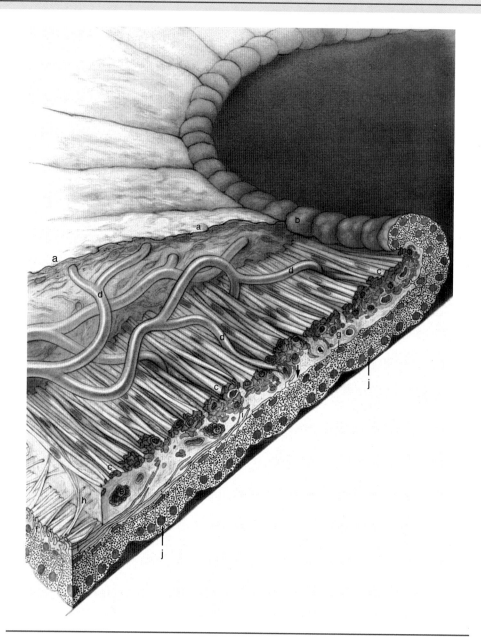

FIGURE 3-6

Pupillary portion of the iris. Dense cellular anterior border layer (*a*) terminates at pigment ruff (*b*) in pupillary margin. Sphincter muscle is at *c*. The arcades (*d*) from the minor circle of the iris extend toward pupil and through sphincter muscle. Sphincter muscle and iris epithelium are close to each other at the pupillary margin. Capillaries, nerves, melanocytes, and clump cells (*e*) are found within and around the muscles. The three to five layers of dilator muscle (*f*) gradually diminish in number until they terminate behind midportion of sphincter muscle (*arrow*), leaving low, cuboidal epithelial cells (*g*) to form the anterior epithelium of pupillary margin. Spurlike extensions from dilator muscle form Michel's spur (*h*) and Fuchs' spur (*i*), which extend anteriorly to blend with sphincter muscle. Posterior epithelium (*j*) is formed by tall columnar cells with basally located nuclei. Its apical surface is contiguous with apical surface of anterior epithelium. (From Hogan MJ, Alvarado JA, Weddell JE: *Histology of the human eye*, Philadelphia, 1971, Saunders.)

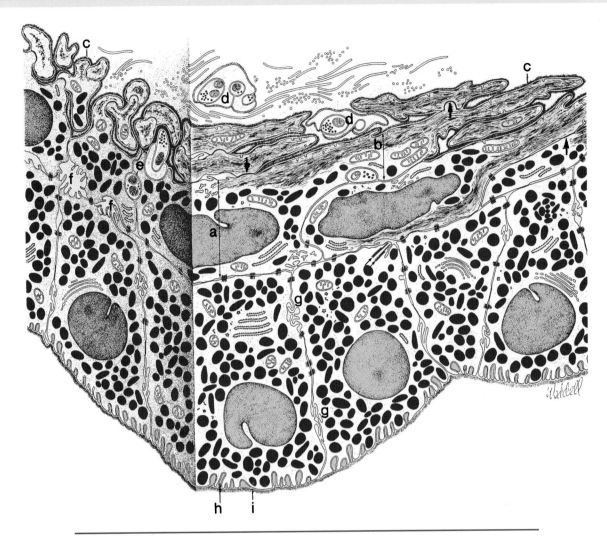

FIGURE 3-7

Posterior epithelial layers. Anterior iris epithelium has two morphologically distinct portions: apical epithelial portion (*a*) and basal muscular portion (*b*). Cytoplasm of basal portion is filled with myofibrils and moderate number of mitochondria. Tonguelike muscular processes overlap, creating three to five layers. Tight junctions (*arrows*), such as those in sphincter muscle, are found between dilator muscle cells. A basement membrane (*c*) surrounds the muscle processes. Unmyelinated nerves and associated Schwann cells (*d*), as well as a few naked axons, innervate sphincter muscle. Axon (*e*) is in close contact with anterior epithelium, separated from it by a space measuring 200 Å wide. Cytoplasm of epithelial portions contains cell organelles, melanin granules, nucleus, and bundles of myofilaments. Most intercellular junctions present here are macula occludens, and only a few desmosomes are present; desmosomes are not found in muscular portion. Apical surface of anterior epithelium is contiguous with that of posterior epithelium. Desmosomes and tight junctions join the two layers, but some areas of separation (*f*) exist between the cells. The spaces so formed are filled with microvilli, and an occasional cilium also is found here (*double arrows*). Posterior pigmented iris epithelium shows lateral interdigitations (*g*) and areas of infolding along its basal surface (*h*). A typical basement membrane (*i*) is found on the basal side as well. Numerous tight junctions and desmosomes occur along lateral and apical walls. Cytoplasm of this epithelium contains numerous melanin granules, measuring approximately 0.8 mm in cross section and up to 2.5 mm in length. Stacks of cisternae of rough-surfaced endoplasmic reticulum, clustered unattached ribosomes, mitochondria, and a Golgi apparatus are typically observed. (From Hogan MJ, Alvarado JA, Weddell JE: *Histology of the human eye*, Philadelphia, 1971, Saunders.)

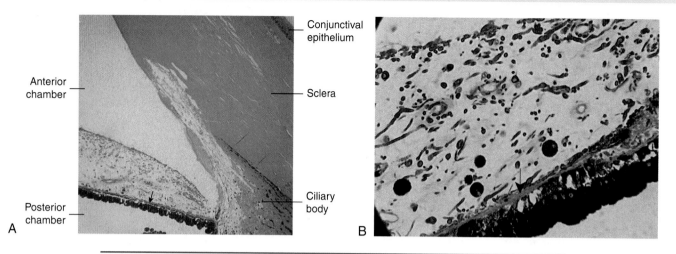

FIGURE 3-8
A, Light micrograph of ciliary portion of iris. Dilator muscle is evident as pink band (*arrow*) anterior to pigmented epithelium. **B,** Light micrograph of epithelial iris layers, strands of dilator (*arrow*) evident above pigmented portion of anterior iris epithelium. In this iris, the anterior iris epithelium is less pigmented than the posterior iris epithelium.

FIGURE 3-9
Surfaces and layers of the iris. Beginning at the upper left and proceeding clockwise, the iris cross-section shows the pupillary (*A*) and ciliary portions (*B*), and the surface view shows a brown iris with its dense, matted anterior border layer. Circular contraction furrows are shown (*arrows*) in the ciliary portion of the iris. Fuchs' crypts (*c*) are seen at either side of the collarette in the pupillary and ciliary portion and peripherally near the iris root. The pigment ruff is seen at the pupillary edge (*d*). The blue iris surface shows a less dense anterior border layer and more prominent trabeculae. The iris vessels are shown beginning at the major arterial circle in the ciliary body (*e*). Radial branches of the arteries and veins extend toward the pupillary region. The arteries form the incomplete minor arterial circle (*f*), from which branches extend toward the pupil, forming capillary arcades. The sector below it demonstrates the circular arrangement of the sphincter muscle (*g*) and the radial processes of the dilator muscle (*h*). The posterior surface of the iris shows the radial contraction furrows (*i*) and the structural folds of Schwalbe (*j*). Circular contraction folds also are present in the ciliary portion. The pars plicata of the ciliary body is at *k*. (From Hogan MJ, Alvarado JA, Weddell JE: *Histology of the human eye*, Philadelphia, 1971, Saunders.)

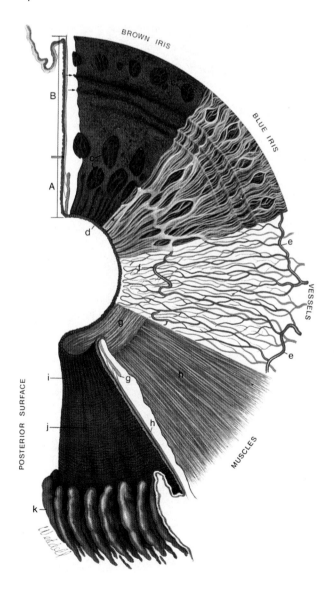

throughout the ciliary zone and continue into the ciliary body as the valleys between the ciliary processes.[1-3] Also found on the posterior surface are circular contraction folds similar to those seen on the anterior surface.

IRIS COLOR

It was once thought that iris color depended on the arrangement and density of connective tissue components in the anterior border layer and stroma, the number of melanocytes, and the size and density of melanin granules within the melanocytes.[6] Studies in which melanocyte counts have been done between irises of various colors and from different races have shown that the number of melanocytes is fairly constant.[7,8] Color seems to be determined by the number of melanin granules within the melanocytes and the area they occupy.[6] The type of melanin present and the arrangement of the connective tissue components can also affect the transmission and reflection of light contributing to iris color.[9] An iris appears blue for the same reason that the sky is blue; the wavelength seen results from light scatter caused by the arrangement and density of the connective tissue components. Other iris colors are caused by the amount of light absorption, which depends on the pigment density within the melanocytes. If the iris is heavily pigmented, the anterior surface appears brown and smooth, even velvety, whereas in a lighter iris, the collagen trabeculae are evident and the color ranges from grays to blues to greens depending on the density of pigment and collagen. A freckle or a nevus is an area of hyperpigmentation, an accumulation of melanocytes, and frequently is seen in the anterior border layer. In all colored irises, the two epithelial layers are heavily pigmented. Only in the albino iris do the epithelial layers lack pigment.[3]

Clinical Comment: Pigmentary Dispersion Syndrome

IN PIGMENTARY DISPERSION SYNDROME pigment granules are shed from the posterior iris surface and are dispersed into the anterior chamber. They can be deposited on the iris, lens, or corneal endothelium or in the trabecular meshwork, where they might compromise aqueous outflow.[4] Significant pigment loss will be evident on transillumination of the iris when the red fundus reflex shows through in the depigmented areas (Figure 3-10).

Clinical Comment: Heterochromia

HETEROCHROMIA of the iris is a condition in which one iris differs in color from the other or portions of one iris differ in color from the rest of the iris. This can be congenital or a sign of uveal inflammation. If congenital, a disruption of the sympathetic innervation may be suspected.[4,10] A history regarding iris coloration should be elicited.

CILIARY BODY

When viewed from the front of the eye, the **ciliary body** is a ring-shaped structure. Its width is approximately 5.9 mm on the nasal side and 6.7 mm on the temporal side.[2] The posterior area of the ciliary body, which terminates at the ora serrata, appears fairly flat, but the anterior

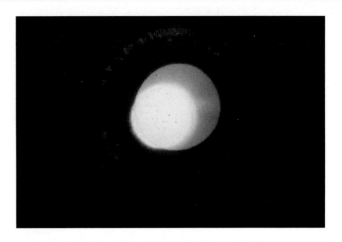

FIGURE 3-10
Retro-illumination of the iris showing defects in the pigmented epithelial layers of the iris. (From Spalton DJ, Hitchings RA, Hunter PA, eds. *Atlas of clinical ophthalmology*, London, 1984, JB Lippincott)

ciliary body contains numerous folds or processes that extend into the posterior chamber. In sagittal section, the ciliary body has a triangular shape, the base of which is located anteriorly; one corner of the base lies at the scleral spur, the iris root extends from the approximate center of the base, and portions of the base border both the anterior and posterior chambers. The outer side of the triangle lies against the sclera, and the inner side lines the posterior chamber and a small portion of the vitreous cavity (Figure 3-11). The apex is located at the ora serrata.

The ciliary body can be divided into two parts: the pars plicata (*corona ciliaris*) and the pars plana (*orbicularis ciliaris*). The **pars plicata** is the wider, anterior portion containing the **ciliary processes** (see Figure 3-10). Approximately 70 to 80 ciliary processes extend into the posterior chamber, and the regions between them are called **valleys of Kuhnt.** A ciliary process measures approximately 2 mm in length, 0.5 mm in width, and 1 mm in height, but there are significant variations in all measurements.[1]

The **pars plana** is the flatter region of the ciliary body. It extends from the posterior of the pars plicata to the **ora serrata,** which is the transition between ciliary body and choroid. The ora serrata has a serrated pattern, the forward-pointing apices of which are called *teeth* or *dentate processes.* The rounded portions that lie between the teeth are called *oral bays* (Figure 3-12, *A*). The dentate processes are elongations of retinal tissue into the region of the pars plana.

The zonule fibers course from the ciliary body to the lens. Some of these fibers insert into the internal limiting membrane of the pars plana region and travel forward through the valleys between the ciliary processes. Some attach to the internal limiting membrane of the valleys of the pars plicata (Figure 3-12, *B*). The ciliary body is

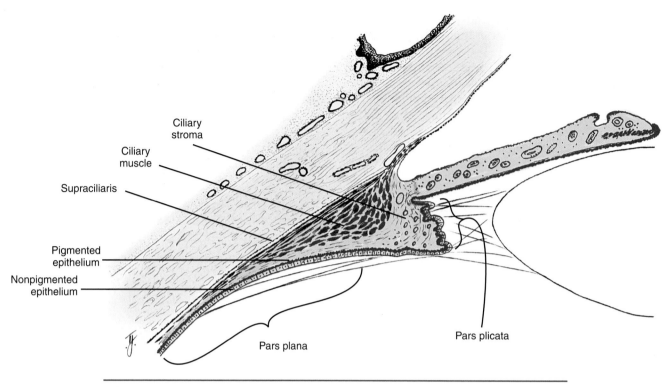

FIGURE 3-11
Partitions and layers of ciliary body.

attached to the vitreous base, which extends forward approximately 2 mm over the posterior pars plana.[1]

SUPRACILIARIS (SUPRACILIARY LAMINA)

The **supraciliaris** is the outermost layer of the ciliary body adjacent to the sclera. Its loose connective tissue is arranged in ribbonlike layers containing pigmented melanocytes, fibroblasts, and collagen bands[1] (Figure 3-13). The arrangement of these bands allows the ciliary body to slide against the sclera without detaching from or stretching the tissue. The arrangement of the supraciliaris allows for the accumulation of fluid within its spaces, which may cause a displacement of the ciliary body from the sclera. Damage to the layer caused by trauma may result in a ciliary body detachment.

CILIARY MUSCLE

The **ciliary muscle** is composed of smooth muscle fibers oriented in longitudinal, radial, and circular directions. Interweaving occurs between fiber bundles and from layer to layer, such that various amounts of connective tissue are found among the muscle bundles.[1] The **longitudinal muscle fibers (of Brücke)** lie adjacent to the supraciliaris and parallel to the sclera. Each muscle bundle resembles

a long narrow V, the base of which is at the scleral spur, whereas the apex is in the choroid. The tendon of origin attaches the muscle fibers to the scleral spur and to adjacent trabecular meshwork sheets. The insertion of the longitudinal ciliary muscle is in the anterior one third of the choroid in the form of stellate-shaped terminations or "muscle stars."[1,2] Inner to the longitudinal muscle fibers, the **radial fibers** form wider, shorter interdigitating Vs that originate at the scleral spur and insert into the connective tissue near the base of the ciliary processes.[1] This layer is a transition from the longitudinally oriented fibers to the circular fibers.

The innermost region of ciliary muscle, **(Müller's) annular muscle,** is formed of circular muscle bundles with a sphincter type of action. These fibers are located near the major circle of the iris. Figure 3-14 shows the relationship between these regions of the ciliary muscle and surrounding structures.

The ciliary muscle is dually innervated by the autonomic nervous system. Parasympathetic stimulation activates the muscle for contraction, whereas sympathetic innervation likely has an inhibitory effect that is a function of the level of parasympathetic activity.[11-13]

CILIARY STROMA

The highly vascularized, loose connective tissue **stroma** of the ciliary body lies between the muscle and the epithelial layers and forms the core of each of the ciliary

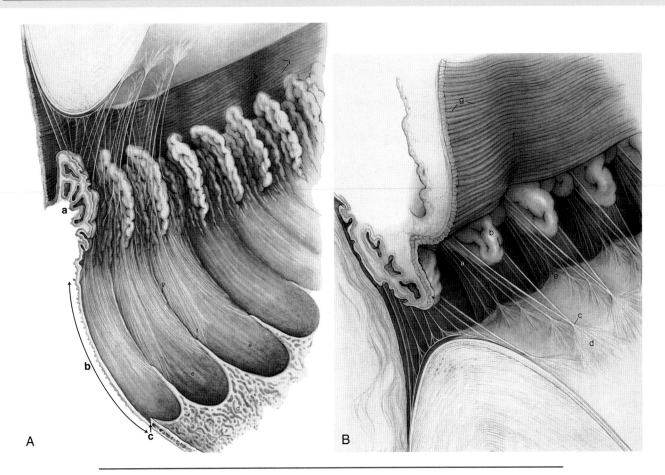

FIGURE 3-12

A, Inner aspect of the ciliary body shows pars plicata (*a*) and pars plana (*b*). Ora serrata is at *c*, and posterior to it, retina exhibits cystoid degeneration (*d*). Bays (*e*) and dentate processes (*f*) of ora are shown; linear ridges or striae (*g*) project forward from dentate processes across pars plana to enter valleys between ciliary processes. Zonular fibers arise from pars plana beginning 1.5 mm from ora serrata. These fibers curve forward from sides of dentate ridges into ciliary valleys, then from valleys to lens capsule. Zonules coming from the valleys on either side of a ciliary process have a common point of attachment on lens. Zonules attach up to 1 mm from the equator posteriorly and up to 1.5 mm from the equator anteriorly. At equatorial border, attaching zonules give a crenated appearance to lens. Ciliary processes vary in size and shape and often are separated from one another by lesser processes. Radial furrows (*h*) and circular furrows (*i*) of peripheral iris are shown. **B,** Anterior view of the ciliary processes showing zonules attaching to lens. Zonules form columns (*a*) on either side of ciliary processes (*b*), which meet on a single site (*c*) as they attach to lens. These two columns form a triangle, the base of which is on ciliary body and apex of which is on lens. Zonules form tentlike structure (*d*) as they become attached to lens capsule. Equatorial surface of lens is crenated (*e*) by attachment of zonule. Iris is pulled upward, revealing its posterior surface containing radial folds (*f*) and circular furrows (*g*). (From Hogan MJ, Alvarado JA, Weddell JE: *Histology of the human eye*, Philadelphia, 1971, Saunders.)

processes; it is continuous with the connective tissue that separates the bundles of ciliary muscle. Anteriorly, the stroma is continuous with iris stroma. It thins in the pars plana, where it continues posteriorly as choroidal stroma. The **major arterial circle of the iris** is located in the ciliary stroma anterior to the circular muscle and near the iris root. This circular artery is formed by the anastomosis of the long posterior ciliary arteries and the anterior ciliary arteries. The stromal capillaries are large and fenestrated, particularly in the ciliary processes, and most are located near the pigmented epithelium.[1]

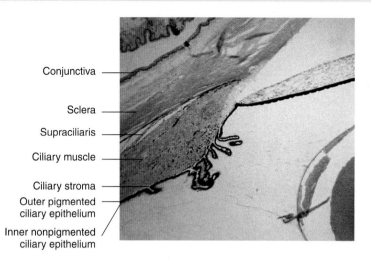

Conjunctiva

Sclera

Supraciliaris

Ciliary muscle

Ciliary stroma

Outer pigmented ciliary epithelium

Inner nonpigmented ciliary epithelium

FIGURE 3-13

Light micrograph of transverse section of the ciliary body, showing detachment from sclera in region of supraciliaris. Ciliary muscle occupies most of ciliary body, stroma is located in center of each process, zonular remnants are evident in posterior chamber between ciliary body and lens equator.

FIGURE 3-14

Ciliary body, including the ciliary muscle and its components. Cornea and sclera have been dissected away, but trabecular meshwork (a), Schlemm's canal (b), and two external collectors (c), as well as scleral spur (d) have been left undisturbed. Three components of ciliary muscle are shown separately, viewed from the outside and sectioned meridionally. Section 1 shows longitudinal ciliary muscle. In section 2, longitudinal ciliary muscle has been dissected away to show radial ciliary muscle. In section 3, only the innermost circular ciliary muscle is shown. Ciliary muscle originates in ciliary tendon, which includes scleral spur (d) and adjacent connective tissue. The cells originate as paired V-shaped bundles. Longitudinal muscle forms long, V-shaped trellises (e) that terminate in epichoroidal stars (f). Arms of V-shaped bundles formed by radial muscle meet at wide angles (g) and terminate in ciliary processes. V-shaped bundles of circular muscle originate at such distant points in ciliary tendon that their arms meet at a very wide angle (h). Iridic portion is shown (i), joining circular muscle cells. (From Hogan MJ, Alvarado JA, Weddell JE: *Histology of the human eye*, Philadelphia, 1971, Saunders.)

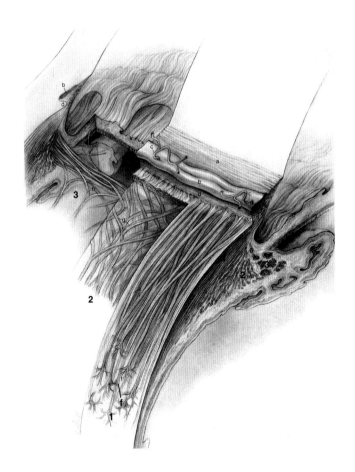

CILIARY EPITHELIUM

Two layers of epithelium, positioned *apex to apex*, cover the ciliary body and line the posterior chamber and part of the vitreous chamber. The two epithelial layers are positioned apex to apex because of invagination of the neural ectoderm in forming the optic cup (see Chapter 7). Intercellular junctions, desmosomes, and tight junctions, connect the two layers.[1] Gap junctions between the apical surfaces provide a means of cellular communication between the layers and are important in the formation of aqueous.[14-17] Both epithelial layers contain cellular components characteristic of cells actively involved in secretion.[18]

The outer layer (i.e., the one next to the stroma) is pigmented and cuboidal, and the cells are joined by desmosomes and gap junctions.[1,14,15,19] *Anteriorly*, the **pigmented ciliary epithelium** is continuous with the anterior iris epithelium (Figure 3-15). *Posteriorly*, it is continuous with the retinal pigment epithelium (RPE) (Figure 3-16). A basement membrane attaches the pigment epithelium to the stroma. This basement membrane is continuous anteriorly with the basement membrane of the anterior iris epithelium and posteriorly with the inner basement membrane portion of Bruch's membrane of the choroid.[1]

The inner epithelial layer (i.e., the layer lining the posterior chamber) is nonpigmented and is composed of columnar cells in the pars plana and cuboidal cells in the pars plicata.[1] The lateral walls of the cells contain extensive interdigitations and are joined, near their apices, by desmosomes, gap junctions, and zonula occludens, which form one site of the blood-aqueous barrier.[3,12-16,19-22]

The **nonpigmented ciliary epithelium** is continuous *anteriorly* with the posterior iris epithelium (see Figure 3-15). It continues *posteriorly* at the ora serrata, where it undergoes significant transformation, becoming neural retina (see Figure 3-16). The metabolically active nonpigmented epithelial cells are involved in active secretion of aqueous humor components and serve as a diffusion barrier between blood and aqueous.[22] The nonpigmented cells have a greater number of mitochondria than the pigmented cells and thus a higher degree of metabolic activity, with a significant role in the active secretion of aqueous humor components.

The basal and basolateral aspects of the nonpigmented cell have numerous invaginations, providing an extensive surface area adjacent to the posterior chamber.[23] The basement membrane covering the nonpigmented epithelium, the internal limiting membrane of the ciliary body, lines the posterior chamber, extends into the invaginations, and is continuous with the internal limiting membrane of the retina.[1,3] The internal limiting membrane in the pars plana region is the attachment site for the zonular fibers and the fibers of the vitreous base.

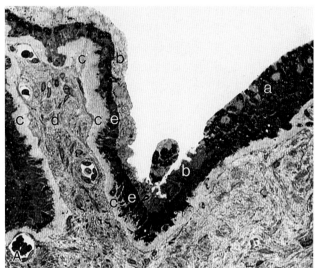

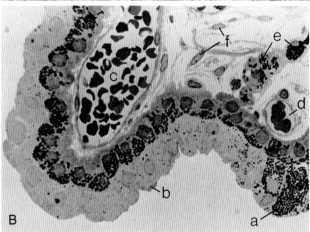

FIGURE 3-15
A, Light micrograph of the ciliary body of an elderly person showing transition of posterior pigmented iris epithelium (*a*) into nonpigmented ciliary epithelium (*b*). Note basement membranelike strip (*c*) interposed between dense collagenous connective tissue layers of this ciliary process (*d*) and pigmented epithelium (*e*). (×500.) **B,** Light micrograph of the ciliary body of a young person showing transition of nonpigmented ciliary body epithelium (*b*) into pigmented posterior iris epithelium. Epithelium reveals increasing numbers of melanin granules until some of the cells become filled with pigment (*a*). Large vein (*c*) and a capillary (*d*) lie in stroma close to pigmented epithelium. Compare stroma of young eye with that in **A.** Some melanocytes (*e*) and fibroblasts (*f*) are seen. (×640.) (From Hogan MJ, Alvarado JA, Weddell JE: *Histology of the human eye*, Philadelphia, 1971, Saunders.)

CHOROID

The **choroid** extends from the ora serrata to the optic nerve and is located between the sclera and the retina, providing nutrients to outer retinal layers (Figure 3-17). It consists primarily of blood vessels. However, a thin

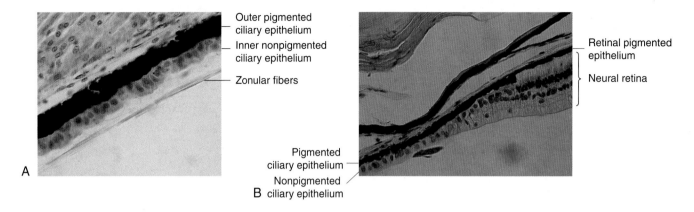

FIGURE 3-16

A, Light micrograph of ciliary epithelial layers in pars plana. **B,** Light micrograph of ora serrata region. Ciliary body at left, retina and choroid at right. Transition from pigmented ciliary epithelium to retinal pigment epithelium and transition from nonpigmented ciliary epithelium to neural retina. (Bright pink artifact is a displaced fragment of the lens.)

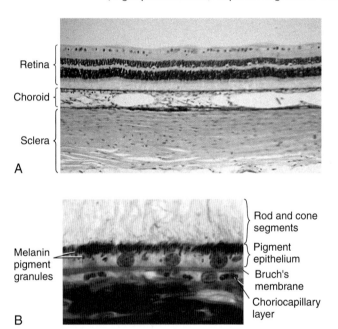

FIGURE 3-17

A, Photomicrograph of section through full thickness of the eye showing retina, choroid, and sclera. **B,** Pigment epithelium. (×1000). (**B** from Krause WJ, Cutts JH: *Concise text of histology,* Baltimore, 1981, Williams & Wilkins.)

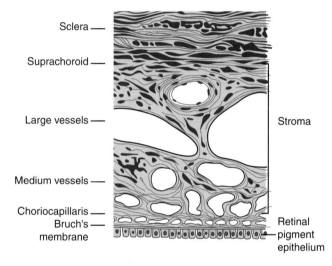

FIGURE 3-18

Histology of choroidal layers.

space or "perichoroidal" space) between the sclera and the choroidal vessels.[1,3] This layer contains components from both sclera (collagen bands and fibroblasts) and choroidal stroma (melanocytes) (Figure 3-18).[1] If the choroid separates from the sclera, part of the suprachoroid will adhere to the sclera and part will remain attached to the choroid.[2] The looseness of the tissue allows the vascular net to swell without causing detachment. The suprachoroidal space carries the long posterior ciliary arteries and nerves from posterior to anterior globe.

connective tissue layer lies on each side of the stromal vessel layer.

SUPRACHOROID LAMINA (*LAMINA FUSCA*)

Thin, pigmented, ribbonlike branching bands of connective tissue—the **suprachoroid lamina** or lamina fusca—traverse a *potential space* (the suprachoroidal

CHOROIDAL STROMA

The **choroidal stroma** is a pigmented, vascularized, loose connective tissue layer containing melanocytes, fibroblasts, macrophages, lymphocytes, and mast cells.

Collagen fibrils are arranged circularly around the vessels, which are branches of the short posterior ciliary arteries. These vessels are organized into tiers, those with larger lumina occupying the outer layer (Haller's layer). They branch as they pass inward, forming the medium-sized vessels (Sattler's layer), which continue branching to form a capillary bed (Figure 3-19). The venules join to become veins that gather in a characteristic vortex pattern in each quadrant of the eye and exit the choroid as four (occasionally five) large **vortex veins.** Choroidal veins contain no valves.[2]

The choroidal vessels are innervated by the autonomic nervous system. Sympathetic stimulation causes vasoconstriction and decreased choroidal blood flow; parasympathetic stimulation causes a nitrous oxide responsive vasodilation, resulting in increased choroidal blood flow.[20]

CHORIOCAPILLARIS

The specialized capillary bed is called the **choriocapillaris** (lamina choroidocapillaris). It forms a single layer of anastomosing, fenestrated capillaries having wide lumina (see Figure 3-19) with most of the fenestrations facing toward the retina.[24] In each, the lumen is approximately three to four times that of ordinary capillaries, such that two or three red blood cells can pass through the capillary abreast, whereas in ordinary capillaries the cells usually course single file.[1] The cell membrane is reduced to a single layer at the fenestrations, facilitating the movement of material through the vessel walls.[25] Occasional pericytes (Rouget cells), which may have a contractile function, are found around the capillary wall.[1,3] Pericytes have the ability to alter local blood flow.[26] The choriocapillaris is densest in the macular area, where it is the sole blood supply for a small region of the retina. The choriocapillaris is unique to the choroid and does not continue into the ciliary body.

BRUCH'S MEMBRANE (BASAL LAMINA)

The innermost layer of the choroid, **Bruch's membrane,** fuses with the retina. It runs from the optic nerve to the ora serrata, where it undergoes some modification before continuing into the ciliary body.[1] Bruch's membrane (or the basal lamina) is a multilaminated sheet containing a center layer of elastic fibers.[27] As seen through an electron microscope, the membrane components, from outer to inner, are the (1) interrupted basement membrane of the choriocapillaris, (2) outer collagenous zone, (3) elastic layer, (4) inner collagenous zone, and (5) basement membrane of the RPE

cells[1,2] (Figure 3-20). Fine filaments from the basement membrane of the RPE merge with the fibrils of the inner collagenous zone, contributing to the tight adhesion between choroid and the outer, pigmented layer of the retina.

At the ora serrata, the basement membrane of the RPE is continuous with the basement membrane of the pigmented epithelium of the ciliary body. The collagenous and elastic layers disappear into the ciliary stroma, and the basement membrane of the choriocapillaris continues as the basement membrane of the ciliary body capillaries.

FUNCTIONS OF UVEA

FUNCTIONS OF IRIS

The iris acts as a diaphragm to regulate the amount of light entering the eye. The two iris muscles are innervated separately: The parasympathetically innervated sphincter muscle is responsible for constriction of the pupil, and the sympathetically innervated dilator muscle causes pupillary enlargement.

FUNCTIONS OF CILIARY BODY

The ciliary body produces and secretes the aqueous humor. Its musculature causes accommodation and can affect aqueous outflow.

Clinical Comment: Accommodation

The ability of the eye to change power and bring near objects into focus on the retina is called **accommodation.** It is accomplished by increasing the power of the lens. Contraction of the longitudinal fibers of the ciliary muscle pulls the choroid forward, and contraction of the circular fibers draws the ciliary body closer to the lens, decreasing the diameter of the ring formed by the ciliary body. This releases tension on the zonule fibers and allows the lens capsule to adopt a more spherical shape. The lens thickens, and the anterior surface curve increases. These changes result in an increase in refractive power, or accommodation. When the ciliary muscle is relaxed, the eye is said to be "at rest" and is used for distance vision. During accommodation, the iris sphincter also contracts, restricting incoming light rays and decreasing spherical aberration.

Ciliary muscle contraction can change the configuration of the trabecular meshwork because some of the longitudinal fibers are attached to trabecular meshwork sheets. This altered configuration can facilitate aqueous movement through the anterior chamber angle structures.[28] Accommodation has been found to cause a decrease in IOP[29] (accommodation is discussed further in Chapter 5).

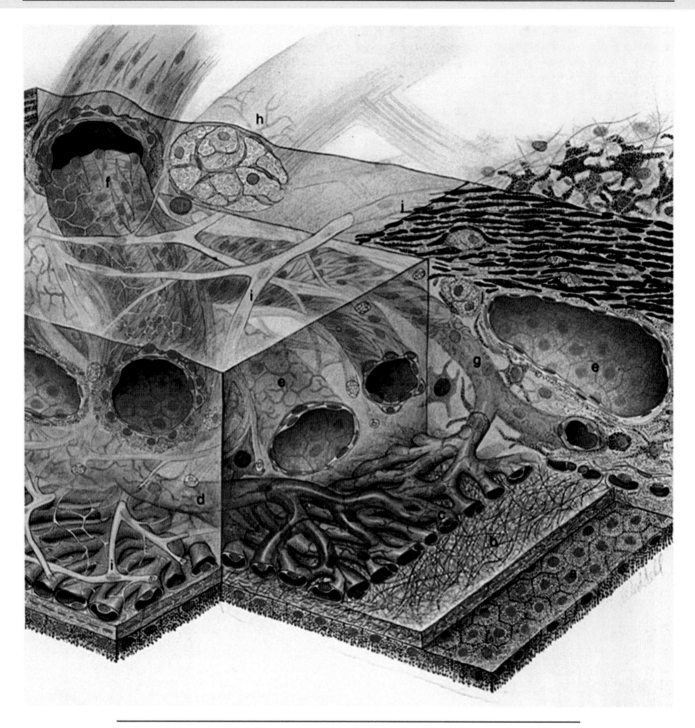

FIGURE 3-19
Drawing of choroidal blood supply and innervation and Bruch's membrane. Pigment epithelium of retina (*a*) is in close contact with Bruch's membrane (*b*). Elastica of Bruch's membrane is blue, and meshes contain collagen fibrils. Choriocapillaris (*c*) forms an intricate network along inner choroid. Venules (*d*) leave choriocapillaris to join vortex system (*e*). Short ciliary artery is shown at *f*, before its branching (*g*) to form choriocapillaris. Short ciliary nerve enters choroid (*h*) and sends ramifying branches into choroidal stroma (*i*). Suprachoroidea (suprachoroid lamina), with its star-shaped melanocytes, is at *j*. (From Hogan MJ, Alvarado JA, Weddell JE: *Histology of the human eye*, Philadelphia, 1971, Saunders.)

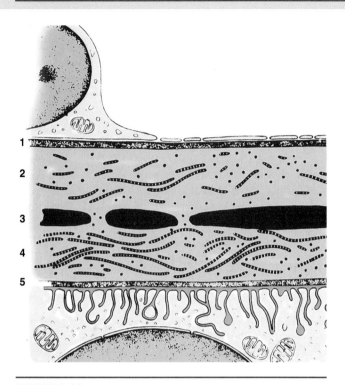

FIGURE 3-20
Layers of Bruch's membrane, delineated on basis of electron microscope studies: *1*, Interrupted basement membrane of choriocapillaris; *2*, outer collagenous zone; *3*, elastic layer; *4*, inner collagenous zone; *5*, basement membrane of retinal pigment epithelial cells. (From Hogan MJ, Alvarado JA, Weddell JE: *Histology of the human eye*, Philadelphia, 1971, Saunders.)

Clinical Comment: Presbyopia

PRESBYOPIA is the loss of the ability to accommodate; it a normal age-related change and the subject of continuing research. In rhesus monkeys, the tendon that attaches the ciliary muscle to the scleral spur shows extensive age-related structural changes: It thickens with age and becomes surrounded by a dense layer of collagen, thus losing its elasticity. This loss of elasticity restricts muscle movement and hampers accommodation.[30] A similar mechanism may be one component of human presbyopia; however, other changes are likely involved including changes involving the lens itself (see Chapter 5).

Aqueous Production

The ciliary body capillaries and the ciliary epithelial layers are significant factors in the production and secretion of aqueous. The stroma within the ciliary processes contains a dense network of fenestrated capillaries, and the number and shape of the processes provides a large surface area for secretion into the posterior chamber. Three mechanisms contribute to production and secretion: diffusion, ultrafiltration, and active secretion.[31] Diffusion occurs when an uneven distribution of molecules exists across a membrane and the molecules move from the higher concentration to the lower concentration. Ultrafiltration occurs as bulk flow across a semipermeable membrane augmented by a hydrostatic pressure. In active secretion molecules are transported across the membrane against a concentration gradient in an energy-utilizing process; active secretion likely accounts for 80% to 90% of aqueous production.[15]

Pressure on the ciliary stroma side of the two-layered epithelia is estimated at greater than 15 mm Hg, providing a driving force that moves solution minus macromolecules across the zonula occludens barrier of the nonpigmented epithelium, thus producing an ionic concentration comparable to blood plasma. An oncotic gradient of approximately 14 mm Hg could move water across the semipermeable membrane of the nonpigmented epithelium from a solution with low concentration of macromolecules (the aqueous) into a higher concentration of macromolecules (blood plasma), counteracting the ultrafiltration process. As these forces are in the opposite direction, it is unclear how great a factor ultrafiltration actually is in aqueous production because it might be offset by water movement back into the ciliary processes.[23]

As molecules exit the blood through the walls of the ciliary capillaries, they move through the stroma and the epithelia. The model of ion movement through these cells is still theoretical; transport mechanisms have been identified but the regulation of those mechanisms is not clear.[23,31-33] The two layers of epithelium are thought to function together as a syncytium due to the extensive gap junctions joining the cells within each layer as well those between the two layers.

The driving force for secretion of the fluid is produced by transepithelial ionic transport across this bilayered ciliary epithelium.[34] Ions enter the basolateral pigmented ciliary epithelium (PE); (Na^+ and Cl^- likely enter by Na^+/H^+ and Cl^-/HCO_3^- exchangers and the $Na^+/K^+/2Cl^-$ cotransporter), then diffuse through the apical membrane into the extracellular fluid, as well as directly into the nonpigmented ciliary epithelium (NPE) through gap junctions.[23,34] The active ATPase pump within the NPE cell accounts for a relatively low concentration of Na^+ in the NPE, creating a driving force for Na^+ movement. The Na^+/H^+ exchange and the $Na^+/K^+/2Cl^-$ transporter maintain the cycle of Na^+ passage.

Ions exit the basolateral membrane of the NPE through ionic pumps, ion channels, and cotransporters into the posterior chamber; the electrical voltage change due to movement of ions can drive increased movement of Na^+ and Cl^- and thus shift water. Potassium ions that were brought into the cell by Na^+/K^+ ATPase pumps are kept circulating by K^+ channels in the basolateral membrane.[34] The coordination of ion pumps, channels, and cotransporters in these two epithelia, as well as aquaporins in the NPE that facilitate water movement, produce the substance secreted into the posterior chamber as

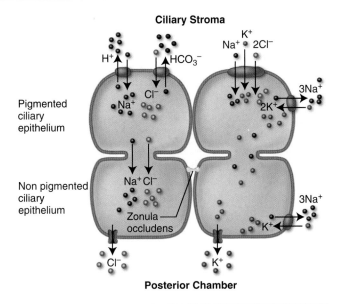

Ciliary Stroma

Pigmented
ciliary
epithelium

Non pigmented
ciliary
epithelium

Zonula
occludens

Posterior Chamber

FIGURE 3-21
Schematic showing possible mechanisms of ion flow through
the PE and NPE.

aqueous humor.[23,35] The current belief is that the movement of Na^+ and Cl^- primarily drives secretion into the posterior chamber with bicarbonate ions having an indirect role by moderating Cl^- flux.[23] Figure 3-21 shows an abreviated schematic of ion flow.

Function and Rate of Production

The aqueous provides nutrients to the avascular cornea and lens. The primary difference between blood plasma and aqueous is in the concentration of ascorbate and of protein. Ascorbate concentration is approximately 20 times higher in aqueous than in blood plasma and must be actively transported into the aqueous. Ascorbate is thus supplied to both cornea and lens and is important as a free radical scavenger helping to guard these tissues against oxidative damage. The protein content in plasma is 200 times greater than in aqueous, a consequence of the tight junctional barrier. The low concentration of protein causes minimal light scatter and thus maximum light transmission is maintained through the aqueous. The aqueous also carries waste products from the cornea and lens and therefore has a high concentration of lactate, a metabolic waste product of the anaerobic glycolysis of the lens and cornea.

Approximately 2.5 μl of aqueous is produced per minute.[15] Aqueous production follows the circadian rhythm with a higher rate during the day, that rate is decreased by about 50% during the night.[23] It is unclear whether the fluctuation of IOP coincides with this production cycle. During sleep circulating epinephrine is decreased which may in part account for the reduction in production but is unlikely the sole factor for the circadian cycle.[36]

Although the ultrafiltration process can be influenced by changes in IOP the effect on the rate of formation is slight.[15] Since active secretion is the primary mechanism for aqueous formation moderate changes in blood pressure have little effect on the rate of formation.[31] Autonomic nerves located within the ciliary body can influence aqueous production by acting on the blood vessels, dilating them and increasing blood volume or decreasing volume by constricting the vessels. Although no anatomic evidence has been found identifying autonomic innervation to the epithelia, animal studies have found some alteration in production volumes in response to manipulations of the autonomic signal. Further information on the effect of aqueous production on intraocular pressure and drug treatments that reduce aqueous production will be found in Chapter 6.

Vitreous Production

Investigators recently have suggested that similar processes may occur in the epithelium of the pars plana region and have a significant role in the production and secretion of various connective tissue macromolecules located in the vitreous body.[37]

Blood-Aqueous Barrier

The **blood-aqueous barrier** selectively controls the secreted substance—aqueous humor. The *fenestrated ciliary body capillaries* permit large molecules to exit the blood. However, the *tight zonular junctions* of the nonpigmented epithelium prevent the molecules from passing between the cells, forcing them instead to pass through the cell to enter the posterior chamber. One of the substances thus controlled is protein. The protein content of aqueous humor is very small compared with that of blood.[38] Proteins pass easily out of the ciliary vessels through the fenestrations but do not pass into the posterior chamber because of the tight junction barrier of the nonpigmented epithelium.[15,39-41]

The iris is freely permeated by the aqueous humor, which readily enters the stroma through the surface crypts.[1] To prevent large molecules from leaking out of the iris blood vessels and altering the content of the aqueous fluid, the iris capillaries have *no fenestrations,* and their endothelial cells maintain the barrier function through their zonula occludens junctions.[21,41-43]

Clinical Comment: Tyndall Phenomenon

Clinical examination of the aqueous with the biomicroscope is accomplished by focusing a conical beam within the anterior chamber and with high magnification and a dark room watching for movement within the beam. In normal aqueous the beam will be invisible, the out-of-focus cornea and lens will be visible in the reflected light, but the aqueous will be dark or "optically empty." If there are particles in the pathway of the beam, light will be reflected and scattered producing the Tyndall phenomenon, making the beam visible within the aqueous.

Cells and flare in the anterior chamber can be indicative of uveal inflammation or infection. A disruption of the zonula occludens between the nonpigmented ciliary cells causes a breakdown of the blood-aqueous barrier and can occur in inflammatory conditions, allowing immune factors and leucocytes into the eye to fight invading microbes, causing cells and flare.[35] This accumulation of material usually appears whitish and if there is significant amount it may settle in the inferior anterior chamber, forming an hypopyon.

Trauma involving a blow to the head or an injury such as whiplash can cause a tear or break at the iris root and result in damaging the iris blood vessel branches entering from the major circle of the iris. Such a hemorrhage will cause blood to enter the anterior chamber and due to gravity will settle inferiorly. This accumulation of blood forms a hyphema.

FUNCTIONS OF CHOROID

The vascular choroid provides nutrients to the outer retina and is an egress for catabolites from the retina, passing through Bruch's membrane into the choriocapillaris. The darkly pigmented choroid absorbs excess light as does the RPE layer. The suprachoroidal space provides a pathway for the posterior vessels and nerves that supply the anterior segment.

With aging, excessive basement membrane (basal lamina) material is deposited in the collagenous zones of Bruch's membrane.[44-46] These deposits in the inner collagenous zone, called **drusen,** can be seen as small, pinhead-sized, yellow-white spots in the fundus (Figure 3-22). The drusen, which contain cellular fragments and an accumulation of basal laminar material, are located outer to the RPE basement membrane and displace the retina inward.[47]

Clinical Comment: Age-Related Macular Degeneration

*Degenerative processes involving the choroid-retina interface in the macular area often are manifested as **age-related macular degeneration (AMD).** AMD is the most common cause of blindness in Western countries.[48] This disease is multifaceted in origin and can involve the presence of multiple or confluent drusen, a thick layer of basal laminar deposit, detachment or atrophy of the RPE, subsequent formation of disciform scars, (Figure 3-23) loss of photoreceptors, and neovascularization.[47,49]*

Metabolites from the choriocapillaris and waste products from the retina must pass through Bruch's membrane. With age, phospholipids accumulate in this membrane, probably because of defective mechanisms in the dephosphorylation process.[45,50-53] Free radicals resulting from oxidative stress have been implicated in these cellular metabolic changes.[54] The accumulation of lipids in Bruch's membrane with increasing age appears to be greater in the central fundus than in the periphery.[55] Bruch's membrane becomes hydrophobic and presents a barrier to water movement, thereby inhibiting the passage of metabolites.[56] If water accumulates between the RPE and Bruch's membrane, displacement and detachment may occur.[52] This process is represented diagrammatically in Figure 3-24.

Loss of nutrients to the highly metabolic retina can cause (1) atrophy of the RPE, followed by loss of photoreceptors,[53,57] or (2) development of a neovascular membrane in an attempt to compensate for the loss of nutrients.[54,56] The new vessels branch from the choriocapillaris and can remain beneath the RPE or can penetrate Bruch's membrane and enter the retina.[54] However, these vessels are fragile, leak, and tend to hemorrhage into retinal tissue.[52,58] Visual loss in AMD results from detachment of the RPE resulting from water accumulation, atrophy of the RPE and photoreceptors, or the presence of a subretinal neovascular membrane.[45,50]

Risk factors associated with AMD include genetics; age; lighter pigmentation of skin, hair, or iris; skin sensitivity to sun; smoking; sun exposure; and cataract surgery.[54,56,59-63] Although these risk factors have been elucidated, their role in AMD is still not seen as causative. The complex interplay among these factors, however, implicates many if not all of them in AMD.

No definitive treatment for AMD exists as yet, but supplementation with antioxidants or minerals (e.g., high doses of vitamins C and E, beta carotene, zinc, lutein, and zeaxanthin) may provide some protective effect or slow the progression to advanced disease in patients with mild AMD.[64,65] However, others question the effectiveness of such supplements in AMD.[66-70] Surgical and drug delivery treatments have been identified to be successful in slowing or eliminating the progression of AMD. Clinical trials continue to seek improved treatment modalities.

BLOOD SUPPLY TO UVEAL TRACT

The short posterior ciliary arteries enter the globe in a circle around the optic nerve, and their branches form the choroidal vessels. The long posterior ciliary arteries and the anterior ciliary arteries join to form the major circle of the iris, which supplies vessels to the iris and ciliary body. The venous return for most of the uvea is through the vortex veins (see Chapter 11 for further information on the blood supply).

UVEAL INNERVATION

Sensory innervation of the uvea is provided through the nasociliary branch from the trigeminal nerve. Sympathetic fibers from the superior cervical ganglion via

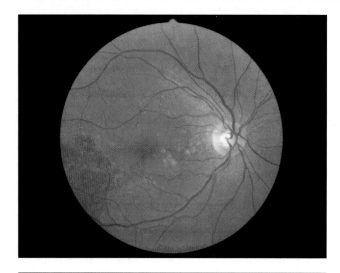

FIGURE 3-22
Fundus photo showing right eye of 49-year-old with scattered retinal drusen. (Courtesy Fraser Horn, OD, Pacific University Family Vision Center, Forest Grove, Ore.)

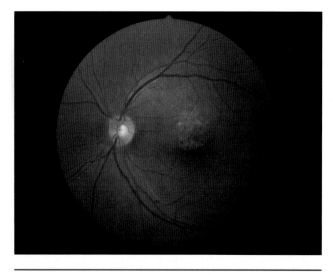

FIGURE 3-23
Fundus photo showing left eye of patient with AMD, confluent drusen, disciform scarring, and pigment mottling in the macular area is evident. (Courtesy Fraser Horn, OD, Pacific University Family Vision Center, Forest Grove, Ore.)

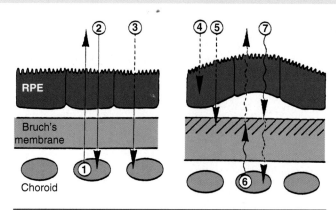

FIGURE 3-24
Summary of implications of lipid accumulation in Bruch's membrane for transport systems operating across retinal pigment epithelium (RPE). In youngest age group: *1,* metabolites pass from choroid through Bruch's membrane across RPE to neural retina; *2,* water moves predominantly from neural retina to choroid; and *3,* progress of catabolism results in accumulation of waste products that are predominantly cleared via the choroid. In older age group: *4,* with increasing age, catabolism results in accumulations (lipofuscin) within RPE; *5,* waste products rich in lipid begin to accumulate within Bruch's membrane; *6,* accumulation of lipid-rich debris within Bruch's membrane may inhibit metabolic input to neural retina; and *7,* presence of a hydrophobic barrier within Bruch's membrane impedes passage of water and may result in detachment of RPE. (From Pauleikhoff D, Harper CA, Marshall J, et al: Aging changes in Bruch's membrane: a histochemical and morphological study, *Ophthalmology* 97[2]:171, 1990.)

AGING CHANGES IN UVEA

IRIS

With age, loss of pigment from the epithelium is evident at the pupillary margin and on transillumination. Pigment deposition may be seen on the iris surface, anterior lens surface, posterior cornea, and trabecular meshwork. The dilator muscle becomes atrophic, and the sphincter muscle becomes sclerotic, making it more difficult to dilate the older pupil pharmacologically.[71]

CILIARY BODY

Although the amount of connective tissue within the layer of ciliary muscle increases with age,[72] there is no significant correlation between loss of ciliary muscle contractile ability and age.[72,73] Ciliary muscle contraction does not diminish with age.[74] The formation of aqueous decreases with age and by age 80 is approximately 25% of what it was; however, the volume of the anterior chamber decreases by about 40%.[36]

the ophthalmic and short ciliary nerves innervate the choroidal blood vessels, and sympathetic fibers from the superior cervical ganglion via the long ciliary nerves innervate the iris dilator and ciliary muscles. Parasympathetic fibers from the ciliary ganglion innervate the ciliary muscle, the iris sphincter muscle, and the choroidal vessels.

CHOROID

The changes that occur in AMD occur throughout the choroid with advancing age. However, only those occurring in the macula significantly affect visual acuity and the patient's daily life. Bruch's membrane increases in thickness with age. Various substances and particles accumulate, decreasing the membrane's permeability to serum proteins, and its capacity to facilitate metabolite exchange with the retina decreases.[75-78] Calcification and deposits in the inner collagenous layer are responsible for the clinical appearance of drusen, which increase in number with age.[56] As lysosomal activity in the RPE decreases with age, atypical material (including *lipofuscin*) may accumulate in Bruch's membrane.[54]

The choriocapillaris decreases in density and diameter, resulting in a decrease in choroidal blood flow, and choroidal thickness decreases in the normal-aging macula.[54,79]

REFERENCES

1. Hogan MJ, Alvarado JA, Weddell JE, editors: *Histology of the human eye*, Philadelphia, 1971, Saunders, p 202.
2. Warwick R: *Wolff's anatomy of the eye and orbit*, ed 7, Philadelphia, 1976, Saunders, p 61.
3. Fine BS, Yanoff M: *Ocular histology*, Hagerstown, Md, 1979, Harper & Row, p 195.
4. Loewenfeld IE: *The pupil: anatomy, physiology, and clinical applications*, Boston, 1999, Butterworth-Heinemann.
5. Bartlett JD, Jaanus SD: *Clinical ocular pharmacology*, ed 3, Boston, 1995, Butterworth-Heinemann, pp 776–915.
6. Imesch PD, Bindley CD, Khademian Z, et al: Melanocytes and iris color. Electron microscopic findings, *Arch Ophthalmol* 114:443, 1996.
7. Wilkerson CL, Syed NA, Fisher MR, et al: Melanocytes and iris color. Light microscopic findings, *Arch Ophthalmol* 114:437–442, 1996.
8. Albert DM, Green WR, Zimbri ML, et al: Iris melanocyte numbers in Asian, African American, and Caucasian irides, *Trans Am Ophthalmol Soc* 101:217–222, 2003.
9. Wakamatsu K, Hu DN, McCormick SA, et al: Characterization of melanin in human iridal and choroidal melanocytes from eye with various colored irides, *Pigment Cell Melanoma Res* 21:97–105, 2007.
10. Catania LJ: *Primary care of the anterior segment*, East Norwalk, Conn, 1988, Appleton & Lange, p 211.
11. Gilmartin B: A review of the role of sympathetic innervation of the ciliary muscle in ocular accommodation, *Ophthalmic Physiol Opt* 6(1):23, 1986.
12. Rosenfield M, Gilmartin B: Oculomotor consequences of beta-adrenoreceptor antagonism during sustained near vision, *Ophthalmic Physiol Opt* 7(2):127, 1987.
13. Gilmartin B, Bullimore MA, Rosenfield M, et al: Pharmacological effects on accommodative adaptation, *Optom Vis Sci* 69(4):276, 1992.
14. Raviola G, Raviola E: Intercellular junctions in the ciliary epithelium, *Invest Ophthalmol Vis Sci* 17:958, 1978.
15. Gabelt BT, Kaufman PL: Aqueous humor dynamics. In Kaufman PL, Alm A, editor: *Adler's physiology of the eye*, ed 10, St Louis, 2003, Mosby, p 237.
16. Raviola G: The structural basis of the blood-ocular barriers, *Exp Eye Res* 25(suppl):27, 1977.
17. Takats K, Kasahara T, Kasahara M, et al: Ultracytochemical localization of the erythrocyte/HepG2-type glucose transporter (GLUT1) in the ciliary body and iris of the rat eye, *Invest Ophthalmol Vis Sci* 32(5):1659, 1991.
18. Eichhorn M, Inada K, Lütjen-Drecoll E: Human ciliary body in organ culture, *Curr Eye Res* 19(4):277, 1991.
19. Raviola G: The fine structure of the ciliary zonule and ciliary epithelium, *Invest Ophthalmol* 10(11):851, 1971.
20. Noske W, Stamm CC, Hirsch M: Tight junctions of the human ciliary epithelium: regional morphology and implications on transepithelial resistance, *Exp Eye Res* 59:141, 1994.
21. Sonsino J, Gong H, Wu P, et al: Co-localization of junction-associated proteins of the human blood—aqueous barrier: occludin, ZO-1 and F-actin, *Exp Eye Res* 71:123, 2002:(abstract).
22. Shiose Y: Electron microscopic studies on blood-retinal and blood-aqueous barriers, *Jpn J Ophthalmol* 14:73, 1970:(abstract).
23. Delamere NA: Ciliary body and ciliary epithelium. In Fischbarg J, editor: *The biology of the eye*, 2006, Elsevier, pp 127–148.
24. Spitzmas M, Reale E: Fracture faces of fenestrations and junctions of endothelial cells in human choroidal vessels, *Invest Ophthalmol* 14:98–107, 1975.
25. Bernstein MH, Hollenberg MJ: Fine structure of the choriocapillaris and retinal capillaries, *Invest Ophthalmol* 4(6):1016, 1965.
26. Chakravarthy U, Gardiner TA: Endothelium-derived agents in pericyte function/dysfunction, *Prog Retin Eye Res* 18(4):511, 1999.
27. Alexander RA, Garner A: Elastic and precursor fibres in the normal human eye, *Exp Eye Res* 36:305, 1983.
28. Ebersberger A, Flugel C, Lütjen-Drecoll E: Ultrastructural and enzyme histochemical studies of regional structural differences within the ciliary muscle in various species, *Klin Monbl Augenheilkd* 203(1):53, 1993:(abstract).
29. Mauger RR, Likens CP, Applebaum M: Effects of accommodation and repeated applanation tonometry on intraocular pressure, *Am J Optom Physiol Opt* 61(1):28, 1984.
30. Tamm E, Lütjen-Drecoll E, Jungkunz W, et al: Posterior attachment of ciliary muscle in young, accommodating, old, presbyopic monkeys, *Invest Ophthalmol Vis Sci* 32:1678, 1991.
31. Bill A: The role of ciliary blood flow and ultrafiltration in aqueous humor formation, *Exp Eye Res* 16:287–298, 1973.
32. Candia OA, Alvarez LJ: Fluid transport phenomena in ocular epithelia, *Prog Retin Eye Res* 27:197–212, 2008.
33. Macri FJ, Cevario SJ: The formation and inhibition of aqueous humor production. A proposed mechanism of action, *Arch Ophthalmol* 96:1664–1667, 1978.
34. Do CW, Civan MM: Species variation in biology and physiology of the ciliary epithelium: similarities and differences, *Exp Eye Res* 88:631–640, 2009.
35. Levin MH, Verkman AS: Aquaporins and CFTR in ocular epithelial fluid transport, *J Membr Biol* 210:205-115, 2006.
36. Mc Laren JW: Measurement of aqueous humor flow, *Exp Eye Res* 88:641–647, 2009.
37. Bishop PN, Takanosu M, Le Goff M, et al: The role of the posterior ciliary body in the biosynthesis of vitreous humour, *Eye* 16:454, 2002.
38. Krause U, Raunio V: Proteins of the normal human aqueous humour, *Ophthalmologica* 159:178, 1969.
39. Smith RS: Ultrastructural studies of the blood-aqueous barrier. I. Transport of an electron-dense tracer in the iris and ciliary body of the mouse, *Am J Ophthalmol* 71:1066, 1971.
40. Varma SD, Reddy VN: Phospholipid composition of aqueous humor plasma and lens in normal and alloxan diabetic rabbits, *Exp Eye Res* 13:120, 1972.
41. Cunha-Vaz JG: The blood-ocular barriers: past, present, and future, *Doc Ophthalmol* 93:149, 1997.

42. Waitzman MB, Jackson RT: Effects of topically administered ouabain on aqueous humor dynamics, *Exp Eye Res* 4:135, 1965.

43. Schlingemann RO, Hofman P, Klooster J, et al: Ciliary muscle capillaries have blood-tissue barrier characteristics, *Exp Eye Res* 66:747, 1998.

44. Sarks SH: Aging and degeneration in the macular region: a clinico-pathological study, *Br J Ophthalmol* 60:324, 1976.

45. van der Schaft TL, Mooy CM, de Bruijn WC, et al: Histologic features of the early stages of age-related macular degeneration. A statistical analysis, *Ophthalmology* 99:278, 1992.

46. Van der Schaft TL, Mooy CM, de Bruijn WC, et al: Immunohistochemical light and electron microscopy of basal laminar deposit, *Graefes Arch Clin Exp Ophthalmol* 232(1):40, 1994.

47. Ramrattan RS, van der Schaft TL, Mooy CM, et al: Morphometric analysis of Bruch's membrane, the choriocapillaris, and the choroid in aging, *Invest Ophthalmol Vis Sci* 35(6):2857, 1994.

48. Leibowitz HM, Krueger DE, Maunder LR, et al: The Framingham Eye Study monograph: an ophthalmological and epidemiological study of cataract, glaucoma, diabetic retinopathy, macular degeneration, and visual acuity in a general population of 2631 adults, 1973–1975, *Surv Ophthalmol* 24:335, 1980.

49. Bressler NM, Bressler SB, Fine SL: Age-related macular degeneration, *Surv Ophthalmol* 32:375, 1988.

50. Sheraidah G, Steinmetz R, Maguire J, et al: Correlation between lipids extracted from Bruch's membrane and age, *Ophthalmology* 100(1):47, 1993.

51. Pauleikhoff D: Drusen in Bruch's membrane. Their significance for the pathogenesis and therapy of age-associated macular degeneration, *Ophthalmologe* 89(5):363, 1992:(abstract).

52. Pauleikhoff D, Harper CA, Marshall J, et al: Aging changes in Bruch's membrane. A histochemical and morphologic study, *Ophthalmology* 97(2):171, 1990.

53. Zarbin MA: Age-related macular degeneration: review of pathogenesis, *Eur J Ophthalmol* 8(4):199, 1998.

54. Ambati J, Ambati BK, Yoo SH, et al: Age-related macular degeneration: etiology, pathogenesis, and therapeutic strategies, *Surv Ophthalmol* 48(3):257, 2003.

55. Holz FG, Sheraidah G, Pauleikhoff D, et al: Analysis of lipid deposits extracted from human macular and peripheral Bruch's membrane, *Arch Ophthalmol* 112(3):402, 1994.

56. Guymer R, Luthert P, Bird A: Changes in Bruch's membrane and related structures with age, *Prog Retin Eye Res* 18(1):59, 1999.

57. Curcio CA, Millican CL, Bailey T, et al: Accumulation of cholesterol with age in human Bruch's membrane, *Invest Ophthalmol Vis Sci* 42:265, 2001.

58. Bailey RN: The surgical removal of a subfoveal choroidal neovascular membrane: an alternative treatment to laser photocoagulation, *J Am Optom Assoc* 64(2):104, 1993.

59. Cruickshanks KJ, Klein R, Klein BE, et al: Sunlight and the 5-year incidence of early age-related maculopathy: the Beaver Dam Eye Study, *Arch Ophthalmol* 119(2):246, 2001.

60. McCarty CA, Mukesh BN, Fu CL, et al: Risk factors for age-related maculopathy: the Visual Impairment Project, *Arch Ophthalmol* 119(10):1455, 2001.

61. Klein R, Klein BE, Jensen SC, et al: The relationship of ocular factors to the incidence and progression of age-related maculopathy, *Arch Ophthalmol* 116(4):506, 1998.

62. Mitchell P, Smith W, Wang JJ: Iris color, skin sun sensitivity, and age-related maculopathy: the Blue Mountains Eye Study, *Ophthalmology* 105(8):1359, 1998.

63. Young RW: The family of sunlight-related eye diseases, *Optom Vis Sci* 71(2):125, 1994.

64. Age-related Eye Disease Study Research Group: A randomized, placebo-controlled, clinical trial of high-dose supplementation with vitamins C and E, beta carotene, and zinc for age-related macular degeneration and vision loss: AREDS report no. 8, *Arch Ophthalmol* 119(10):1417, 2001.

65. Gale CR, Hall NF, Phillips DI, et al: Lutein and zeaxanthin status and risk of age-related macular degeneration, *Invest Ophthalmol Vis Sci* 44:2461, 2003.

66. Smith W, Mitchell P, Webb K, et al: Dietary antioxidants and age-related maculopathy: the Blue Mountains Eye Study, *Ophthalmology* 106(4):761, 1999.

67. Flood V, Smith W, Wang JJ: Dietary antioxidant intake and incidence of early age-related maculopathy: the Blue Mountains Eye Study, *Ophthalmology* 109(12):2272, 2002.

68. Kuzniarz M, Mitchell P, Flood VM, et al: Use of vitamin and zinc supplements and age-related maculopathy: the Blue Mountains Eye Study, *Ophthalmic Epidemiol* 9(4):283, 2002.

69. Bone RA, Landrum JT, Guerra LH, et al: Lutein and zeaxanthin dietary supplements raise macular pigment density and serum concentrations of these carotenoids in humans, *J Nutr* 133(4):922, 2003.

70. Klein R, Klein BE, Tomany SC, et al: Ten-year incidence and progression of age-related maculopathy: the Beaver Dam Eye Study, *Ophthalmology* 109:1767, 2002.

71. Oates DC, Belcher CD: Aging changes in trabecular meshwork, iris, and ciliary body. In Albert DM, Jakobiec FA, editors: *Principles and practice of ophthalmology*, Philadelphia, 1994, Saunders, p 697.

72. Pardue MT, Sivak JG: Age-related changes in human ciliary muscle, *Optom Vis Sci* 77(4):204, 2000.

73. Strenk SA, Semmlow JL, Strenk LM, et al: Age-related changes in human ciliary muscle and lens: a magnetic resonance imaging study, *Invest Ophthalmol Vis Sci* 40(6):1162, 1999.

74. Strenk SA, Strenk LM, Guo S: Magnetic resonance imaging of aging, accommodating, phakic, and pseudophakic ciliary muscle diameters, *J Cataract Refract Surg* 32:1792–1798, 2006.

75. Moore DJ, Clover GM: The effect of age on the macromolecular permeability of human Bruch's membrane, *Invest Ophthalmol Vis Sci* 42:2970, 2001.

76. Moore DJ, Hussain AA, Marshall J: Age-related variation in the hydraulic conductivity of Bruch's membrane, *Invest Ophthalmol Vis Sci* 36(7):1290, 1995.

77. Ruberti JW, Curcio CA, Millican CL, et al: Quick-freeze/deep-etch visualization of age-related lipid accumulation in Bruch's membrane, *Invest Ophthalmol Vis Sci* 44:1753, 2003.

78. Huang JD, Presley JB, Chimento MF, et al: Age-related changes in human macular Bruch's membrane as seen by quick-freeze-deep-etch, *Exp Eye Res* 85:202–218, 2007.

79. Ramrattan RS, van der Schaft TL, Mooy CM, et al: Morphometric analysis of Bruch's membrane, the choriocapillaris, and the choroid in aging, *Invest Ophthalmol Vis Sci* 35(6):2857, 1994.

The innermost coat of the eye is a neural layer, the retina, located between the choroid and the vitreous. It includes the macula, the area at the posterior pole used for sharpest acuity and color vision. The retina extends from the circular edge of the optic disc, where the nerve fibers exit the eye, to the ora serrata. It is continuous with the epithelial layers of the ciliary body, with which it shares embryologic origin. The retina is derived from neural ectoderm and consists of an outer pigmented layer, derived from the outer layer of the optic cup, and the neural retina, derived from the inner layer of the optic cup (see Chapter 7). The pigmented layer is tightly adherent to the choroid throughout, but the neural retina is attached to the pigmented epithelium and thus to the choroid only in a peripapillary ring around the disc and at the ora serrata. Although it contains millions of cell bodies and their processes, the neural retina has the appearance of a thin, transparent membrane.

The retina is the site of transformation of light energy into a neural signal. It contains the first three cells (photoreceptor, bipolar, and ganglion) in the visual pathway, the route by which visual information from the environment reaches the brain for interpretation. Photoreceptor cells transform photons of light into a neural signal through the process of phototransduction, then transfer this signal to bipolar cells, which in turn synapse with ganglion cells, which transmit the signal from the eye. Other retinal cells—horizontal cells, amacrine cells, and interplexiform neurons—modify and integrate the signal before it leaves the eye. This chapter discusses these cells and the detailed anatomy of the retina; the remainder of the visual pathway is described in Chapter 13.

RETINAL HISTOLOGIC FEATURES

Under light microscopy, the retina has a laminar appearance in which 10 layers are evident (Figure 4-1). Closer examination reveals that these are not all "layers," but rather a single layer of pigmented epithelium and three layers of neuronal cell bodies, between which lie their processes and synapses. This section describes the epithelial layer and the types and functions of the neural cells; the next section discusses the components of each of the 10 so-called retinal layers.

RETINAL PIGMENT EPITHELIUM

The **retinal pigment epithelium (RPE),** the outermost retinal layer, is a single cell thick and consists of pigmented hexagonal cells. These cells are columnar in the area of the posterior pole and are even longer, narrower, and more densely pigmented in the macular area.[1] The cells become larger and more cuboidal as the layer nears the ora serrata, where the transition to the pigmented epithelium of the ciliary body is located. Because of the orientation of the embryologic cells, the basal aspect of the cell is adjacent to the choroid and the apical surface faces the neural retina. The basal aspect contains numerous infoldings and is adherent to its basement membrane, which forms a part of Bruch's membrane of the choroid; therefore, its attachment to the choroid is strong. Despite its close association with the choroid, the RPE is considered a part of the retina because it is from the same embryologic germ cell layer—neural ectoderm.

The RPE cells contain numerous melanosomes, pigment granules, that extend from the apical area into the middle portion of the cell and somewhat obscure the nucleus, which is located in the basal region. Pigment density differs in various parts of the retina and in individual cells, which can give the fundus a mottled appearance when viewed with the ophthalmoscope. In the retina, melanin is densest in the RPE cells located in the macula and at the equator.[2] Other pigmented bodies, lipofuscin granules, contain degradation products of phagocytosis, which increase in number with age.[1,3-7] The cell cytoplasm also contains smooth and rough endoplasmic reticulum, Golgi apparatus, mitochondria, and numerous lysosomes.

The apical portion of an RPE cell consists of microvilli that extend into the layer of photoreceptors, enveloping the specialized outer segment tips (Figure 4-2). However, no intercellular junctions connect the RPE and photoreceptor cells. A potential space separates the epithelial cell and the photoreceptor.[1] This subretinal space[8] is a remnant of the gap formed between the two layers of the optic cup after invagination of the optic vesicle (see Chapter 7).

Terminal bars consisting of zonula occludens and zonula adherens join the RPE cells near their apices.[1] Desmosomes are present throughout the layer, and gap junctions between the cells allow for electrical coupling,

FIGURE 4-1

A, Layers of the retina. *1,* Retinal pigment epithelial layer; *2,* photoreceptor layer; *3,* external limiting membrane; *4,* outer nuclear layer; *5,* outer plexiform layer; *6,* inner nuclear layer; *7,* inner plexiform layer; *8,* ganglion cell layer; *9,* nerve fiber layer; *10,* internal limiting membrane. Only photoreceptors (rods and one cone), bipolar cells, ganglion cells, and fibers of Müller cells (m) are illustrated. Numbers refer to 10 retinal layers. (From Leeson CR, Leeson S: *Histology,* Philadelphia, 1976, Saunders.) **B,** Photomicrograph of same area. At top is inner portion of choroid with choriocapillaris (arrow).

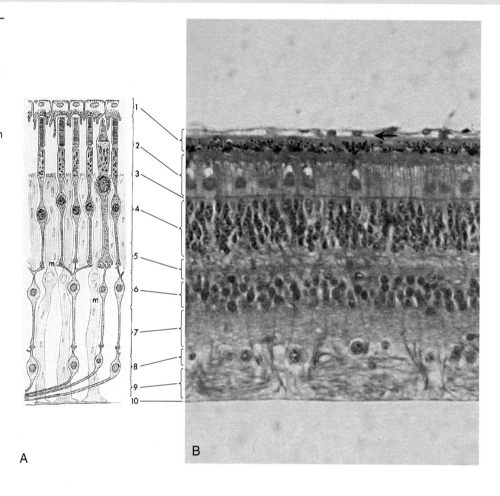

A

B

providing a low-resistance pathway for the passage of ions and metabolites.[9]

PHOTORECEPTOR CELLS

Photoreceptor cells, the rods and cones, are special sense cells containing photopigments that absorb photons of light. The cells originally were named for their shapes, but the name does not always reflect the shape, particularly in the cone population. More important in the designation of a rod or cone is the level of illumination in which each is active. Rods are more active in dim illumination, and cones are active in well-lit conditions. Visual pigments in the photoreceptors are activated on excitation by light.

Retinal Pigment Epithelium-Neuroretinal Interface

Several factors are involved in maintaining the close approximation between the photoreceptor cell layer and the RPE layer. Passive forces, such as intraocular pressure (IOP), osmotic pressure,[10-12] fluid transport across the RPE,[13,14] and presence of the vitreous,[15] help preserve the position of the neural retina. Interdigitations between the RPE microvilli and the rod and cone outer segments provide a physical closeness between the two entities.[1] The material that occupies the extracellular space between the two layers likely provides adhesive forces.[16-18]

An unstructured, amorphous material was once thought to occupy the extracellular space between the RPE cells and the photoreceptors, and to surround the outer and inner segments of the photoreceptors. More recent studies have described an organized honeycomb-like structure, the **interphotoreceptor matrix (IPM),** which is composed of proteins and glycosaminoglycans.[19] The outer segments are surrounded completely by the IPM and extend through openings in its meshwork. The constituents of the IPM domains around rods differ from those around cones; those surrounding cones are described as a "matrix sheath."[19-21] The domains are believed to be bound together laterally, forming a highly coherent structural unit.[19] The IPM constituents are bound

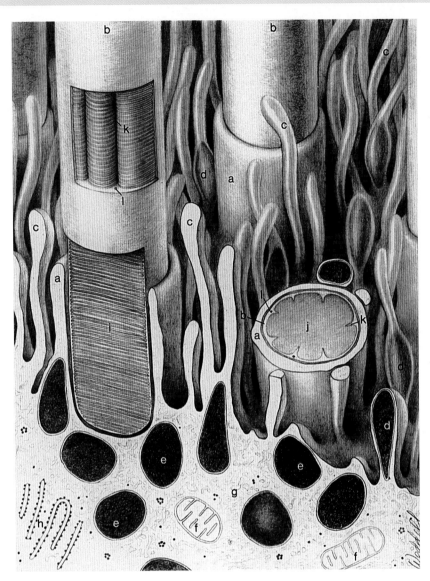

FIGURE 4-2
Three-dimensional drawing of relationship between outer segments of rods and cells of retinal pigment epithelium (RPE). Thick sheaths (*a*) of RPE enclose external portions of rod outer segments (*b*). Numerous fingerlike villous processes (*c*) are found between photoreceptors and contain pigment granules (*d*). Apical portion of RPE layer of cells at bottom contains numerous pigment granules (*e*); mitochondria (*f*); a well-developed, smooth-surfaced endoplasmic reticulum (*g*); a poorly developed, rough-surfaced endoplasmic reticulum (*h*); and scattered free ribosomes. Stacks of rod outer segment discs are depicted in meridional section (*i*) and in cross section (*j*). Periphery of discs shows scalloping (*k*). Microtubules originating in basal body of rod cilium extend externally into outer segment; one such microtubule is shown in cross section (*l*). (From Hogan MJ, Alvarado JA, Weddell JE: *Histology of the human eye*, Philadelphia, 1971, Saunders.)

tightly to both the epithelial cells and the photoreceptor cells, and may exceed the strength of the RPE cells. In laboratory experiments, a forceful separation between these two layers often ruptures the RPE cell, leaving remnants of pigment attached to the photoreceptors.[3,22] The adhesive mechanism is attributed to molecular bonds within this extracellular material.[16,18,22-24]

The IPM provides a means for the exchange of metabolites[25] and for interactions between the two layers.[26] In addition, the IPM may be partly responsible for orienting the photoreceptor outer segments for optimal light capture.[17] Despite these apparent forces, the interface between the RPE and the photoreceptor layer is the common location of separation in a retinal detachment.

Clinical Comment: Retinal Detachment

*When a **retinal detachment** occurs, the separation usually lies between the RPE cells and the photoreceptors because no intercellular junctions join these cells. The RPE cells remain attached to the choroid and cannot be separated from it without difficulty. Bruch's membrane contains fibronectin and laminin, large adhesive glycoproteins with many binding sites that help maintain the adherence of RPE cells to the membrane.[27] Fluid can accumulate within the subretinal space separating the photoreceptors from the nutrients supplied by the choroid; if the layers are not repositioned quickly, the affected area of photoreceptor cells will necrose. An argon laser often is used to photocoagulate the border of a detachment, producing scar tissue. These act like a "spot weld" and prevent the detachment from enlarging and facilitates the repositioning of the photoreceptors.*

Composition of Rods and Cones

Rods and cones are composed of several parts, starting nearest the RPE: (1) the outer segment, containing the visual pigment molecules for the conversion of light into a neural signal; (2) a connecting stalk, the cilium; (3) the inner segment, containing the metabolic apparatus; (4) the outer fiber; (5) the cell body; and (6) the inner fiber, which ends in a synaptic terminal (Figure 4-3).

Outer Segment

The **outer segment** is made up of a stack of membranous discs (600 to 1000 per rod)[2] and is enclosed by the plasmalemma of the cell. Each disc is a flattened membrane sac with a narrow intradisc space; the discs are stacked on top of one another and are separated by an extradisc space. Visual pigment molecules are located within the disc membrane. A biochemical change is initiated within these molecules when they are activated by a photon of light. The tip of the outer segment is oriented toward the RPE, and the base is oriented toward the inner segment.

Cilium

A connecting stalk, or **cilium,** extends from the innermost disc, joining the outer segment with the inner segment and acting as a conduit between them (Figure 4-4). It is a modified cilium consisting of a series of nine pairs of tubules from which the central pair, usually present in motile cilia, is missing. The plasmalemma around the outer segment is continuous across the cilium with that of the inner segment.

Inner Segment

The **inner segment** contains cellular structures and can be divided into two parts. The ellipsoid is nearer the outer segment and contains the numerous mitochondria necessary for the many energy-dependent photoreceptor processes. The part closer to the cell body, which is sometimes called the myoid, contains other cellular organelles, such as the endoplasmic reticulum and Golgi apparatus; protein synthesis is concentrated in this area.[28] The term "myoid," however, is derived from a similar area in amphibians that contains a contractile structure that produces orientational movements of the outer segments of the cones.[29] The human myoid does not have contractile properties,[30] although the axis of the inner and outer segments is oriented toward the exit pupil of the eye, maximizing the ability of the photoreceptor to capture light. The radial orientation becomes more evident in cells located farther from the macula.[8,31,32]

Outer Fiber, Cell Body, and Inner Fiber

The **outer fiber** extends from the inner segment to the **cell body,** the portion containing the nucleus. The **inner fiber** is an axonal process containing microtubules and

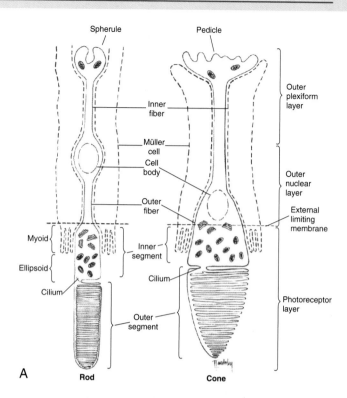

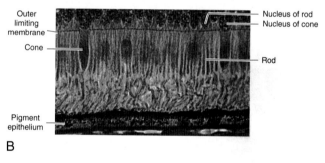

FIGURE 4-3

A, Photoreceptor cells. Portions of Müller cells (*dotted lines*) are shown adjoining the rods and cones. The retinal layers listed to the right indicate the layers in which the parts of the photoreceptor are located. **B,** Retina. (×1000.) (**B** from Krause WJ, Cutts JH: *Concise text of histology,* Baltimore, 1981, Williams & Wilkins.)

runs inward from the cell body, ending in specialized synaptic terminals that contain synaptic vesicles. The photoreceptor nerve endings synapse with bipolar and horizontal cells.

Rod and Cone Morphology

Rods

The plasmalemma, enclosing the rod outer segment, is separate from the disc membrane except for a small region at the base where invaginations of the plasmalemma form discs, the intradisc space of which is continuous with the extracellular space (see Figure 4-3, *A*). The remainder of the discs form sacs that are closed at

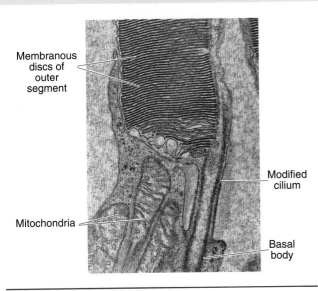

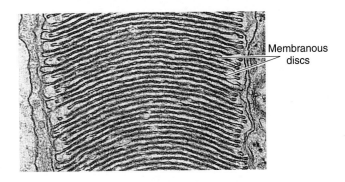

FIGURE 4-5
Cone outer segment. (Transmission electron microscope; ×56,000.) (From Krause WJ, Cutts JH: *Concise text of histology*, Baltimore, 1981, Williams & Wilkins.)

FIGURE 4-4
Junction of outer and inner segment of rod. (Transmission electron microscope; ×45,000.) (From Krause WJ, Cutts JH: *Concise text of histology*, Baltimore, 1981, Williams & Wilkins.)

both ends and are free of attachment to the surrounding membrane and adjacent discs.[8,33] The discs are fairly uniform in width, and the photosensitive pigment rhodopsin is located within the disc membrane.

Young[28] applied a pulse of radiolabeled amino acids, which were incorporated into the disc components. He observed that the band of radioactivity moved from the inner segment, where protein is synthesized, into newly assembled discs in the outer segment. The labeled discs moved from the base to the tip, and the label was finally seen in phagosomes of the RPE cells. This study established that components of disc membranes are produced in the inner segment and move along the connecting stalk to be incorporated into discs at the outer segment base.[28] The discs gradually are displaced outward by the formation of new discs and, as they reach the tip, are sloughed off, taken up by the RPE cells, and phagocytosed.[34,35] This process, the **rod outer segment renewal system,** appears to involve active processes in both the RPE and the outer segment.[28,36] The discs apparently are shed regularly, with most of the shedding occurring in the early morning.[37-40]

The rod inner and outer segments are approximately the same width. The inner segment is joined to the cell body by the relatively long and narrow *outer* fiber. The *inner* fiber extends from the cell body and terminates in a rounded, pear-shaped structure called a **spherule** (see Figure 4-3, *A*). The internal surface of the spherule is invaginated forming a synaptic complex that contains bipolar dendrites and horizontal cell processes.[41,42] Rods release the neurotransmitter glutamate.

Cones

As in the rod, the outer segment of the cone is enclosed by a plasmalemma, but in this case the plasma membrane is continuous with the membranes forming most of the discs, and the discs are not separated easily from one another[43] (Figure 4-5). In many cones the discs at the base are wider than those at the tip, giving the characteristic cone shape, although some cone outer segments have a shape similar to the rod.

The cone outer segment is shorter than that of the rod and may not reach the RPE layer. However, tubular processes protrude from the apical surface of the epithelial cell to surround the cone outer segment.[44] One of three visual pigment molecules is contained within the disc membrane, and each pigment molecule is activated by the absorption of light in a specific range in the color spectrum. The peak absorptions occur at 420 nm (blue), 531 nm (green), and 588 nm (red).

Early studies of cone outer segment renewal theorized that the formation of discs at the cone base was not uniform and sequential because radiolabeled protein appeared to be distributed throughout the outer segment membrane, not merely in the disc membranes.[35,45] More recently, electron-microscope studies suggest that formation of new discs does occur at the base, but because of the more extensive connections with the surrounding plasmalemma, the labeled molecules are able to diffuse throughout the cone outer segment membrane rather than being confined to discs, as occurs in the rods.[43] Investigations continue into the mechanism by which the discs become narrower as they approach the tip.[46] Cone discs too are shed periodically, often at the end of the day, and are phagocytosed by the RPE.[40,43,47,48] The factors that regulate the cycle of disc shedding are still under investigation.

The shape of the inner segment also contributes to the cone shape. The ellipsoid area of the cone is wider and contains more mitochondria than the rod.[1] The outer fiber is short and stout and may even be absent in the cone; thus, cone nuclei lie outer to rod nuclei. The inner fiber terminates in a broad, flattened structure called a **pedicle,** which has several invaginated areas within its flattened surface (see Figure 4-3, *A*). Cone pedicles have three types of synaptic contacts. Triads are found within the invaginations; contacts with bipolar cells occur on the flat surfaces; and gap junctions are located on the lateral expansions (telodendria) of the pedicle and permit electrical communication between adjacent rods or cones.[8,49]

As with rods, the neurotransmitter released by cones is glutamate.

BIPOLAR CELLS

The **bipolar cell** is the second-order neuron in the visual pathway. The nucleus of the bipolar cell is large and contains minimal cell body cytoplasm. Its dendrite synapses with photoreceptor and horizontal cells, and its axon synapses with ganglion and amacrine cells; glutamate is its neurotransmitter. Bipolar cells relay information from photoreceptors to horizontal, amacrine, and ganglion cells and receive extensive synaptic feedback from amacrine cells.[50] Their dendrites also have contact with interplexiform neuron processes.[51] Eleven types of bipolar cells have been classified on the basis of morphology, physiology, and dendritic contacts with photoreceptors;[51] all types except the rod bipolar cell are associated with cones.

Only one type of **rod bipolar cell** has been identified. It has a relatively large body and several spiky dendrites, usually arising from a single, thick process. Rod bipolar cells begin to appear 1 mm from the fovea and continue into the periphery. These are the only bipolar cells that contact rods.[1,51] The expanse of the dendritic tree widens and the reach of the axonal terminals increases in the rod bipolar cells located in peripheral retina compared with those in central retina. The dendrites of a single rod bipolar cell contact 15 to 20 rods in central retina and up to 80 rods in the periphery, improving sensitivity.[51,52] Often two dendrites lie within the spherule invagination flanked by two horizontal cell processes (Figure 4-6). The rod bipolar axon is large and unbranched, and rarely synapses directly with ganglion cells but instead synapses with amacrine processes, which then signal ganglion cells.[53] This synaptic arrangement allows a ganglion cell to carry information from both the rod and the cone pathway.[53]

The midget bipolar cell has a relatively small body and can be either flat or invaginating. Dendritic terminals of the **flat midget bipolar cell** end in a flat expansion and make contact only with the flat area of the

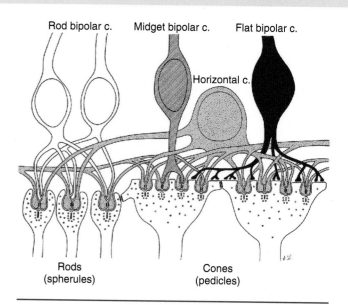

FIGURE 4-6

Rod spherule and cone pedicle and their synapses. Rod and cone bipolar cells show extensive contacts. Horizontal cells also make synapses with both rods and cones. Interconnections are shown between rod spherules and cone pedicles. (From Hogan MJ, Alvarado JA, Weddell JE: *Histology of the human eye,* Philadelphia, 1971, Saunders.)

cone pedicle. In central retina, each flat midget bipolar cell contacts only one cone so its dendritic "bouquet" is small—the size of a single cone pedicle. In peripheral retina, each flat midget bipolar cell has two or three dendritic clusters and thus each cell contacts two or three neighboring cones.[51,54] A single cone pedicle may have as many as 500 contacts on its flat surface.[2] The axon of the flat midget bipolar cell has many endings and synapses with ganglion cells of all types.[1]

The **invaginating midget bipolar cell** is similar to the flat midget bipolar cell, but its dendritic processes are located within the pedicle invaginations, usually in groupings called a triad. A **triad** consists of a single central bipolar dendrite flanked by two horizontal cell processes within an invagination in the cone pedicle (see Figure 4-6). In central retina, the dendritic bouquet of an invaginating midget bipolar cell is the size of a single cone pedicle, implying that each cone is innervated by only one invaginating bipolar cell. Each pedicle can have 12 to 25 triads.[2] In peripheral retina, each bipolar cell may have up to three such dendritic expansions, with the capacity to contact several pedicles.[51] The axon of the invaginating midget bipolar cell synapses with the dendrite of a single midget ganglion cell and with amacrine processes.[1]

The two types of **diffuse cone bipolar cells** are designated type a and type b, called "flat bipolars" and "brush bipolars" by Polyak.[55] In the central retina, the diffuse cone bipolar cell contacts approximately five neighboring cones, and in the periphery, each contacts 10 to 15 neighboring cones. The location of the axon terminal differentiates the two types.[51]

The **blue cone bipolar cell** synapses with up to three cone pedicles.[56] It differs from diffuse cone bipolar cells in that it contacts widely spaced rather than neighboring cones.[51]

The **giant cone bipolar cell** derives its name from the extent of its dendritic tree. The major dendrite branches into three trees, and then clusters of processes branch from these, each group being the size of a cone pedicle. The two types, designated diffuse and bistratified, differ only in the location of their axon terminations.[51,57]

Figure 4-7 shows several of the bipolar cell types.

GANGLION CELLS

The next cell in the visual pathway, the third-order neuron, is the **ganglion cell.** Ganglion cells can be bipolar (e.g., a single axon and a single dendrite) or multipolar (a single axon and more than one dendrite).[58] Cell size varies greatly, with some large cell bodies measuring 28 to 36 μm.[51] The various methods used to classify ganglion cells make classification rather confusing.

An older, broad classification groups ganglion cells into three types. *W* cells project to the midbrain, carrying information for the pupillary response and reflexive eye movements. *Y* cells project to the lateral geniculate nucleus (LGN), with some having collateral branches that travel to the midbrain, perhaps with pupillary information. *X* cells primarily respond in visual discrimination and project to the LGN.[2]

Ganglion cells have also been classified on the basis of cell body size, branching characteristics, termination of dendrites, and the expanse of the dendritic tree.[51] Figure 4-8 shows several types of ganglion cells, both central and peripheral. These ganglion cell types are designated G3 to G23 (not all numbers are represented).

Another designation classifies ganglion cells based on the lateral geniculate nucleus layer in which they terminate. P cells terminate in the parvocellular layers. The **P1 ganglion cell,** also called the midget ganglion cell, is the most common P cell. This relatively small cell has a single dendrite and can be differentiated into two types, according to the stratification of the dendritic branching.[51] Certain P1 midget cells are connected to only one midget bipolar cell, invaginating or flat, which in turn might be linked to a single cone receptor,[59] providing a channel that processes high-contrast detail and color resolution. This situation is likely to occur in the fovea. A convergent pathway occurs in some P1 cells that receive input from two bipolar axons.

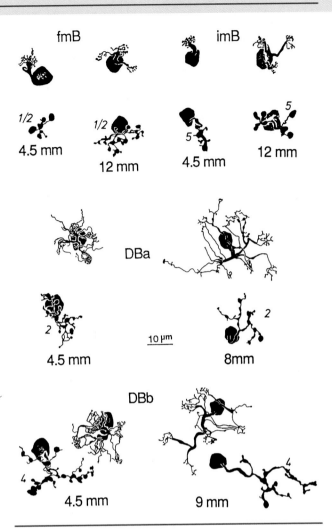

FIGURE 4-7
Camera lucida drawings of cone bipolar cells of the human retina as seen in whole-mount Golgi preparations (scale bar = 10 mm). Each cell is drawn at two levels: dendritic tree in outer plexiform layer (OPL) (*top*) and axon terminal in inner plexiform layer (IPL) (*bottom*). Stratification of axon terminal according to five strata of IPL is given by adjacent italicized number. Positions on retina in millimeters of eccentricity are indicated for each cell illustrated. Midget bipolar cells, fmB and imB varieties, are indicated above diffuse small-field bipolar types, DBa and DBb. See text for further details. (From Kolb H, Linberg KA, Fisher SK: Neurons of the human retina: a Golgi study, *J Comp Neurol* 318:150, 1992.)

The **P2 ganglion cell** also terminates in the parvocellular layers but has a densely branched, compact dendritic tree that spreads horizontally. These cells can be differentiated into two types depending on the location of the dendrite termination.[51]

The **M-type ganglion cell** projects to the magnocellular layers of the LGN. The M cell has coarse dendrites (because of its shape can also be called a parasol ganglion cell) with spiny features, and the dendritic tree enlarges from central to peripheral retina.[51]

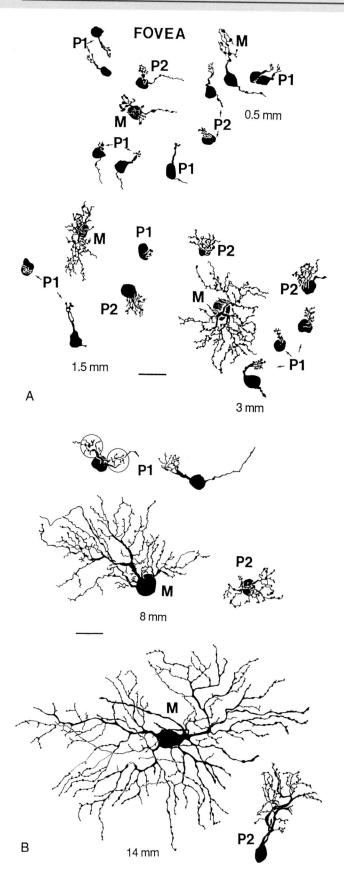

FIGURE 4-8
A, Ganglion cells (P1, P2, and M) of foveal and central human retina (scale bar = 25 mm). Three types can be distinguished on dendritic tree size when they occur adjacent to one another. P1 ganglion cells have a minute dendritic tree at the fovea, which expands to be no more than a small bouquet of varicosities 9 to 12 mm across ×3 mm of eccentricity. P2 ganglion cells have dendritic trees approximately double the size of P1 cells. M ganglion cells average three times the size of P2 cells in dendritic extent. All three types occur as "a" and "b" subtypes, dependent on levels of their dendritic trees in sublamina a or sublamina b of inner plexiform layer. **B,** Ganglion cells (P1, P2, and M) of middle and far peripheral retina (scale bar = 25 mm). These cells exhibit continuation (in relation to part A) of their increasing dendritic tree sizes at greater eccentricities. Many P1 cells in this region have two dendritic heads (*circled*). Others are normal, single-headed P1 cells, reaching a maximum dendritic tree size of 25 mm. P2 and M cells occur into far periphery and are distinguished clearly by both cell body size and dendritic tree size. (From Kolb H, Linberg KA, Fisher SK: Neurons of the human retina: a Golgi study, *J Comp Neurol* 318:147, 1992.)

Each ganglion cell has a single axon, which emerges from the cell body and turns to run parallel to the inner surface of the retina; the axon releases glutamate at its synaptic cleft. The axons come together at the optic disc and leave the eye as the optic nerve. The termination for approximately 90% of these axons is the lateral geniculate nucleus; the other 10% project to subthalamic areas involved in processes such as the pupillary reflexes and the circadian rhythm.[2,51]

The photoreceptor cells, bipolar cells, and ganglion cells carry the neural signal in a three-step pathway through the retina. The neural signal is modified within the retina by other cells that create intraretinal cross-connections, provide feedback information, or integrate retinal function.[1]

HORIZONTAL CELLS

The **horizontal cell** transfers information in a horizontal direction parallel to the retinal surface. It has one long process, or axon, and several short dendrites with branching terminals; the processes spread out parallel to the retinal surface, and all terminate in the outer plexiform layer (Figure 4-9). Horizontal cells synapse with photoreceptors, bipolar cells, and other horizontal cells. Horizontal cells are joined to each other by an extensive network of gap junctions. One type of horizontal cell synapses only within a cone pedicle in the special triad junction. Horizontal cells can contact bipolar cells lying some distance from the photoreceptor that activated the horizontal cell. Horizontal cells can effect an inhibitory

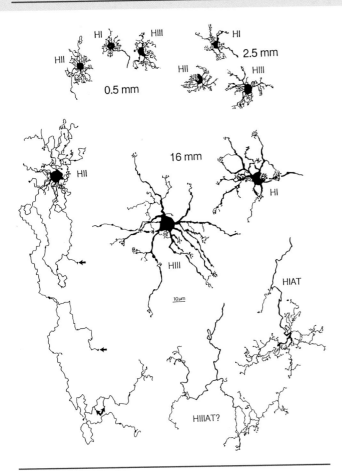

FIGURE 4-9

Whole-mount views of horizontal cells of human retina (scale bar = 10 mm). Cells of fovea (0.5 mm) are small and difficult to distinguish into the three types but still recognizable to the trained eye. By 2.5 mm of eccentricity, HI, HII, and HIII cell types are discernible from one another. In peripheral retina (16 mm), HIII is clearly larger than HI and has an asymmetric dendritic field. HII cells have a "woolly" appearance that distinguishes them readily from HI and HIII cells. Short, curled axon of HII type gives rise to occasional terminals (*arrows*). HI axon terminal ends as fan-shaped structure with many "lollipop" terminals (HIAT), whereas a finer, more loosely clustered terminal is putatively assigned to HIII horizontal cell type HIIIAT. (From Kolb H, Linberg KA, Fisher SK: Neurons of the human retina: a Golgi study, *J Comp Neurol* 318:147, 1992.)

response, thus playing a role in the complex process of visual integration.[57,60]

Three types of horizontal cells have been differentiated: HI, HII, and HIII. **HI** cells have dendrites that synapse with 7 to 18 cones as lateral elements in triads and a large, thick axon ending in a fan-shaped expanse of terminals that end in rod spherules more than 1 mm away.[61] All the **HII** processes (dendrites and axons) apparently contact cones and might be specific for blue cones.[51] **HIII cells** have a large dendritic tree that synapses with many cones, (9 to 12 in the macular area and 20 to 25 in the periphery) not all of which are neighboring; evidence suggests that these horizontal cells avoid blue cones, thus being selective for red and green.[51,62] The termination of the HIII axon has not yet been determined but probably contacts both rods and cones.[60] Horizontal cells provide inhibitory feedback to photoreceptors or inhibitory feed forward to bipolar cells.[61] Horizontal cells can modulate the cone response but are not thought to influence that of the rod.[53,61]

AMACRINE CELLS

The **amacrine cell** has a large cell body, a lobulated nucleus, and a single process with extensive branches that extend into the inner plexiform layer. The process, which has both dendritic and axonal characteristics and carries information horizontally, forms complex synapses with axons of bipolar cells, dendrites and the soma of ganglion cells; with processes of interplexiform neurons; and with other amacrine processes.[1,63] Because of the extremely broad spread of its process, the amacrine cell plays an important role in modulating the information that reaches the ganglion cells.[57]

As many as 30 to 40 different amacrine cell types may be described as stratified or diffuse. They can also be classified into four groups—narrow field, small field, medium field, and large field—according to the extent of coverage by their intertwined branching processes. Each of these groups can be subdivided into different types according to the level of the retinal layer in which their nerve endings terminate.[51,64]

One of the most widely studied amacrine types is the **AII cell** (that is Roman numeral 2), a narrow-field type (Figure 4-10). The AII cells are the conduit by which the rod signal reaches ganglion cells.[64] An AII cell may receive input from as many as 300 rods through 80 rod bipolar cells.[31] The AII cell then synapses with a ganglion cell and may also relay information from the rod pathway to the cone pathway.

Wide-field amacrine (A17) cells form reciprocal synapses with rod bipolar cells and appear to modify the signal transmitted from rod bipolar to AII cells.[51] Most amacrine cells contain the inhibitory neurotransmitter gamma-aminobutyric acid (GABA) or glycine, and have both presynaptic and postsynaptic endings.[2,64] Amacrine cells are joined to one another via gap junctions,[64] and some cells have been found to combine information from rod and cone pathways before innervating a ganglion cell.[59]

INTERPLEXIFORM NEURONS

The **interplexiform neuron** has a large cell body and is found among the layer of amacrine cells. The processes extend into both synaptic layers and convey information

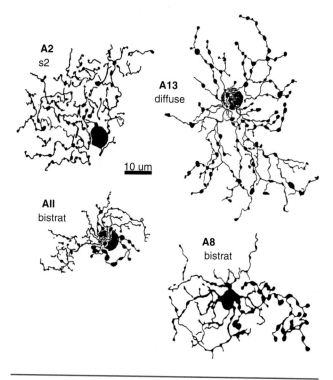

A2
s2

A13
diffuse

10 um

AII
bistrat

A8
bistrat

FIGURE 4-10
Whole-mount view of amacrine cells. (From Kolb H: Amacrine cells of the mammalian retina: neurocircuitry and functional roles, *Eye* 11:904, 1997.)

between these layers (Figure 4-11), apparently providing feedback from inner to outer retinal layers.[51,57] Some of their nerve endings are presynaptic and some are post-synaptic to amacrine processes or amacrine cell bodies in the inner plexiform layer. Interplexiform neurons are presynaptic to rod or cone bipolar cells in the outer plexiform layer.[2,8,65]

NEUROGLIAL CELLS

Neuroglial cells, although not actively involved in the transfer of neural signals, provide structure and support and have a role in the neural tissue reaction to injury or infection. Types of neuroglial cells found in the retina include Müller cells, microglial cells, and astrocytes.

Müller Cells

Müller cells are large neuroglial cells that extend throughout much of the retina. There are 10 million Müller cells in the mammalian retina.[66] They play a supportive role, providing structure. The apex of the Müller cell is in the photoreceptor layer, whereas the basal aspect is at the inner retinal surface. Cellular processes form a reticulum among the retinal cell bodies and fill in most of the space of the retina not occupied by neuronal elements

(Figure 4-12). Müller cells ensheathe dendritic processes within the synaptic layers, giving structural support, and their processes envelop most ganglion axons.[67]

Neuronal cell bodies and their processes appear to reside in tunnels within the Müller cell.[52] Delicate apical villi, *fiber baskets (of Schultze)*, terminate between the inner segments of the photoreceptors.[1,29] On light microscopy, Müller cell processes can be seen passing through the layer containing the nerve fibers of the ganglion cells, perpendicular to the retinal surface. An expanded process, called the endfoot, along the basal aspect of the Müller cell contributes to the membrane separating the retina from the vitreous, and extensions of Müller cells wrap around blood vessels.[1] The pervasiveness of the Müller cell results in very little extracellular space in the retina (see Figure 4-12). Besides providing structure, the Müller cell acts as a buffer by regulating the concentration of potassium ions (K^+); they help maintain the extracellular pH by absorbing metabolic waste products[68]; they recycle GABA and glutamate, removing them from the extracellular space; and Müller cells metabolize, synthesize, and store glycogen.[69-71]

Microglial Cells and Astrocytes

Microglial cells are wandering phagocytic cells and might be found anywhere in the retina. Their number increases in response to tissue inflammation and injury.

Astrocytes are star-shaped fibrous cells found in the inner retina, usually in the nerve fiber and ganglion cell layers. These perivascular cells form an irregular supportive network that encircles nerve fibers and retinal capillaries.[1] They may contribute to the internal limiting membrane as well as perform some of the same functions as the Müller cells.[72]

TEN RETINAL LAYERS

The "10-layered" arrangement of the retina is actually a remarkable organization of alternate groupings of the retinal neurons just described and their processes. Traditionally, descriptive names were given to these so-called layers, and these designations are still in use today (Figure 4-13).

1. Retinal pigment epithelium
2. Photoreceptor cell layer
3. External limiting membrane
4. Outer nuclear layer
5. Outer plexiform layer
6. Inner nuclear layer
7. Inner plexiform layer
8. Ganglion cell layer
9. Nerve fiber layer
10. Internal limiting membrane

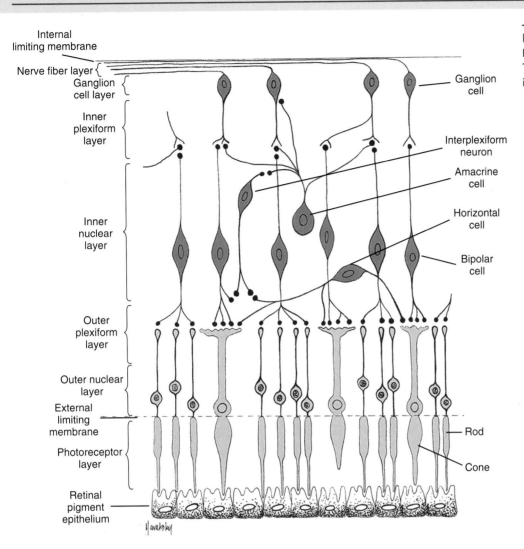

Internal limiting membrane

Nerve fiber layer

Ganglion cell layer

Inner plexiform layer

Inner nuclear layer

Outer plexiform layer

Outer nuclear layer

External limiting membrane

Photoreceptor layer

Retinal pigment epithelium

Ganglion cell

Interplexiform neuron

Amacrine cell

Horizontal cell

Bipolar cell

Rod

Cone

FIGURE 4-11
Retinal cells and synapses. The 10 retinal layers are indicated.

RETINAL PIGMENT EPITHELIUM

The **RPE** consists of a single layer of pigmented cells, as previously discussed. There are 4 to 6 million RPE cells, and each cell interacts with 30 to 40 photoreceptors.[37,73,74] There is little cell division in the layer. The RPE is an active area with several functions that will be described in a later section.

PHOTORECEPTOR LAYER

The **photoreceptor layer** contains the outer and inner segments of rods and cones. Projections from the apical surface of Müller cells extend into the photoreceptor layer and separate the inner segments.

EXTERNAL LIMITING MEMBRANE

The **external limiting membrane (ELM, outer limiting membrane)** is not a true membrane but is actually composed of *zonula adherens* junctions between photoreceptor cells and between photoreceptors and Müller cells at the level of the inner segments. On light microscopy, the so-called membrane appears as a series of dashes, resembling a fenestrated sheet through which processes of the rods and cones pass. This band of zonula adherens has the potential to act as a metabolic barrier restricting the passage of some large molecules.[8,75]

OUTER NUCLEAR LAYER

The **outer nuclear layer (ONL)** contains the rod and cone cell bodies; the cone cell body and nucleus are larger than those of the rod. Cone outer fibers are very short, and therefore the cone nuclei lie in a single layer close to the external limiting membrane; cell bodies of the rods are arranged in several rows inner to the cone cell bodies. The ONL is 8 to 9 cells thick on the nasal edge of the optic disc and 4 rows thick at the temporal edge and is thickest in the fovea, where it contains approximately 10 layers of cone nuclei.[2]

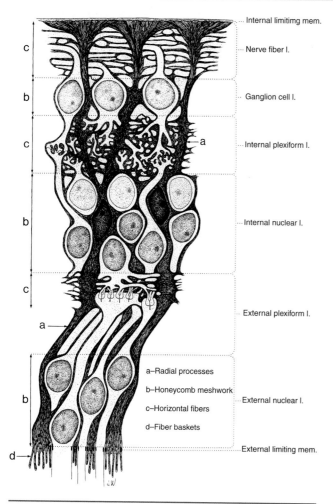

c — Internal limitimg mem.

— Nerve fiber l.

b — Ganglion cell l.

c — a — Internal plexiform l.

b — Internal nuclear l.

c —
a — External plexiform l.

a–Radial processes
b–Honeycomb meshwork — External nuclear l.
c–Horizontal fibers
d–Fiber baskets

b —

d — External limiting mem.

FIGURE 4-12
Structure of the Müller cell (dark gray). *mem.,* membrane; *l.,* layer. (From Hogan MJ, Alvarado JA, Weddell JE: *Histology of the human eye*, Philadelphia, 1971, Saunders.)

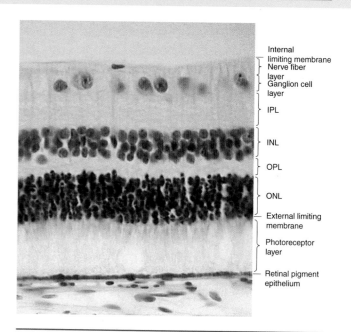

Internal limiting membrane
Nerve fiber layer
Ganglion cell layer
IPL
INL
OPL
ONL
External limiting membrane
Photoreceptor layer
Retinal pigment epithelium

FIGURE 4-13
Light micrograph of full-thickness view of the retina.

OUTER PLEXIFORM LAYER

The **outer plexiform layer (OPL;** also **outer synaptic layer)** has a wide external band composed of inner fibers of rods and cones and a narrower inner band consisting of synapses between photoreceptor cells and cells from the inner nuclear layer. Rod spherules and cone pedicles synapse with bipolar cell dendrites and horizontal cell processes in the OPL. Many of these synapses consist of invaginations in the photoreceptor terminal; invaginations are deep in the spherule but more superficial in the pedicle.[8] In these junctures the photoreceptor element contains a membranous plate, the synaptic ribbon[8,59] (Figure 4-14). The invaginating synapse generally has three postsynaptic processes and is called a triad. The lateral elements are horizontal cell processes and are deep within the invagination, a bipolar dendrite is the center process (see Figure 4-6). Invaginating

midget bipolar cells are involved in cone triads, and all cones have at least one invaginating midget bipolar and one flat midget bipolar contact.[8]

Synaptic contacts also occur outside invaginating synapses in the OPL. Horizontal cells make synaptic contact with bipolar dendrites and contact other horizontal cell processes via gap junctions.[61,76] Bipolar dendrites synapse with photoreceptor cell endings; a single photoreceptor can have contact with more than one bipolar dendrite. The relatively long axon of the interplexiform neuron makes numerous synaptic connections with processes entering photoreceptor terminals.[65,77]

Desmosome-like attachments called *synaptic densities* are located within the arrangement of interwoven, branching, bipolar dendrites and horizontal cell processes in the OPL. These synaptic densities are seen as a series of dashed lines on light microscopy and resemble a discontinuous membrane, termed the **middle limiting membrane.** This "membrane" demarcates the extent of the retinal vasculature[29] and may prevent retinal exudates and hemorrhages from spreading into the outer retinal layers.[52]

INNER NUCLEAR LAYER

The **inner nuclear layer (INL)** consists of the cell bodies of horizontal cells, bipolar cells, amacrine cells, interplexiform neurons, Müller cells, and sometimes displaced ganglion cells. The nuclei of the horizontal cells are located next to the outer plexiform layer, where their processes synapse. The nuclei of the amacrine cells are located next to the inner plexiform layer, where their processes terminate. The bipolar cell has its dendrite in the

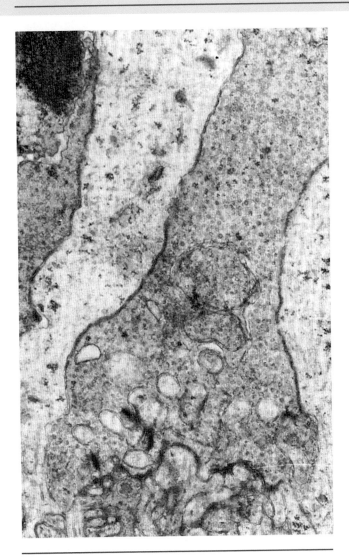

FIGURE 4-14
Electron micrograph of cone pedicle. Note dark linear bodies (synaptic ribbons) in pedicle. (×20,000.) (From Leeson CR, Leeson ST: *Histology*, Philadelphia, 1976, Saunders.)

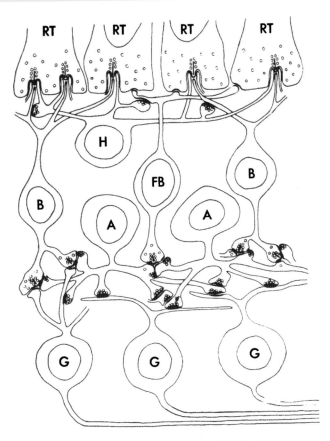

FIGURE 4-15
Arrangements of synaptic contacts found in vertebrate retinas. In outer synaptic layer, processes from bipolar (B) and horizontal cells (H) penetrate into invaginations in receptor terminals (RT) and terminate near synaptic ribbons (lamellae) of receptor. Processes of flat bipolar cells (FB) make superficial contacts on bases of some receptor terminals. Horizontal cells make conventional synaptic contacts onto bipolar dendrites and other horizontal cell processes (not shown). Because horizontal cells usually extend farther laterally in outer synaptic layer than do bipolar dendrites, distant receptors presumably can influence bipolar cells via horizontal cells. In the inner synaptic layer, two basic synaptic pathways are suggested. Bipolar terminals may contact one ganglion cell dendrite and one amacrine process at ribbon synapses (*left side*) or two amacrine cell (A) processes (*right side*). When the latter arrangement predominates in a retina, numerous conventional synapses between amacrine processes (serial synapses) are observed, and ganglion cells (G) are contacted mainly by amacrine processes (*right*). Amacrine processes in all retinas make synapses of conventional type back onto bipolar terminals (reciprocal synapses). (From Dowling JE: Organization of vertebrate retinas, *Invest Ophthalmol* 9:655, 1970.)

outer plexiform layer and its axon in the inner plexiform layer (Figure 4-15). The interplexiform neuron also has processes in both synaptic layers. It is thought to receive input in the inner plexiform layer and project it to the outer plexiform layer.[65] The retinal vasculature of the deep capillary network is located in the inner nuclear layer.

INNER PLEXIFORM LAYER

The **inner plexiform layer (IPL**; also **inner synaptic layer)** consists of synaptic connections between the axons of bipolar cells and dendrites of ganglion cells. The IPL contains the synapse between the second-order and third-order neuron in the visual pathway (see Figure 4-15). Generally, the axon of the invaginating midget bipolar cell ends in the *inner* half of the IPL, and the axon of the flat midget bipolar cell ends in the

outer half of the IPL.[51,54] Synapses also occur between (1) amacrine processes and bipolar axons, (2) amacrine processes and ganglion cell bodies and dendrites, (3) amacrine cells, and (4) amacrine cells and interplexiform neurons (Figure 4-16). The processing of motion

it is 2 cells thick. Although lying side by side, ganglion cells are separated from each other by glial processes of Müller cells.[72] Displaced amacrine cells, which send their processes outward, may be found in the ganglion cell layer, as may some displaced Müller cell bodies and astroglial cells.[8] Toward the ora serrata, the number of ganglion cells diminishes, and the nerve fiber layer thins.

NERVE FIBER LAYER

The **nerve fiber layer (NFL**; also *stratum opticum*) consists of ganglion cell axons. Their course runs parallel to the retinal surface; the fibers proceed to the optic disc, turn at a right angle, and exit the eye through the lamina cribrosa as the optic nerve. The fibers generally are unmyelinated within the retina. The NFL is thickest at the margins of the optic disc, where all the fibers accumulate. The group of fibers that radiate to the disc from the macular area is called the *papillomacular bundle.* This important grouping of fibers carries the information that determines visual acuity.

The retinal vessels, including the superficial capillary network, are located primarily in the NFL but may lie partly in the ganglion cell layer. Processes of Müller cells are common in the NFL, where they ensheathe vessels and nerve fibers.

Clinical Comment: Retinal Hemorrhages

HEMORRHAGES from retinal vasculature have a characteristic appearance. Because of the arrangement of the nerve fibers, the blood pools in a feathered pattern called a flame-shaped hemorrhage, which is indicative of the NFL location. Hemorrhages in the inner nuclear layer usually appear rounded and often are called dot or blot hemorrhages (Figure 4-17).

INTERNAL LIMITING MEMBRANE

The **internal limiting membrane (inner limiting membrane)** forms the innermost boundary of the retina. The outer retinal surface of this membrane is uneven and is composed of extensive, expanded terminations of Müller cells (often called footplates) covered by a basement membrane. The inner or vitreal surface is smooth. The connection between this membrane and the vitreous is still under investigation and may actually occur at a biochemical level (see Chapter 6); only in the periphery are vitreal fibers incorporated into the internal limiting membrane.[52]

Anteriorly, the internal limiting membrane of the retina is continuous with the internal limiting membrane of the ciliary body. It is present over the macula but undergoes modification at the optic disc, where processes from astrocytes replace those of the Müller cells.[58]

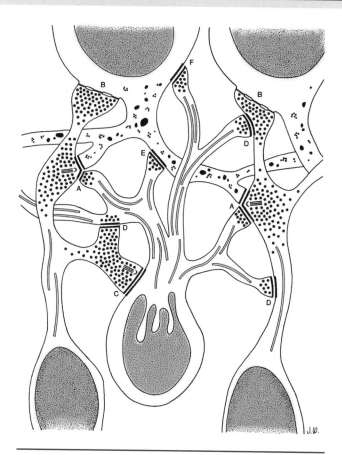

FIGURE 4-16
Synaptic contacts among bipolar, amacrine, and ganglion cells in inner plexiform layer. Bipolar axonal endings: **A**, axodendritic endings at a dyad; **B**, axosomatic ending on ganglion cell; **C**, bipolar axon-amacrine soma contact. Amacrine cell contacts with other cells; **D**, axoaxonal contact between bipolar and amacrine cell processes; **E**, axodendritic contact between amacrine and ganglion cell; **F**, axosomatic contact between amacrine cell process and soma of ganglion cell. (From Hogan MJ, Alvarado JA, Weddell JE: *Histology of the human eye,* Philadelphia, 1971, Saunders.)

detection and changes in brightness, as well as recognition of contrast and hue begin in this layer.[78]

Ribbon synapses in the IPL involve contact among a bipolar axon and a pair of postsynaptic processes, which may be amacrine or ganglion.[8,79] A reciprocal synapse, thought to be inhibitory, involves the second contact of an amacrine process with a bipolar axon, providing negative feedback.[52] Gap junctions between amacrine cells are also located in the IPL. Some displaced amacrine and ganglion cell bodies may also be seen.

GANGLION CELL LAYER

The **ganglion cell layer** is generally a single cell thick except near the macula, where it might be 8 to 10 cells thick, and at the temporal side of the optic disc, where

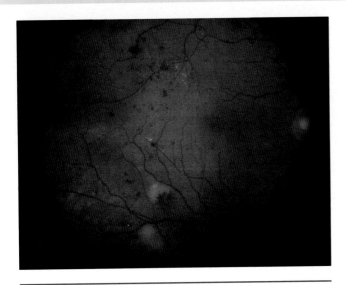

FIGURE 4-17
Fundus photo, OD, from patient with nonproliferative diabetic retinopathy exhibiting scattered dot and blot hemorrhages. (Courtesy Pacific University Family Vision Center, Forest Grove, Ore.)

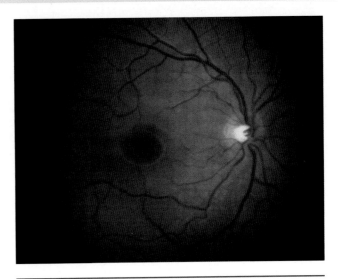

FIGURE 4-18
Normal fundus of the right eye of a teenager. The sheen from the internal limiting membrane is visible as a macular reflection. (Courtesy Pacific University Family Vision Center, Forest Grove, Ore.)

Clinical Comment: Fundus View of the Internal Limiting Membrane

Reflections from the internal limiting membrane produce the retinal sheen seen with the ophthalmoscope. In younger persons, this membrane gives off many reflections and appears glistening; the sheen is less evident in older individuals (Figure 4-18).

RETINAL FUNCTION

Light passes through most of the retinal layers before reaching and stimulating the photoreceptor outer segment discs. The neural flow then proceeds back through the retinal elements in the opposite direction of the incident light. The efficient and accurate performance of the retina is not hampered by this seemingly reversed situation.

PHYSIOLOGY OF THE RPE

The RPE fosters the health of the neural retina and the choriocapillaris in several ways. First, the zonula occludens joining the RPE cells are part of the blood-retinal barrier and selectively control movement of nutrients and metabolites from the choriocapillaris into the retina and removal of waste products from the retina into the choriocapillaris.[80] (In this regard, the RPE is analogous to the epithelium of the choroid plexus in the ventricles of the brain.)

A proposed model for RPE ion transport is shown in Figure 4-19. Ion movement occurs by Na^+/K^+ ATPase pumps, $Na^+/K^+/2Cl^-$ and $Na^+/2HCO_3^-$ cotransporters, Na^+/H^+ and Cl^-/HCO_3^- exchangers, and gated and ungated ion channels.[81] A proton-lactate-water cotransporter moves a significant amount of lactate (the product of anaerobic metabolism) across the RPE layer.[81,82] Water passage occurs through aquaporins and Cl^- and K^+ are thought to be the primary ions driving the movement of water.[83] Glucose transporters located in both the apical and basal membrane maintain a steady supply of glucose to the active photoreceptors.

Second, the RPE cells phagocytose fragments from the continual shedding of the photoreceptor outer segment discs; numerous lysosomes within each RPE cell enable it to ingest as many as 2000 discs daily.[84] Undigested material accumulates as deposits of lipofuscin.[81] Recently, a substance (A2E) has been identified in lipofuscin deposits that appears to inhibit RPE degradation of the outer segment remnants and contributes to RPE cell death.[85] Third, the RPE metabolizes and stores vitamin A, one of the components of photopigment molecules[86,87]; it is the site for part of the biochemical process in the rod disc renewal system.[84] Fourth, the cells contribute to the formation of the IPM between the RPE layer and the photoreceptors.[75,88] Fifth, the RPE produces growth factors that drive certain cellular processes. It secretes vascular endothelial growth factor (VEGF), which helps maintain choriocapillaris function. However, the over-production of VEGF could

Rod and cone outer segments

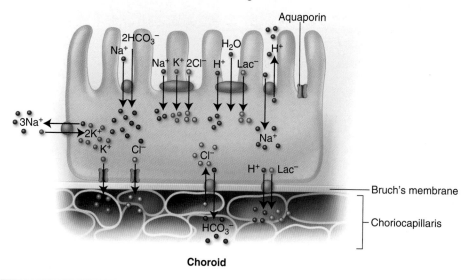

FIGURE 4-19
Proposed model showing RPE ion transport.

result in neurovascularization, and so the RPE also produces an antiangiogenic factor, pigment epithelial derived factor (PEDF); the balance between these contributes to healthy function.[80] Sixth, pigment granules within the RPE cells absorb light, thereby reducing excess light scatter.

The relationship between the RPE and the photoreceptors is a reciprocal one. When either layer dysfunctions the other is ultimately affected. Retinal degenerative diseases and dystrophies often cause changes in the RPE that are clinically visible.

Clinical Comment: Retinal Degenerations

RETINITIS PIGMENTOSA is an autosomal dominant retinal dystrophy, resulting in a progressive loss of RPE and photoreceptor function. Both rods and cones undergo apoptosis. Rods remain functional only in the far periphery and cones remain functional in the fovea, causing a ringlike scatomatous visual field defect. As the RPE degenerates, pigment migrates into the sensory retina, and accumulates around blood vessels in a characteristic bone-spicule pattern (Figure 4-20).

Stargardt's macular dystrophy is a hereditary autosomal recessive disorder, resulting in vision loss occurring at an early age. A defect has been identified in a gene that directs the production of a protein that facilitates transport to and from photoreceptor cells. Early in the disease the RPE degenerates and as the disease progresses, lipofuscin-like deposits accumulate in the macular area (Figure 4-21). These deposits are yellow and fleck-shaped. Eventually the RPE atrophies and changes

to the photoreceptors follow. Vision loss is progressive and by age 50, 50% of patients affected can have reduction of visual acuity to 20/200 or worse [89]

Best's disease, also called vitelliform macular dystrophy, is a rare autosomal dominant disorder. This disease also occurs because of a malfunctioning transport protein resulting in deposits between the RPE and neural retina.[90] It usually presents in childhood as a striking yellow or orange egg yolklike elevated lesion in the macula (Figure 4-22).

SCOTOPIC AND PHOTOPIC VISION

In dim light the detection by rods predominates and in bright light, color detection takes precedence. Rods are extremely sensitive in poorly lit conditions (scotopic vision), when cones are least responsive. In **scotopic vision,** the light-sensitive retina allows detection of objects at low levels of illumination. Its ability to recognize fine detail is poor, however, and color vision is absent; objects are seen in shades of gray.[60]

Cone activity dominates in **photopic vision,** when the retina is responsive to a broader range of light wavelengths. Bright illumination is necessary for the sharp visual acuity and color discrimination of photopic vision. Cones are designated, depending on the wavelength that they absorb, as red (588 nm), green (531 nm), or blue (420 nm).[91]

NEURAL SIGNALS

The neural signal generated by photoreceptors is modified and processed within the complex synaptic pathway through which it passes. There is a greater convergence

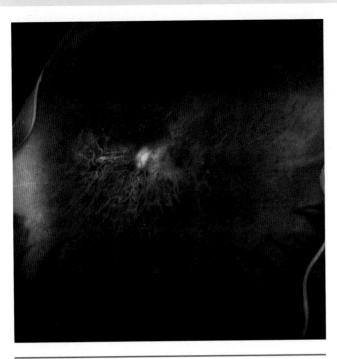

FIGURE 4-20
Optomap® (Marlborough, MA) showing fundus of patient with retinitis pigmentosa; bone spicule-shaped deposits of pigment are evident in sensory retina. Extent of retinal vasculature can be seen. (Courtesy of Fraser Horn, O.D., Pacific University Family Vision Center, Forest Grove, Ore.)

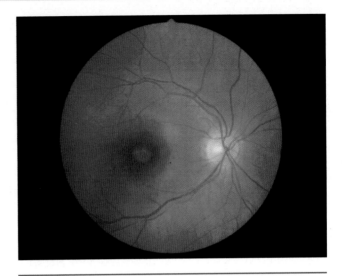

FIGURE 4-21
Photo showing right fundus of 20-year-old patient with Stargardt's macular dystrophy, RPE degeneration and lipofuscin deposittion in the macular area. VA is reduced to 20/80. (Courtesy of JP Lowery, O.D., Pacific University Family Vision Center, Forest Grove, Ore.)

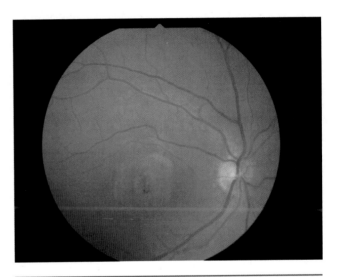

FIGURE 4-22
Photo showing right fundus of patient with Best's disease; tissue disruption and mottling are evident in macular area. (Courtesy of James Kundart, O.D. and Jennifer Schumacher, Pacific University Family Vision Center, Forest Grove, Ore.)

of rods than of cones onto a ganglion cell. The ratio of rods to ganglion cells is high in most retinal regions, resulting in tremendous sensitivity for the detection of light and motion. It is estimated that 75,000 rods drive 5000 rod bipolar cells and 250 AII amacrine cells before converging onto a single ganglion cell.[92] A relatively small number of cones drive the cone bipolar cell, and a small number of cone bipolar cells drive a single ganglion cell. In some situations, there is a 1:1 ratio between cones and ganglion cells, reflecting the significant amount of detail that the cone population can discriminate.[1] A single midget bipolar dendrite may contact only one cone pedicle, and its axon then synapses on a single midget ganglion cell.[92] The cone pathway involves a three-neuron chain, whereas the rod pathway involves a four-neuron chain because of the amacrine cell inclusion.[2]

Ganglion cell axons can be thought of as "carrying information in processing streams," such that certain types of information are directed toward specific destinations.[8] One major target is the lateral geniculate nucleus, wherein some axons terminate in the parvocellular layers, which process wavelength, shape, fine detail, and resolution of contrast. Other axons end in the magnocellular layers, which discern movements and flickering light but have poor wavelength sensitivity.[93] Visual information terminating in the midbrain is important in the autonomic control of the ciliary and iris muscles. Other centers that receive visual information can influence motor pathways that control eye, head, and neck movements.

Clinical Comment: Electroretinogram (ERG)

An electroretinogram is a recording of the electrical response of the retina to light stimulus, which may be a flash of light or a light pattern. It can be measured in a clinical setting and can be useful diagnostically in differentiating certain retinal diseases.

NUMBER AND DISTRIBUTION OF NEURAL CELLS

In 1935, Østerberg[94] estimated the cell count in the retina at 110 million to 125 million rods and 6.3 million to 6.8 million cones. More recent research indicates that there are 80 million to 110 million rods and 4 million to 5 million cones.[95,96] The density of rods is greater than that of cones except in the macular region, where cones are concentrated; rods are absent from the foveola,[15] the macular center (Figure 4-23). Rod density is greatest in an area concentric with the fovea, beginning approximately 3 mm (7 degrees) from it.[52,60] The number of both types of photoreceptors diminishes toward the ora serrata.

There are approximately 35.68 million bipolar cells[97] and 1.12 million to 2.22 million ganglion cells.[98] The signals from numerous photoreceptors converge at one ganglion cell, indicating integration and refinement of the initial response of the photoreceptor cells.

PHYSIOLOGY OF THE NEURAL RETINA

The complex structure of the retina contains millions and millions of neurons and synapses, and has been extensively investigated in studies of cats, rabbits, and monkeys. Although most knowledge of the retinal circuitry is based on animal models, visual scientists have found much of the information to be applicable to the human retina.

Retinal Synapses

Information transmission between retinal neurons occurs by ion channel activity at gap junctions or by neurotransmitter release in chemical synapses. The gap junction is an electrical synapse, allowing current to pass directly between cells, ensuring a rapid rate of signal transmission; no chemical mediator is necessary. Gap junctions are found between photoreceptor and photoreceptor, between photoreceptor and horizontal cell, between horizontal cells, and between a bipolar axon and an amacrine process.[8]

Chemical synapses contain synaptic vesicles that release a neurotransmitter from the presynaptic terminal

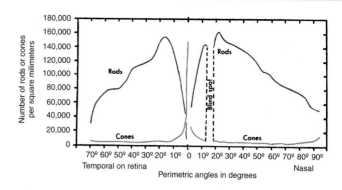

FIGURE 4-23

Distribution of rods and cones in human retina. Instead of retinal distances, Østerberg's values[84] for corresponding perimetric angles are given. Although approximate only, especially at higher angles, such values are more useful in practice than are distances on the retina. Note that distribution of rods and cones on nasal side in and near the fovea, not given on this graph, would be approximately the same as distribution on temporal side of retina, which is seen to the left of vertical, passing through 0 degrees on the angle scale. (From Pirenne M: *Vision and the eye*, London, 1948, Pilot Press.)

into the synaptic cleft. The transmitter binds to specific sites on the postsynaptic membrane, eliciting an excitatory or inhibitory change in that neuron. In the OPL synapses occur either on the flat part of the pedicle or in invaginations in spherules and pedicles. The synapses in the invaginations are often ribbon synapses; ribbon synapses allow for fast and sustained neurotransmitter release. An electron-dense bar, surrounded by a large number of synaptic vesicles, extends into the cytoplasm perpendicular to the pre-synaptic membrane. The ribbonlike structure seems to guide the vesicles to a release site on the pre-synaptic membrane, causing sustained release. Calcium ion channels facilitate vesicle fusion with the membrane and promote high-speed release. Ten times more vesicles per second are released at a ribbon synapse than at a conventional synapse.[27] Triads are ribbon junctions, located in the OPL, that have three postsynaptic processes; dyads are ribbon synapses found in the IPL with two postsynaptic processes. Although visual interpretation occurs in the striate cortex, there is significant organization and processing of neural signals in excitatory and inhibitory circuits within the retina. The process is extremely complex and most current understanding is based on animal studies.

Neurotransmitters

Glutamate is the excitatory neurotransmitter released by photoreceptors, bipolars, and ganglion cells. Glycine and GABA are inhibitory neurotransmitters released from amacrines; it is unclear what neurotransmitter horizontal cells secrete. In addition to neurotransmitters, neuromodulators are chemicals that can alter neuron transmission. They are released by retinal cells into the extracellular space but not necessarily by synaptic vesicles at the synaptic cleft; they include dopamine, nitric oxide, and retinoic acid. An example of a neuromodulator effect: Dopamine can change the conductance of gap junctions between horizontal cells and modulate responses to changes in background illumination.[99,100]

Phototransduction

Phototransduction, the process by which a photon of light is changed to an electrical signal, occurs in the photoreceptors. Visual pigments in the photoreceptor outer segment absorb light, initiating the process of vision. A series of biochemical changes follow and the cell hyperpolarizes, which starts an electrical current flow through the retina. The signal passes to bipolar and horizontal cells, some organization and processing occurs, with more organization and processing occurring as the signal is transferred to amacrine and ganglion cells. Once a ganglion cell is activated, its axon carries the message to the brain.

A **visual pigment (photopigment)** consists of two parts, a membrane protein, called an opsin, and a chromophore. The **opsin** forms a long helix that loops back and forth across the membrane bilayer seven times; the **chromophore** is the molecule that actually absorbs the photon, and is contained within the looped protein. **11-*cis*-retinal** is the chromophore present in all photoreceptors; it is a derivative of vitamin A. The seven-looped opsin determines the wavelength absorbed by a photoreceptor. The photopigment in rods is arranged in the disc membranes and its protein is **rhodopsin**. In cones the photopigment is located throughout the continuous plasma membrane whose deep infoldings form the cone discs.[45] The protein opsin in L-cone cells is red sensitive and in M-cones is green sensitive. The structure of these two photopigments differs by only a few amino acids, and the genes for them are located in a tandem array on the X-chromosome. Blue sensitive S-cones (comprising only 5% to 10% of the cone population) are structurally different.[78]

The photoreceptor is in the **depolarized** state when it is not stimulated by light. As neurons usually do in the depolarized state, the photoreceptor secretes its neurotransmitter. During depolarization, voltage-gated Ca^{++} channels are open and calcium ions facilitate the process by which the vesicles containing glutamate merge with the cell membrane, enabling the release of neurotransmitter into the synaptic cleft.[78,101] Thus, **in the dark the photoreceptor terminal is continually releasing glutamate.** The depolarized state occurs because of an ion circuit within the photoreceptor. The photoreceptor outer segment is permeable to Na^+; the cGMP-gated cationic channels in the outer segment membrane are kept

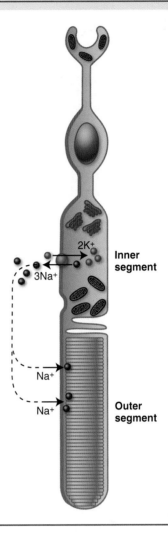

FIGURE 4-24

Photoreceptor dark current. The dotted lines represent the dark current; Na^+ enters the outer segment through ligand-gated channels, ions pass through the cilium, Na^+ is extruded by Na^+K^+ ATPase pumps in the cell membrane of the inner segment. The cell membrane potential in the dark is approximately –40 mV.

open because of a high concentration of cytoplasmic cGMP. Na^+ moves into the outer segment, through the open channels and the ions pass easily into the inner segment through the cilium, where Na^+ is extruded by Na^+/K^+ ATPase pumps (Figure 4-24). This circuit (caused by Na^+ moving into the outer segment and exiting the inner segment), is called the **dark current.** In this state the photoreceptor is depolarized with a membrane potential of approximately –40 mV.

Within a picosecond of light activating the visual pigment, a biochemical cascade occurs that results in a decrease in the concentration of cGMP closing the Na^+ channels.[78] The inside of the cell increases in negativity due to the continued loss of Na^+ through the pumps in the inner segment membrane and the cell becomes

hyperpolarized; the membrane potential approaches −75 mV. The change in potential is graded, the level of hyperpolarization depends on the amount of light absorbed and the number of visual pigment molecules activated. The magnitude of the hyperpolarization determines the change in the amount of transmitter released, either slowing or stopping the flow.[78] Once the level of cGMP is restored, the ion channels open and the cell once again becomes depolarized and releases glutamate. The amount of transmitter released by the photoreceptor decreases as the amount of light absorbed increases.

In the rod, the process of phototransduction begins with the absorption of a photon of light that causes the breaking of a double bond in 11-*cis*-retinal forming the isomer all-*trans*-retinal. A sequence of conformational changes in rhodopsin results and several intermediaries are formed. Activated metarhodopsin II stimulates transducin, the G-protein of visual transduction, and is then transformed into inactive metarhodopsin III; finally all-*trans*-retinal dissociates from the photopigment.[27] The visual pigment is now said to be bleached. The phototransduction cascade causes the decrease of cGMP, leading to hyperpolarization of the photoreceptor.

All-*trans*-retinal moves from the disc lumen into the cytoplasm where it is reduced to all-*trans*-retinol. The photoreceptor cannot re-isomerize the molecule, so it must be transported by specific carrier proteins within the interphotoreceptor matrix (IPM) to the RPE.[81] These cells contain the enzymes that convert all-*trans*-retinol to 11-*cis*-retinol and finally oxidize it back to11-*cis*-retinal; 11-*cis*-retinal is then transported back through the IPM to be incorporated into the photopigment. In the cone recycling process, some animal models indicate that the Müller cell has a role in the visual cycle by taking up all-*trans*-retinol and re-isomerizing it to 11-cis-retinol, which is then transported back to the cone and oxidized to 11-*cis*-retinal and incorporated into the photopigment.[102,103] The steps of the rod renewal system are well known, but those of the cone renewal system are still unclear.

Information Processing

Once the photoreceptor is activated and the message begins its circuit through the retinal neurons, organization and processing will take place prior to the signal exiting the eye. Since a million ganglion cells receive input from over a hundred million photoreceptors, there must be a systematic process to control and relay photoreceptor messages. Retinal neurons have been given designations as ON cells or OFF cells as a means to describe the processing schematic.

Retinal neurons are named ON or OFF cells by the light condition when the cell is depolarized. A cell that is depolarized with *light OFF* is called an **OFF cell** and

a cell that is depolarized with *light ON* is called an **ON cell.** Since all photoreceptors depolarize in the dark, all photoreceptors are OFF cells.

Glutamate will cause a bipolar cell to either depolarize or hyperpolarize depending on the type of receptor present in the plasma membrane of the bipolar dendrite.[104,105] Bipolar cells with *ionotropic* receptors in their membrane respond to glutamate with a depolarization and are **OFF bipolars** and bipolar cells that have *metabotropic* receptors in their membrane respond to glutamate with a hyperpolarization and are **ON bipolars.**[104,105] The neurotransmitter at the axon terminal in bipolar cells is also glutamate (Glu) and bipolars release Glu when they are in the depolarized state.

When a photoreceptor is *depolarized* (thus it is in the dark, light is OFF) it is releasing Glu. When Glu binds to the *ionotropic* receptor on a bipolar dendrite, cation channels are opened in the cell membrane, causing the bipolar cell to depolarize and release Glu.[106] This is an OFF bipolar because it is depolarized in the dark. When Glu binds to the *metabotropic* receptors on a bipolar cell dendrite, a decrease of cGMP occurs, closing cation channels in the cell membrane and causing the bipolar cell to hyperpolarize, resulting in a decrease of glutamate release.[107] This is an ON bipolar because it is hyperpolarized in the dark.

When the photoreceptor is *hyperpolarized* (light is ON), Glu release is reduced or stopped. The lack of Glu at the ionotropic receptor causes the Glu-gated cationic channels in the bipolar membrane to close. The OFF bipolar cell hyperpolarizes, reducing its release of neurotransmitter.[106] When Glu is reduced or no longer present, the lack of Glu at the *metabotropic* receptor signals a cGMP cascade, cGMP increases, cGMP-gated cation channels open, and the ON bipolar depolarizes, which increases its neurotransmitter release.[107]

Succinctly put: The OFF bipolar depolarizes in dark and hyperpolarizes in light. The ON bipolar depolarizes in light and hyperpolarizes in dark.

Some current literature uses other terms. OFF bipolars are also called *hyperpolarizing bipolar cells (HBCs)* and ON bipolars are also called *depolarizing bipolar cells (DBCs).* (This terminology reflects the state of the bipolar when the light is on.) Recognize that the ON or OFF designation does not imply that the bipolar itself is responding to the light condition; only photoreceptors do that.

Generally, the ON bipolar dendrite synapses within a photoreceptor invagination and the OFF bipolar dendrite synapses only with cones and on the flat part of the pedicle. Each cone in central retina contacts both an ON and an OFF midget bipolar.[78] All rod bipolars are ON cells (Figure 4-25).

Bipolar axons end in the IPL. One synaptic configuration is a dyad, which consists of a synapse between a

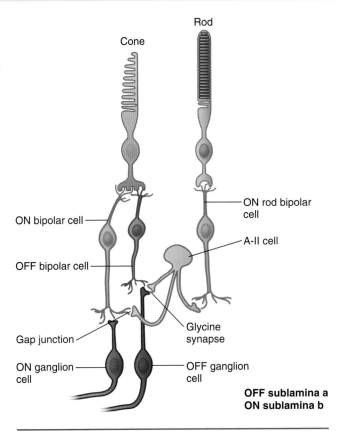

Rod

Cone

ON bipolar cell

OFF bipolar cell

Gap junction

ON ganglion cell

ON rod bipolar cell

A-II cell

Glycine synapse

OFF ganglion cell

**OFF sublamina a
ON sublamina b**

FIGURE 4-25
Schematic of ON and OFF bipolar pathways. OFF bipolar dendrite synapses on flat part of cone, ON bipolar dendrite synapses within photoreceptor invagination; OFF bipolar axon terminates in sublamina a, ON bipolar axon terminates in sublamina b; All amacrine cell relays rod signals to both ON and OFF ganglion cells.

bipolar axon and two post synaptic elements, either two amacrine processes or one amacrine process and one ganglion dendrite. ON and OFF bipolar axons terminate in different tiers of the IPL. OFF bipolars synapse in the outer tier, sublamina a (nearest the INL), and ON bipolars synapse in the inner tier, sublamina b, closest to the ganglion cell layer.[78] Rod bipolars do not synapse with ganglion cells directly but with amacrine cells; thus the rod signal must pass through a four neuron chain (see Figure 4-25).

Bipolar cells transfer information to retinal ganglion cells, which are the first cells in the visual pathway to respond with an action potential. Once a threshold is reached, the ganglion cell responds and a signal is sent to higher CNS locations. All other retinal neurons give graded responses, the intensity of which is determined by the intensity of the stimulus.

The P ganglion cells terminate in the parvocellular layers of the LGN, are associated with cone bipolar cells, and carry color information. The P1 cells, also called

midget ganglion cells are concentrated in central retina, and constitute 80% of the ganglion cell population.[78] M ganglion cells project to the magnocellular layers of the LGN. They have also been called parasol ganglion cells because of their large spreading dendritic trees. Because they have such expansive processes and cover a large area of retina, they can respond rapidly to moving or changing stimuli.

The *vertical* connections through the retina have been described, but horizontal and amacrine cells interconnect in a *horizontal* direction. They link one region of retina with another allowing a signal sent by a photoreceptor to be influenced by a signal from a photoreceptor in a different retinal location, thus modifying the message.

Horizontal cells communicate with other horizontal cells through gap junctions and receive excitatory input through chemical synapses from photoreceptors. Horizontal cells provide inhibitory feedback to photoreceptors and inhibitory feed forward to bipolars.[78]

In the dark, while the photoreceptor is continuously releasing the excitatory neurotransmitter glutamate, its horizontal cells are depolarized. With light stimulation the photoreceptor hyperpolarizes and transmitter release is reduced. Ligand-gated channels close in the horizontal cell membrane, causing it to hyperpolarize.[108] The amplitude and duration of the response depends on the strength of the photoreceptor hyperpolarization, and thus on the intensity and duration of the light stimulus.[92,108] Because horizontal cells are joined by gap junctions a great number of horizontal cells can be affected when just one is influenced by a photoreceptor.

The mechanism by which the inhibitory message is passed from the horizontal cell to the cone is not fully understood. It was once thought that the horizontal cell released the inhibitory neurotransmitter GABA. Subsequent studies have raised doubts that GABA is a major player in the feedback process from horizontal cells.[99,109] It is speculated (based on animal models) that a change in the horizontal cell polarization causes a current change in the extracellular potential in the synaptic cleft within an invagination. This could affect the Ca^{++} channels in the synaptic membrane of the cone influencing the synaptic vesicle release of Glu without actually changing the cone membrane potential. The change in neurotransmitter release would affect the bipolar dendrites within the invagination and in some cases might reverse their reaction.[99,108,109]

Amacrine cells also carry information in a *horizontal* direction. There are 40 different types but the circuitry of only a few has been established. Amacrine cells are generally inhibitory and release either GABA or glycine. Amacrine processes make conventional synapses with bipolar axons and with ganglion cell dendrites or soma.

The conventional chemical synapse with bipolar cell axons are feedback synapses; synapses on ganglion cells are feed-forward synapses.[110] Amacrine cells also synapse with other amacrine cells.

The narrow-field rod amacrine cell, AII, releases glycine. It is the intermediary between the rod bipolar and the ganglion cell. An AII amacrine cell gathers information from about 300 rods.[78] The AII provides connection between the ON and OFF pathways. The AII receives information from a rod bipolar axon (an ON cell) in sublamina b of the IPL, and relays information by a conventional synapse to an OFF cone bipolar in sublamina a, thereby influencing an OFF ganglion cell. The AII also carries rod information to an ON cone bipolar axon through gap junctions in sublamina b and influences an ON ganglion cell.[61] AII amacrine cells, whose processes are joined by gap junctions, form a weak electrical syncytium.[78]

The A17 amacrine cells are wide-field diffusely branching cells. They appear to interconnect rod bipolar cells but do not appear to make synapses with other amacrines nor ganglion cells.[110] A single A17 amacrine cell can receive input from as many as 1000 rod bipolars.[110] They are thought to amplify signals in dim illumination.

The A18 amacrine cell is a wide-field amacrine with an extensive dendritic tree. It seems to have a role in the regulation of scotopic vision flow, and in modulating retinal adaptation to differing light conditions. It can interfere with the AII amacrine synapse with cone bipolar cells, and effectively reduce the size of the receptive field.[92] The A18 releases dopamine, which can disrupt the gap junctions that forms the syncytium of AII amacrines. Dopamine released by the A18 amacrine may also have some function in the circadian cycle.[111]

Interplexiform neurons have processes in both the OPL and the IPL and convey signals between these layers, that is, from *inner* retina to *outer*. They might secrete dopamine as their transmitter but further details about their physiology is lacking.[112]

Receptive Fields

ON and OFF cells provide two information processing channels for differentiating light and dark signals. Flat bipolars are the start of the OFF channel and invaginating bipolars are the start of the ON channel. The ON and OFF channels in the cone pathway begin at the photoreceptor-bipolar connection because cones synapse with both ON and OFF bipolar cells. In the rod pathway, because a rod synapses only with an ON bipolar, the competing channels begin with the AII amacrine cell.

Retinal processing can be described in terms of receptive fields. A **receptive field** consists of the area in the visual field or the area of the retina that, when stimulated, elicits a response in a retinal neuron. The receptive field for a particular bipolar cell consists of those photoreceptor cells with which it is in direct contact, and all the photoreceptors and horizontal cells that can influence it. Because neighboring horizontal cells are joined by gap junctions, the receptive field is consequently enlarged beyond its dendritic tree.

Retinal receptive fields are arranged in a center-surround pattern. When light activates cells in the *center* of the field, a given response occurs. When light falls on the *surround* (the annular region immediately around the center), an antagonistic response occurs. The response by the cells in the surround inhibits the response from the cells in the center. This pattern is seen at the level of the bipolar cells, the ganglion cells, and in the LGN and the striate cortex. When cells in the surround are activated, the signal coming from the center cell is changed to the opposite response. The center-surround response occurs in part due to lateral inhibition by horizontal cells and because of amacrine cell activity on bipolar axon terminals.[113]

The center-surround configuration allows a neuron to not only respond to a direct message but to gather information from neighboring areas providing details about the bigger picture that then influences that neuron. This process aides in the detection of edges and in the recognition of contrast, and it maximizes retinal contrast sensitivity through a wide range of background illuminations.[78]

A circular receptive field can be either ON-center/OFF surround or OFF-center/ON surround. When light falls on the annular region, the message from the center is inhibited: i.e., when an ON-center cell is stimulated, it sends its ON message, but when cells in its surround are also stimulated, the ON-center cell will be inhibited and the ON message is not sent, and instead an OFF message is recognized; the converse occurs if the surround of an OFF-center cell is stimulated the message sent from the center will be an ON message.

Light and Dark Adaptation

The visual system is highly specialized for the detection and analysis of patterns of light; by visual adaptation, it can modify its capacity to respond at extremely high and low levels of illumination. The level of background illumination can affect both the ease and the speed with which a photoreceptor responds. When a significant change in light level occurs, adaptation can be prolonged; it can take 30 minutes for the retina to adapt fully when going from bright sunlight to complete dark (*dark adaptation*). At first only cones are functioning, but since they are now in the dark they are not stimulated and the rods take some time to reach maximum function. *Light adaptation*, going from complete dark to bright light, takes approximately 5 to 10 minutes; the cones reach their functional mode much more quickly than do rods. The state of adaptation (sensitivity) of a photoreceptor is regulated by Ca^{++}, which can influence the concentration of cGMP, the messenger that controls gated ion channels in the photoreceptor membrane.[78]

Circadian Rhythm

The circadian rhythm is the light/dark or wake/sleep cycle, which usually extends over a period of 24 hours. It is under the direction of pineal melatonin secretion, which is influenced by the suprachiasmatic nucleus, the master biologic clock located in the hypothalamus.[114] A special population of ganglion cells that contain melanopsin has been identified; they are photosensitive and can respond directly to light. It is estimated that there are 3000 of these ganglion cells dispersed across the retina.[115,116] Their axons project to the suprachiasmatic nucleus and help in synchronizing the circadian rhythm to the wake/sleep cycle.[78,116] Neuromodulators, such as dopamine, secreted by the interplexiform neuron and the amacrine A18 cells, may also have some role in regulating the circadian rhythm.[113]

Retinal Metabolism

The extensive network of continual intracellular communication requires extensive energy utilization by retinal tissue. The primary source of energy is provided by glucose metabolism. Glucose moves out of the blood and into retinal tissue via facilitated diffusion; glucose transporters are located on both the apical and basal membranes of the retinal pigmented epithelial cell and on the endothelium of retinal capillaries.[27] The retina can switch from glycolysis to oxidative metabolism depending on need, but even under normal physiologic conditions the retina has a high rate of anaerobic glycolysis.[78] The monophosphate pathway is particularly active in photoreceptors for rhodopsin regeneration and ribose production for nucleotide synthesis.[27] Müller cells store glycogen, providing a ready source for glucose. Because energy requirements are high, oxygen consumption is high. Capillary blood flow in retinal tissue has been measured in primates and is approximately 60 ml/min/100 g of tissue, similar to the flow in the brain.[117] Oxygen utilization by photoreceptors is 3 to 4 times higher than other CNS neurons.[27] Because oxygen must diffuse from the choriocapillars to the inner segments where the mitochondria are located, blood flow is significantly higher in the choriocapillaris, i.e., approximately 2000 ml/min/100 g of tissue.[116] In dark, the photoreceptors consume so much oxygen that the oxygen tension in the tissue is near zero and the photoreceptors are operating under near ischemic conditions.[78]

REGIONS OF RETINA

The retina is often described as consisting of two regions: peripheral and central. The peripheral retina is designed for detecting gross form and motion, whereas the central area is specialized for visual acuity. In area, the periphery makes up most of the retina, and rods dominate. The central retina is rich in cones, has more ganglion cells per area than elsewhere, and is a relatively small portion of the entire retina.

Clinical Comment: Peripheral Vision

When the eyes are looking straight ahead, the object of interest is imaged on the macular area in the central retina, and the rest of the field that is in view, sometimes described as that seen "out of the corner of one's eye," is focused on more peripheral retinal regions. Detail and color of those objects in the central area of vision are evident, but the objects in the periphery are less clear. The periphery is quite sensitive to change, and even slight movement in the more peripheral areas often stimulates the retina and frequently elicits a turning of the eye or head toward the motion.

CENTRAL RETINA

Macula Lutea

The **macula lutea** appears as a darkened region in the central retina and may seem to have a yellow hue because of the xanthophyll pigments, lutein, and zeaxanthin.[52,118] These pigments are located throughout the retina, but the greatest concentration is in the macula. The pigments are primarily located in the photoreceptor inner fibers but are also found in the rod outer segments.[78,118,119] The newborn has little if any of these pigments, but they gradually accumulate from dietary sources. These pigments apparently act as filters, absorbing short wavelength visible light to reduce chromatic aberration but may also have an antioxidant effect, suggesting a protective role against UVR damage.[118] The macula lutea is approximately 5.5 mm in diameter; its center is approximately 3.5 mm lateral to the *edge* of the disc and approximately 1 mm inferior to the *center* of the disc. The pigment epithelial cells are taller and contain more pigment than cells elsewhere in the retina, contributing to the darkness of this area. However, the density of the pigment varies greatly from person to person.[58] The choroidal capillary bed also is thicker in the macula lutea than elsewhere.

Useful color vision occupies an area approximately 9 mm in diameter, the center of which is the macula lutea.[8] The entire macular region consists of the foveola, the fovea, and the parafoveal and perifoveal areas (both are annular regions) (Figure 4-26). These areas are described and delineated on the basis of histologic findings, with consideration given to the number and rows of cells in the nuclear layers. However, these areas are not easily differentiated on viewing the living retina.

Clinical Comment: Terminology

> The terms used to describe the macular area differ between the histologist and the clinician. The histologist uses the word fovea to describe what a clinician would name macula, and the histologist calls the foveola that which a clinician would name the fovea. The term **macula** is purely a clinical one and usually refers to the area of darker coloration that is approximately the same size as the optic disc; clinically, the term **fovea** then refers to the very center of this area. The **posterior pole** is another term used in clinical descriptions of the fundus. There is no universal agreement regarding its definition, and its usage varies from clinician to clinician.[29]

Fovea (Fovea Centralis)

The shallow depression in the center of the macular region is the **fovea,** or central fovea of the retina *(fovea centralis retinae)*. This depression is formed because the retinal neurons are displaced, leaving only photoreceptors in the center. The fovea has a horizontal diameter of approximately 1.5 mm. The curved wall of the depression is known as the *clivus*, which gradually slopes to the floor, the *foveola*. The fovea has the highest concentration of cones in the retina; estimates vary from 199,000 to 300,000 cones per square millimeter.[96,120] The number falls off rapidly as one moves away from the fovea in all directions. In this area of the retina, specialized for discrimination of detail and color vision, the ratio between cone cells and ganglion cells approaches 1:1.[8] In more peripheral areas of the retina, which are sensitive to light detection but have poor form discrimination, there is a high ratio of rods to ganglion cells.

Within the fovea is a *capillary-free zone* 0.4 to 0.5 mm in diameter (Figure 4-27).[121] The lack of blood vessels in this region allows light to pass unobstructed into the photoreceptor outer segment.

The only photoreceptors located in the center of the fovea are cones. These are tightly packed, and the outer segments are elongated, appearing rodlike in shape yet containing the visual pigments of the cone population. The external limiting membrane is displaced vitreally because of the lengthening of the outer segments. This *rod-free region* has a diameter of approximately 0.57 mm[1] and represents approximately 1 degree of visual field.[120] Most of the other retinal elements are displaced, allowing

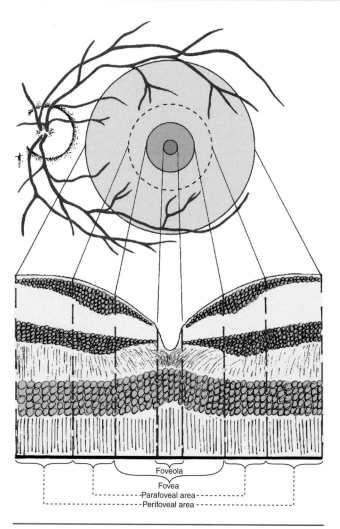

FIGURE 4-26
Schematic showing regions of retina and corresponding histologic architecture.

light to reach the photoreceptors directly without interference of other retinal cells (Figure 4-28).

The cells of the inner nuclear layer and ganglion cell layer are displaced laterally and accumulate on the walls of the fovea. The photoreceptor axons become longer as they deviate away from the center; these fibers are called Henle's fibers. They must take an oblique course to reach the displaced bipolar and horizontal cells (Figure 4-29). This region of the OPL is known as **Henle's fiber layer.**[1] The retinal layers and the foveal indentation are clinically evident with a CRT view of the retina (Figure 4-30).

Foveola

The diameter of the foveola is approximately 0.35 mm. At the foveola, the retina is approximately 0.13 mm thick, compared with 0.18 mm at the equator and

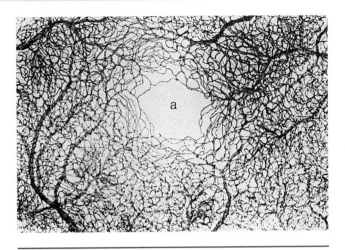

FIGURE 4-27
Capillary bed of macular region, with capillary-free zone (*a*) in its center. (×42.5.) (From Hogan MJ, Alvarado JA, Weddell JE: *Histology of the human eye*, Philadelphia, 1971, Saunders.)

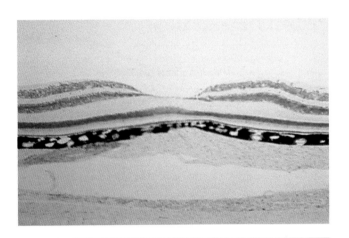

FIGURE 4-28
Light micrograph of the foveal region. The indentation caused by the absence of several retinal layers is evident.

0.11 mm at the ora serrata.[1] The **foveola** contains the densest population of cones that have the smallest cross-sectional diameters of all the photoreceptors.[8]

The layers present in the foveola are the (1) RPE, (2) photoreceptor layer, (3) external limiting membrane, (4) ONL (which contains about 10 rows of cone nuclei), (5) Henle's fiber layer, and (6) the internal limiting membrane. Moving laterally along the sides of the fovea, the other layers of the retina are increasingly represented. Müller cell processes are found throughout the macular, foveal, and foveolar areas.

Clinical Comment: Central Foveal Reflex

When the direct ophthalmoscope light shines directly into the fovea, it reflects a pinpoint of light called the **central foveal reflex.** *This pinpoint reflection is caused by the parabolic shape formed by the clivus. Because the shape of the fovea is not always exactly parabolic, the reflection may vary in sharpness and regularity from person to person. The fovea is the site at which the object of interest is imaged. In younger persons the sheen from the internal limiting membrane sometimes is seen as a circular macular reflex (see Figure 4-18).*

Clinical Comment: Metamorphopsia

The axis of the photoreceptor outer segment is oriented to accomplish capture of incident light rays. If a disruption occurs so that the outer segment is no longer oriented toward the exit pupil, vision may be altered. With macular edema, the orientation of the photoreceptors is changed, and metamorphopsia can often be elicited with an Amsler grid.[122]

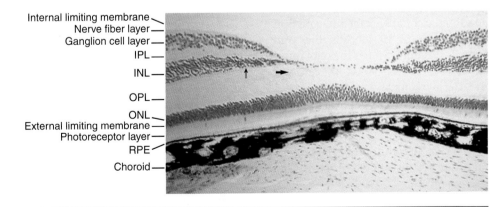

Internal limiting membrane
Nerve fiber layer
Ganglion cell layer
IPL
INL
OPL
ONL
External limiting membrane
Photoreceptor layer
RPE
Choroid

FIGURE 4-29
Light micrograph of foveal region. Layers present in the center of the foveal area are RPE, photoreceptor layer, external limiting membrane, outer nuclear layer, Henle fiber layer (note oblique orientation of fibers at heavy arrow), a few scattered nuclei from inner nuclear layer, internal limiting membrane. Light arrow shows middle limiting membrane within outer plexiform layer.

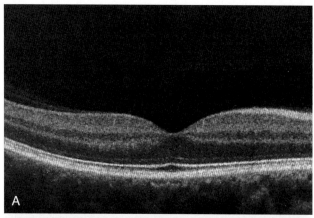

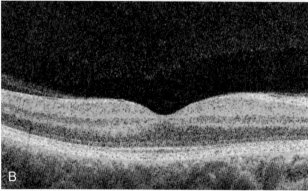

FIGURE 4-30
Ocular coherence tomography (OCT) scan of right macular area, retinal layers can be visualized; foveal indentation clearly evident (A black and white; B color). (Courtesy of Ami Halvorson, O.D., Pacific University Family Vision Center, Forest Grove, Ore.)

Parafoveal and Perifoveal Areas

The annular zone surrounding the fovea can be divided into an inner parafoveal area and an outer perifoveal area (see Figure 4-26). The **parafoveal area** contains the largest accumulation of retinal bipolar and ganglion cells. The inner nuclear layer can be 12 cells thick and the ganglion cell layer 7 cells thick.[52,58] At the maximum density of ganglion cells there can be 40,000 cells per square millimeter.[78] The **perifoveal area** begins where the ganglion cell layer is four cells thick and ends where it is one cell thick. Within the perifoveal area, the fibers of Henle's fiber layer revert to the usual orientation seen in the outer plexiform layer. The width of the parafoveal area is 0.5 mm and of the perifoveal area, 1.5 mm.[1]

PERIPHERAL RETINA

Approaching the retinal periphery, rods disappear and are replaced by malformed cones, the nuclear layers merge with the plexiform layers, and finally, the neural retina becomes a single layer of irregular columnar cells that continue as the nonpigmented epithelium of the ciliary body. The RPE is continuous with the outer pigmented epithelium of the ciliary body, and the internal limiting membrane continues as the internal limiting membrane of the ciliary body. There are few blood vessels in peripheral retina.

The **ora serrata** is the peripheral termination of the retina and lies approximately 5 mm anterior to the equator of the eye.[123] Its name derives from the scalloped pattern of bays and dentate processes (see Chapter 3); the retina extends further anteriorly on the medial side of the eye. The ora serrata is approximately 2 mm wide and is the site of transition from the complex, multi-layered neural retina to the single, nonpigmented layer of ciliary epithelium.[123] A firm attachment between the retina and vitreous, the vitreous base, extends several millimeters posterior to the ora serrata.

Clinical Comment: Peripheral Retinal Degeneration

Cystic spaces and atrophied areas are often found in peripheral retina, and their incidence increases with age. One cause for these changes is the poor blood supply in the extreme retinal periphery.[52,58] Some conditions affecting the peripheral retina are normal, age-related changes, and others might predispose the affected individual to more serious conditions, necessitating periodic, routine, dilated-fundus examinations.

OPTIC DISC

The **optic disc**, or **optic nerve head**, is the site where ganglion cell axons accumulate and exit the eye. It is slightly elongated vertically. The horizontal diameter of the disc is approximately 1.7 mm and the vertical diameter approximately 1.9 mm.[124] The number of nerve fibers appears to be positively correlated with the size of the optic nerve head; larger discs have relatively more fibers than smaller discs. Smaller discs may demonstrate optic nerve head crowding.[124,125] Fiber number decreases with age.[98]

The optic disc lacks all retinal elements except the nerve fiber layer and an internal limiting membrane. It is paler than the surrounding retina because there is no RPE. The pale-yellow or salmon color of the optic disc is a combination of the scleral lamina cribrosa and the capillary network. In some individuals, the openings of the lamina cribrosa may be visible through the transparent nerve fibers.

Because the disc contains no photoreceptor cells, light incident on the disc does not elicit a response; thus it represents the **physiologic blind spot**. A depression in the surface of the disc, the **physiologic cup**, varies greatly in size and depth, according to embryologic development (Figure 4-31).

Normally, the disc margins are flat and in the same plane as the retina, swelling only toward the vitreous in optic nerve head edema. Various types of crescents or rings are observed around the optic disc margin. In almost all individuals, the disc edges are emphasized by a white rim of scleral tissue, which separates the optic nerve from the choroid. Different configurations in the anatomic arrangement at the disc border produce the pigmented crescent often seen outer to the scleral crescent. The RPE may not extend to the edge of the disc, and the darkly pigmented choroid might be evident. Irregular areas of hypopigmentation and hyperpigmentation of the RPE are common near the disc.[126,127]

The optic disc serves as the site of entry for the central retinal artery and the exit site for the central retinal vein.

Clinical Comment: Optic Disc Assessment

The color of the disc, configuration and depth of the physiologic cup, cup-to-disc ratio, and appearance of the rim tissue and disc borders are assessed during an ocular health examination.

Clinical Comment: Papilledema

PAPILLEDEMA *is edema of the optic disc secondary to an increase in intracranial pressure (ICP).[128] As ICP increases, pressure within the meningeal sheaths around the optic nerve slows axoplasmic flow in the ganglion fibers, causing fluid to accumulate within the fibers so that they swell.[129,130] This accumulation of fluid is seen at the disc as an elevation of the nerve head with blurring of the disc margins (Figure 4-32). This condition is or will become bilateral. The central retinal vein may also be compromised, with hemorrhages becoming evident in the nerve fiber layer in the vicinity of the disc.*

Edema of the optic disc from any other cause is referred to as simply "edema of the optic disc."

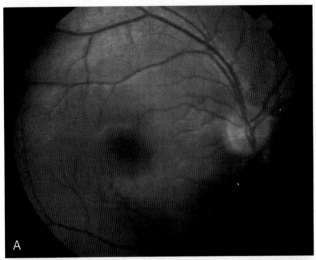

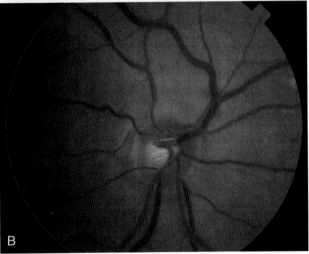

FIGURE 4-31
Variability in the normal cup-to-disc ratios. A, Normal fundus of right eye of young adult. Cup is small and shallow, reflection from internal limiting membrane is evident. **B,** Normal fundus of right eye showing large, deep normal cup. (Courtesy Pacific University Family Vision Center, Forest Grove, Ore.)

RETINAL BLOOD SUPPLY

The outer retinal layers receive nutrition from the choroidal capillary bed; metabolites diffuse through Bruch's membrane and the RPE into neural retina. The **central retinal artery** provides nutrients to inner retinal layers. The artery enters the retina through the optic disc, usually slightly nasal of center, and branches into a superior and inferior retinal artery, each of which divides further into nasal and temporal branches. These vessels continue to bifurcate (see Figure 4-31). The nasal branches run a relatively straight course toward the ora serrata, but the temporal vessels arch around the macular area en route to the periphery. The vessels are located in the nerve fiber layer just below the transparent internal limiting membrane.

Two capillary networks are formed. The *deep* capillary network lies in the inner nuclear layer near the outer plexiform layer, and the *superficial* capillary network is in the nerve fiber layer or ganglion cell layer.[58] The retina outer to the outer plexiform layer is avascular, and the outer plexiform layer is thought to receive its nutrients from both retinal and choroidal vessels. The middle limiting membrane usually is regarded as the border between the choroidal and retinal supplies.

A capillary-free zone directly surrounds the retinal vessels, and in the fovea, as mentioned, an area approximately 0.5 mm in diameter is free of all retinal vessels.[1,29] Retinal vessels are said to be "end vessels" because they do not anastomose with any other system

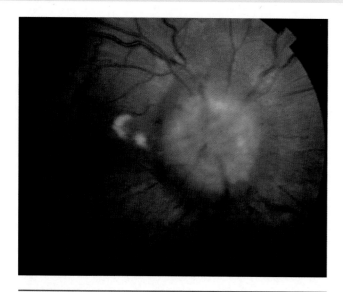

FIGURE 4-32
Papilledema of right eye. Note obvious elevation of the optic nerve head. Note that the plane of focus is at the retinal surface—the retinal vessels are clear, the optic nerve head surface is blurred. (Courtesy Pacific University Family Vision Center, Forest Grove, Ore.)

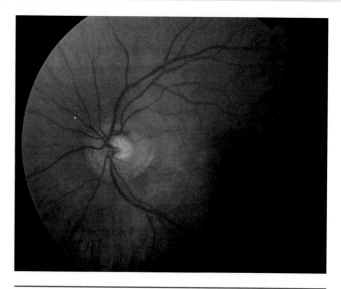

FIGURE 4-33
Fundus of left eye. Choroidal vessels are evident as lightly colored bands deeper than the retinal vessels. (Courtesy Pacific University Family Vision Center, Forest Grove, Ore.)

of blood vessels.[58] Retinal vessels terminate in delicate capillary arcades approximately 1 mm from the ora serrata.[29] The retinal capillaries are made up of a single layer of unfenestrated endothelium surrounded by a basement membrane and an interrupted layer of pericytes.[29,58,131] **Pericytes** are cells with a contractile function that facilitate blood flow.[132] The endothelial cells are one part of the blood-retinal barrier because they are joined by zonula occludens.[80,133,134]

A dense peripapillary network of capillaries, radially arranged around the optic nerve head, follows the arcuate course of the nerve fibers as they enter the disc.[135]

A **cilioretinal artery** is a vessel that enters the retina from the edge of the disc but has its origin in the choroidal vasculature. Such a vessel, that nourishes the macular area, is found in approximately 15% to 20% of the population (see Figure 11-4).[136] A cilioretinal artery can maintain the viability of the macula if blockage of the central retinal artery occurs. Smaller, less significant cilioretinal vessels can be found in 25% of the population.[136]

BLOOD-RETINAL BARRIER

It is important that light entering the eye have few obstacles in its pathway to the photoreceptor outer segments. The **blood-retinal barrier** prevents components of blood plasma that might impede light from entering retinal tissue. There are several factors to consider in the function of this barrier: (1) the choriocapillaris is

fenestrated allowing large molecules to exit into choroidal tissue; these molecules can usually pass through Bruch's membrane easily; (2) the *zonula occludens* junctions joining the RPE cells prevent such molecules from moving into retinal tissue; and (3) the retinal capillaries are *not* fenestrated and their endothelium contains *zonula occludens* that prevent large molecule exit from retinal vessels.

Clinical Comment: Fundus View of Vessels

The retinal blood vessels are readily visible with the ophthalmoscope, and because the vessel walls are transparent, the clinician actually is seeing the column of blood within the vessel. The lighter-colored blood is the oxygenated blood of the artery, whereas the venous deoxygenated blood is slightly darker. The artery generally lies superficial to the vein. With aging and some disease processes, such as hypertension, the arterial wall may thicken and constrict the vein at a crossing; this is called arteriovenous nicking.

In some individuals, the pigmented choroid and its vessels are visible through the retina, and the choroidal vessels appear as flattened ribbons (Figure 4-33).

AGING CHANGES IN RETINA

Normal aging is a slow, continuous process that may predispose to pathologic changes. It may be unclear, however, where normal aging changes stop and disease processes begin.

Because an estimated 33% to 50% of central nervous system neurons are lost during a lifetime, the number of retinal neurons will decrease, with ganglion cell loss especially noted in the fovea.[137] The number of nerve fibers in the optic nerve decreases, and the fibers are replaced with connective tissue as they degenerate.[138-140] Some studies report a decrease in foveal cones with age[141]; others do not.[142] Rod density declines with age,[142] but no decrease is evident in scotopic sensitivity.[143] Some bipolar dendrites and horizontal cell processes lengthen and extend into the ONL.[144] The number of astroglial cells is reduced.[145]

The number of retinal pigmented epithelial cells is reduced from 4000/mm^2 to 2000/mm^2; other changes in the RPE layer include pleomorphism, atrophy, depigmentation, and hyperplasia.[2,81,146] Lipofuscin accumulates throughout life in the RPE and the cone inner segments and may be linked to a decrease in the lysosomal activity of enzymes in the metabolically active RPE.[2,146-148]

Peripapillary chorioretinal atrophy, usually evident as a pale, temporal crescent, is an age-related degeneration of RPE and Bruch's membrane, and may be caused by attenuation of the peripapillary circulation.[149] With age there is a decrease in neuroretinal rim tissue, and the vertical optic cup diameter and the area of the optic cup both increase; these factors need to be considered when assessing the optic nerve head for glaucoma.[150]

Müller cells become hypertrophic with age.[138,139]

Degenerative processes, such as paving stone degeneration, peripheral reticular degeneration, and cystoid degeneration occur in peripheral retina, probably linked to a decrease in blood supply. Retinal vessels become narrower, which may diminish blood flow.

Clinical Comment: Visible Changes

Aging changes in the retina may be clinically observable. The foveal reflex dims because the internal limiting membrane thickens. The fundus color fades because RPE melanin and choroidal pigmentation are lost, making the choroidal vessels more prominent and giving the fundus a tigroid (striped) or tessellated appearance. The accumulations of debris in drusen are located in Bruch's membrane of the choroid but are observed as pinpoint deposits in the retina.

Clinical Comment: Alzheimer's Disease

Some speculate that early changes in the retina might be diagnostic in patients with Alzheimer's disease. Some investigators report a reduction in NFL thickness related to retinal dysfunction,[151-153] with the greatest reduction in the foveal region.[153] Others have not found a reduction in NFL thickness.[154] Evaluating the nerve fiber layer can be difficult but is becoming more accurate with improvements in technology. An extensive loss of neurons throughout the retina, particularly ganglion cells and glial cells, has been histologically documented in specimens from patients with Alzheimer's disease.[155] An increased cup-to-disc ratio and decreased rim tissue have also been observed in these patients.[156]

REFERENCES

1. Hogan MJ, Alvarado JA: Retina. In Hogan MJ, Alvarado JA, Weddell JE, editors: *Histology of the human eye*, Philadelphia, 1971, Saunders, p 393.
2. Sharma RK, Ehinger BEJ: Development and structure of the retina. In Kaufman PL, Alm A, editors: *Adler's physiology of the eye*, ed 10, St Louis, 2003, Mosby, p 319.
3. Young RW: Pathophysiology of age-related macular degeneration, *Surv Ophthalmol* 31:291, 1987.
4. Ko MK, Lee WR, McKechnie NM, et al: Post-traumatic hyperlipofuscinosis in the human retinal pigment epithelium, *Br J Ophthalmol* 75(1):54, 1991.
5. Feeney-Burns L, Hilderbrand ES, Eldridge S: Aging human RPE: morphometric analysis of macular, equatorial, and peripheral cells, *Invest Ophthalmol Vis Sci* 25:195, 1984.
6. Weiter JJ, Delori FC, Wing GL, et al: Retinal pigment epithelial lipofuscin and melanin and choroidal melanin in human eyes, *Invest Ophthalmol Vis Sci* 27:145, 1986.
7. Guymer R, Luthert P, Bird A: Changes in Bruch's membrane and related structures with age, *Prog Retin Eye Res* 18(1):59, 1999.
8. Cohen AI: The retina. In Hart MJ Jr, editor: *Adler's physiology of the eye*, ed 9, St Louis, 1992, Mosby, p 579.
9. Hudspeth AJ, Yee AG: The intercellular junctional complexes of retinal pigment epithelia, *Invest Ophthalmol* 12:354, 1973.
10. Fatt I, Shantinath K: Flow conductivity of retina and its role in retinal adhesion, *Exp Eye Res* 12:218, 1971.
11. Kita M, Marmor MF: Systemic mannitol increases the retinal adhesive force in vivo, *Arch Ophthalmol* 109:1449, 1991.
12. Yao XY, Moore KT, Marmor MF: Systemic mannitol increases retinal adhesiveness measured in vitro, *Arch Ophthalmol* 109:275, 1991.
13. Marmor FM, Abdul-Rahim AS, Cohen DS: The effect of metabolic inhibitors on retinal adhesion and subretinal fluid resorption, *Invest Ophthalmol Vis Sci* 19:893, 1980.
14. Kita M, Marmor MF: Effects on retinal adhesive force in vivo of metabolically active agents in the subretinal space, *Invest Ophthalmol Vis Sci* 33:1883, 1992.
15. Foulds WS: The vitreous in retinal detachment, *Trans Ophthalmol Soc U K* 95:412, 1975.
16. DeGuillebon H, Zanberman H: Experimental retinal detachment: biophysical aspects of retinal peeling and stretching, *Arch Ophthalmol* 87:545, 1972.
17. Hollyfield JG, Varner HH, Rayborn ME, et al: Retinal attachment to the pigment epithelium, *Retina* 9:59, 1989.
18. Hageman GS, Marmor MF, Yao XY, et al: The interphotoreceptor matrix mediates primate retinal adhesion, *Arch Ophthalmol* 113(5):655, 1995.
19. Hollyfield JG, Varner HH, Rayborn ME: Regional variation within the interphotoreceptor matrix from fovea to the retinal periphery, *Eye* 4:333, 1990.
20. Hollyfield JG, Rayborn ME, Landers RA, et al: Insoluble interphotoreceptor matrix domains surround rod photoreceptors in the human retina, *Exp Eye Res* 51:107, 1990.
21. Mieziewska K: The interphotoreceptor matrix, a space in sight, *Microsc Res Tech* 35(6):463, 1996.

22. Marmor MF, Yao XY, Hageman GS: Retinal adhesiveness in surgically enucleated human eyes, *Retina* 14(2):181, 1994.

23. Nicolaisson B Jr: Connections between the sensory retina and the retinal pigment epithelium, *Acta Ophthalmol (Copenh)* 63:68, 1985.

24. Lazarus HS, Hageman GS: Xyloside-induced disruption of interphotoreceptor matrix proteoglycans results in retinal detachment, *Invest Ophthalmol Vis Sci* 33:364, 1992.

25. Sigleman J, Ozanics V: Retina. In Jakobiec FA, editor: *Ocular anatomy, embryology, and teratology*, Philadelphia, 1982, Harper & Row, p 441.

26. Tombran-Tink J, Shivaram SM, Chader GJ, et al: Expression, secretion, and age-related downregulation of pigment epithelium-derived factor, a serpin with neurotrophic activity, *J Neurosci* 15(7, pt 1):4992, 1995.

27. Picaud S: Retinal biochemistry. In Adler's physiology of the eye Kaufman PL Alm A, editor: St Louis, 2003, Mosby, pp 382–408.

28. Young RW: The renewal of the photoreceptor cell outer segments, *J Cell Biol* 33:61, 1967.

29. Fine BS, Yanoff M: The retina. In Fine BS, Yanoff M, editors: *Ocular histology*, ed 2, Hagerstown, Md, 1979, Harper & Row, p 59.

30. Fine BS, Zimmerman LE: Observations on the rod and cone layer of the retina. A light and electron microscopic study, *Invest Ophthalmol* 2:446, 1963.

31. Laties A, Liebman P, Campbell C: Photoreceptor orientation in the primate eye, *Nature* 218:172, 1968.

32. Laties A, Enoch J: An analysis of retinal receptor orientation. I. Angular relationship of neighboring photoreceptors, *Invest Ophthalmol* 10:69, 1971.

33. Arikawa K, Molday LL, Molday RS, et al: Localization of peripherin/RDS in the disk membranes of cone and rod photoreceptors: relationship to disk membrane morphogenesis and retinal degeneration, *J Cell Biol* 116(3):659, 1992.

34. Young RW, Bok D: Participation of the retinal pigment epithelium in the rod outer segment renewal process, *J Cell Biol* 42:392, 1969.

35. Young RW: The renewal of rod and cone outer segments in rhesus monkey, *J Cell Biol* 49:303, 1971.

36. Bok D: Retinal photoreceptor-pigment epithelium interactions, *Invest Ophthalmol Vis Sci* 26:1659, 1985.

37. Young RW: Shedding of discs from rod outer segments in the rhesus monkey, *J Ultrastruct Res* 34:190, 1971.

38. LaVail MM: Rod outer segment disk shedding in rat retina: relationship to cyclic lighting, *Science* 194:1071, 1976.

39. Basinger S, Hoffman R, Matthews M: Photoreceptor shedding is initiated by light in the frog retina, *Science* 194:1074, 1978.

40. Young RW: The daily rhythm of shedding and degradation of rod and cone outer segment membranes in the chick retina, *Invest Ophthalmol Vis Sci* 17:105, 1976.

41. Migdale K, Herr S, Klug K, et al: Two ribbon synaptic units in rod photoreceptors of macaque, human, and cat, *J Comp Neurol* 455(1):100, 2003:(abstract).

42. Kolb H, Famiglietti EV: Rod and cone pathways in retina of cat, *Invest Ophthalmol Vis Sci* 15:935, 1976.

43. Anderson DH, Fisher SK, Steinberg RH: Mammalian cones: disc shedding, phagocytosis, and renewal, *Invest Ophthalmol Vis Sci* 17:117, 1978.

44. Walls GL: Human rods and cones, *Arch Ophthalmol* 12:914, 1934.

45. Young RW: A difference between rods and cones in the renewal of outer segment protein, *Invest Ophthalmol* 8:222, 1969.

46. Eckmiller MS: Distal invaginations and the renewal of cone outer segments in anuran and monkey retinas, *Cell Tissue Res* 260:19, 1990.

47. Steinberg RH: Phagocytosis by pigment epithelium of human retinal cones, *Nature* 25:305, 1974.

48. O'Day WT, Young RW: Rhythmic daily shedding of outer segment membranes by visual cells in the goldfish, *J Cell Biol* 76:593, 1978.

49. Raviola E, Gilula NB: Intramembrane organization of specialized contacts in the outer plexiform layer of the retina: a freeze-fracture study in monkey and rabbits, *J Cell Biol* 65:192, 1975.

50. Ayoub GS, Matthews G: Substance P modulates calcium current in retinal bipolar neurons, *Vis Neurosci* 8(6):539, 1992.

51. Kolb H, Linberg KA, Fisher SK: Neurons of the human retina: a Golgi study, *J Comp Neurol* 318(2):147, 1992.

52. Park SS, Sigelman J, Gragoudas ES: The anatomy and cell biology of the retina. In Tasman W, Jaeger EA, editors: *Duane's foundations of clinical ophthalmology*, vol 1, Philadelphia, 1994, Lippincott.

53. Bloomfield SA, Dacheux RF: Rod vision: pathways and processing in the mammalian retina, *Prog Retin Eye Res* 20(3):351, 2001.

54. Boycott BB, Hopkins JM: Cone bipolar cells and cone synapses in the primate retina, *Vis Neurosci* 7(1-2):49, 1991.

55. Polyak SL: *The retina*, Chicago, 1941, Chicago University Press.

56. Mariani AP: Bipolar cells in the monkey retina selective for cones likely to be blue sensitive, *Nature* 308:184, 1984.

57. Witkorsky P: Functional anatomy of the retina. In Tasman W, Jaeger EA, editors: *Duane's foundations of clinical ophthalmology*, vol 1, Philadelphia, 1994, Lippincott.

58. Warwick R: The eyeball. In Warwick R, editor: *Eugene Wolff's anatomy of the eye and orbit*, ed 7, Philadelphia, 1976, Saunders, p 99.

59. Kolb H, Dekorver L: Midget ganglion cells of the parafovea of the human retina: a study by electron microscopy and serial section reconstructions, *J Comp Neurol* 303(4):617, 1991.

60. Hart M: Visual adaptation. In Hart WM Jr, editor: *Adler's physiology of the eye*, ed 9, St Louis, 1992, Mosby, p 523.

61. Kolb H, Fernandez E, Nelson R: *The organization of the vertebrate retina*, Webvision (website). Webvision.med.utah.edu/. Accessed March 22, 2011.

62. Kolb H, Ahuelt P, Fisher SK, et al: Chromatic connectivity of the three horizontal cell types in the human retina, *Invest Ophthalmol Vis Sci* 30(suppl):348, 1989.

63. Dowling JE, Boycott BB: Neural connections of the retina: fine structure of the inner plexiform layer, *Cold Spring Harb Symp Quant Biol* 30:393, 1965.

64. Kolb H: Amacrine cells of the mammalian retina: neurocircuitry and functional roles, *Eye* 11:904, 1997.

65. Linberg KA, Fisher SK: Ultrastructure of the interplexiform cell of the human retina, *Invest Ophthalmol Vis Sci* 24(suppl):259, 1983.

66. Sarthy V, Ripps H: Structural organization of retinal glia. In: *The retinal Müller cell: structure and function*, New York, 2001, Kluwer Academic/Plenum Press.

67. Ogden TE: Nerve fiber layer of the primate retina: thickness and glial contents, *Vision Res* 23:581, 1983.

68. Newman E, Reichenback A: The Müller cell: a functional element of the retina, *Trends Neurosci* 19(8):307, 1996.

69. Kuwabara T, Cogan D: Retinal glycogen, *Arch Ophthalmol* 66:680, 1961.

70. Newman EA: Membrane physiology of retina glial (Müller) cells, *J Neurosci* 5:2225, 1985.

71. Reichenbach A, Stolzenburg JU, Eberhardt W, et al: What do retinal Müller (glial) cells do for their neuronal "small siblings"? *J Chem Neuroanat* 6(4):201, 1993.

72. Ramírez JM, Triviño A, Ramírez AI, et al: Structural specializations of human retinal glial cells, *Vision Res* 36(14):2029, 1996.

73. LaCour M: The retinal pigment epithelium. In Kaufman PL, Alm A, editors: *Adler's physiology of the eye*, ed 10, St Louis, 2003, Mosby, p 348.

74. Panda-Jonas S, Jonas JB, Jakobczyk-Zmija M: Retinal pigment epithelial cell count, distribution, and correlations in normal human eyes, *Am J Ophthalmol* 121:181, 1996.

75. Zinn KM, Benjamin-Henkind J: Retinal pigment epithelium. In Jakobiec FA, editor: *Ocular anatomy, embryology, and teratology*, Philadelphia, 1982, Harper & Row, p 533.

76. Usui S, Kamiyama Y, Ishii H, et al: Reconstruction of retinal horizontal cell responses by the ionic current model, *Vision Res* 36(12):1711, 1996:(abstract).

77. Kolb H: Organization of the outer plexiform layer of the primate retina: electron microscopy of Golgi-impregnated cells, *Philos Trans R Soc Lond B Biol Sci* 258:261, 1970.

78. la Cour M, Ehinger B: The Retina. *The biology of the eye, Fischbarg J, ed. Amsterdam, the Netherlands*, 2006, Elsevier, pp 195–252.

79. Dowling JE, Boycott BB: Organization of the primate retina: electron microscopy, *Proc R Soc Lond B Biol Sci* 166:80, 1966.

80. Cunha-Va JG: The blood-ocular barriers: past, present, and future, *Doc Ophthalmol* 93:149, 1997.

81. la Cour M, Tezel T: The retinal pigment epithelium. In Fischbarg J, ed. *The biology of the eye*, 2006, Elsevier, 253–271.

82. la Cour M, Lin H, Kenyon E, et al: Lactate transport in freshly isolated human fetal retinal pigment epithelium, *Invest Ophthalmol Vis Sci* 35:434–442, 1994.

83. Strauss O: The retinal pigment epithelium in visual function, *Physiol Rev* 85:845–881, 2005.

84. Young RW: Renewal systems in rods and cones, *Ann Ophthalmol* 843-854 , 1973.

85. Sparrow JR, Nakanishi K, Parish CA: The lipofuscin fluorophore A2E mediates blue light-induced damage to retinal pigmented epithelial cells, *Invest Ophthalmol Vis Sci* 41:1981-1989, 2000.

86. Bok D: The retinal pigment epithelium: a versatile partner in vision, *J Cell Sci Suppl* 17:189, 1993.

87. Grierson I, Hiscott P, Hogg P, et al: Development, repair and regeneration of the retinal pigment epithelium, *Eye* 8(pt 2):255, 1994.

88. Martini B, Pandey R, Ogden TE, et al: Cultures of human retinal pigment epithelium. Modulation of extracellular matrix, *Invest Ophthalmol Vis Sci* 33(3):516, 1992.

89. Wiggs JL: Molecular genetics of selected ocular disorders. In Yanoff M, Duker JS, editors: *Ocular pathology (e-book)*, St Louis, 2008, Mosby.

90. Altawel M: *Best disease*, eMedicine (website): http://emedicine.medscape.com/article/1227128-overview. Accessed March 22, 2011.

91. Marks WB, Dobelle WH, MacNichol EF Jr: Visual pigments of single primate cones, *Science* 43:1181, 1964.

92. Kolb H: The architecture of functional neural circuits in the vertebrate retina, *Invest Ophthalmol Vis Sci* 35(5):2385, 1994.

93. Horton JC: The central visual pathways. In Hart WM Jr, editor: *Adler's physiology of the eye*, ed 9, St Louis, 1992, Mosby, p 728.

94. Østerberg GA: Topography of the layer of rods and cones in the human retina, *Acta Ophthalmol (Copenh)* 6:1, 1935.

95. Farber DB, Flannery JG, Lolley RN, et al: Distribution patterns of photoreceptors, protein, and cyclic nucleotides in the human retina, *Invest Ophthalmol Vis Sci* 26:1558, 1985.

96. Curcio CA, Sloan KR, Kalina RE, et al: Human photoreceptor topography, *J Comp Neurol* 292:497, 1990.

97. Oppel O: Untersuchungen Über Die Retinaganglien und Optikusfasern. In Rohen JW, editor: *The structure of the eye*, vol 2, Stuttgart, Germany, 1965, Verlag, p 97.

98. Jonas JB, Gusek GC, Naumann GO: Optic disc, cup, and neuroretinal rim size, configuration and correlations in normal eyes, *Invest Ophthalmol Vis Sci* 29:1151, 1988.

99. Twig G, Levy H, Perlman I: Color opponency in horizontal cells of the vertebrate retina, *Prog Retin Eye Res* 22:31–68, 2003.

100. Kolb H: How the retina works, *Am Sci* 91:28–35, 2003.

101. Barnes S, Kelly ME: Calcium channels at the photoreceptor synapse, *Adv Exp Med Biol* 514:465–476, 2002.

102. Arshavsky VY: Like night and day: rods and cones have different pigment regeneration pathways, *Neuron* 36:1–3, 2002.

103. Muniz A, Villazana-Espinoza ET, Hatch AL, et al: A novel cone visual cycle in the cone-dominated retina, *Exp Eye Res* 83:175–184, 2007.

104. Boycott B, Wässle H: Parallel processing in the mammalian retina, *Invest Ophthalmol Vis Sci* 40:1313–1327, 1999.

105. Wässle H, Boycott BB: Functional architecture of the mammalian retina, *Physiol Rev* 71:447–480, 1991.

106. Slaughter MM, Miller RF: An excitatory amino acid antagonist blocks cone input to sign-conserving second-order retinal neurons, *Science* 219:1230–1232, 1983.

107. Dhingra A, Jiang M, Wang TL, et al: Light response of retinal ON bipolar cells requires a specific splice variant of Galpha(o), *J Neurosi* 22:4878–4884, 2002.

108. Fahrenfort I, Klooster J, Sjoerdsma T, et al: The involvement of glutamate-gated channels in negative feedback from horizontal cells to cones, *Prog Brain Res* 147:219–229, 2005.

109. Kamermans M, Spekreijse H: The feedback pathway from horizontal cells to cones. A mini review with a look ahead, *Vision Res* 39:2449–2468, 1999.

110. Kolb H, Nelson R: Functional neurocircuitry of amacrine cells in the cat retina. Neurocircuitry of the retina: *a Cajal memorial Eds. Gallego, A. Gouras, P*, New York, 1985, Elsevier Press, pp 215–232.

111. Jensen RJ, Daw NW: Effects of dopamine and its agonists and antagonists on the receptive field properties of ganglion cells in the rabbit retina, *Neuroscience* 17:837–855, 1986.

112. Dowling JE: Retinal neuromodulation: the role of dopamine, *Vis Neurosci* 7:87–97, 1991.

113. Wu SM: Intracellular light responses and synaptic organization of the vertebrate retina. In Kaufman PL, Alm A, editors: *Adler's physiology of the eye*, ed 10, St Louis, 2003, Mosby, pp 422–438.

114. Reppert SM, Weaver DR, Rivkees SA, et al: Putative melatonin receptors in human biological clock, *Science* 242:78–81, 1988.

115. Turner PL, Manister MA: Circadian photoreception: ageing and the eye's important role in systemic health, *Br J Ophthalmol* 92:1439–1444, 2008.

116. Berson M: Phototransduction in ganglion-cell photoreceptors, *Pflugers Arch* 454:849–855, 2007.

117. Gioffi GA, Grandtam E, Alm A: Ocular circulation In: Adler's physiology of the eye. In Kaufman PL, Alm A, editors: ed 10, St Louis, 2003, Mosby, pp 747–784.

118. Rapp LM, Maple SS, Choi JH: Lutein and zeaxanthin concentrations in rod outer segment membranes from perifoveal and peripheral human retina, *Invest Ophthalmol Vis Sci* 41:1200, 2000.

119. Nussbaum JJ, Pruett RC, Delori FC: Historic perspectives. Macular yellow pigment. The first 200 years, *Retina* 1(14):296, 1981.

120. Ahnelt PK: The photoreceptor mosaic, *Eye* 12:531, 1998.

121. Yamada E: Some structural features of the fovea centralis in the human retina, *Arch Ophthalmol* 82:151, 1969.

122. Kanski JJ: *Clinical ophthalmology*, ed 3, London, 1994, Butterworth- Heinemann, p 383.

123. Pei TF, Smelser GK: Some fine structural features of the ora serrata region in primate eyes, *Invest Ophthalmol Vis Sci* 7:672, 1968.

124. Jonas JB, Schmidt AM, Müller-Bergh JA, et al: Human optic nerve fiber count and optic disc size, *Invest Ophthalmol Vis Sci* 33(6):1992, 2012.

125. Quigley HA, Brown AE, Morrison JD, et al: The size and shape of the optic disc in normal human eyes, *Arch Ophthalmol* 108(1):51, 1990.

126. Hogan MJ, Alvarado JA, Weddell JE, editors: *Histology of the human eye*, Philadelphia, 1971, Saunders, pp 523.

127. Fantes FE, Anderson DR: Clinical histologic correlation of human peripapillary anatomy, *Ophthalmology* 96(1):20, 1989.

128. Alexander LJ: Diseases of the optic nerve. In Bartlett JD, Jaanus SD, editors: *Clinical ocular pharmacology*, ed 2, Butterworth, 1989, Boston, p 690.

129. Hayreh SS: Optic disc edema in raised intracranial pressure. Associated visual disturbances and their pathogenesis, *Arch Ophthalmol* 95:1566, 1975.

130. Wirtschafter JD, Rizzo FJ, Smiley BC: Optic nerve axoplasm and papilledema, *Surv Ophthalmol* 20:157, 1977.

131. Cogan DG, Kuwabara T: The mural cell in perspective, *Arch Ophthalmol* 78:133, 1967.

132. Chakravarthy U, Gardiner TA: Endothelium-derived agents in pericyte function/dysfunction, *Prog Retin Eye Res* 18(4):511, 1999.

133. Shakib M, Cunha-Vaz JG: Studies on the permeability of the blood-retinal barrier. IV. Junctional complexes of the retinal vessels and their role in the permeability of the blood-retinal barrier, *Exp Eye Res* 5:229, 1966.

134. Bernstein MH, Hollenberg MJ: Fine structure of the choriocapillaris and retinal capillaries, *Invest Ophthalmol* 4(6):1016, 1965.

135. Henkind P: Radial peripapillary capillaries of the retina, II. Anatomy-human and comparative, *Br J Ophthalmol* 51:115, 1967.

136. Hayreh SS: The central artery of the retina: its role in the blood supply of the optic nerve, *Br J Ophthalmol* 47:651, 1963.

137. Gao H, Hollyfield JG: Aging of the human retina. Differential loss of neurons and retinal pigment epithelial cells, *Invest Ophthalmol Vis Sci* 33:1–17, 1992.

138. Paasche G, Gärtner U, Germer A, et al: Mitochondria of retina Müller (glial) cells: the effects of aging and of application of free radical scavengers, *Ophthalmic Res* 32:229, 2000.

139. Bringmann A, Biedermann B, Schnurbusch U, et al: Age- and disease-related changes of calcium channel-mediated currents in human Müller glial cells, *Invest Ophthalmol Vis Sci* 14:2791, 2000.

140. Dohlman CL, McCormick AQ, Drance SM: Aging of the optic nerve, *Arch Ophthalmol* 98:2053, 1980.

141. Yuodelis C, Hendrickson A: A qualitative and quantitative analysis of the human fovea during development, *Vision Res* 26:847, 1986.

142. Curcio CA: Photoreceptor topography in ageing and age-related maculopathy, *Eye* 15(3):376, 2001.

143. Jackson GR, Owsley C, Cordle EP, et al: Aging and scotopic sensitivity, *Vision Res* 38:3655, 1998.

144. Eliasieh K, Liets LC, Chalupa LM: Cellular reorganization in the human retina during normal aging, *Invest Ophthalmol Vis Sci* 48:2824–2830, 2007.

145. Ramírez JM, Ramírez AI, Salazar JJ, et al: Changes of astrocytes in retinal ageing and age-related macular degeneration, *Exp Eye Res* 73:601, 2001.

146. Yoo SH, Adamis AP: Retinal manifestations of aging, *Int Ophthalmol Clin* 38(1):95, 1998.

147. Boulton M, Dayhaw-Barker P: The role of the retinal pigment epithelium: topographical variation and ageing changes, *Eye* 15:384, 2001.

148. Sparrow JR, Boulton M: RPE lipofuscin and its role in retinal pathobiology, *Exp Eye Res* 80:595–606, 2005.

149. Curcio CA, Saunders PL, Younger PW, et al: Peripapillary chorioretinal atrophy: Bruch's membrane changes and photoreceptor loss, *Ophthalmology* 107:334, 2000.

150. Garway-Heath DF, Wollstein G, Hitchings RA: Aging changes of the optic nerve head in relation to open angle glaucoma, *Br J Ophthalmol* 81(10):840, 1997.

151. Parisi V, Restuccia R, Fattapposta F, et al: Morphological and functional retinal impairment in Alzheimer's disease patients, *Clin Neurophysiol* 112(10):1860, 2001.

152. Hedges TR III, Perez Galves S, Speigelman D, et al: Retinal nerve fiber layer abnormalities in Alzheimer's disease, *Acta Ophthalmol Scand* 74(3):271, 1996.

153. Blanks JC, Schmidt SY, Torigoe Y, et al: Retinal pathology in Alzheimer's disease. II. Regional neuron loss and glial changes in GCL, *Neurobiol Aging* 17(3):385, 1996.

154. Justino L, Kergoat M, Bergman H, et al: Neuroretinal function is normal in early dementia of the Alzheimer type, *Neurobiol Aging* 22(4):691, 2001.

155. Blanks JC, Torigoe Y, Hinton DR, et al: Retinal pathology in Alzheimer's disease. I. Ganglion cell loss in foveal/parafoveal retina, *Neurobiol Aging* 17(3):377, 1996.

156. Tsai CS, Ritch R, Schwartz B, et al: Optic nerve head and nerve fiber layer in Alzheimer's disease, *Arch Ophthalmol* 109:199, 1991.

5 *Crystalline Lens*

The crystalline lens is an avascular, transparent elliptic structure that aids in focusing light rays on the retina. The lens is located within the posterior chamber, anterior to the vitreous chamber and posterior to the iris (Figure 5-1). The lens is suspended from the surrounding ciliary body by zonular fibers. It is malleable, and ciliary muscle contraction can cause a change in lens shape, increasing the dioptric power of the eye. The mechanism that causes an increase in lens power is accommodation, which allows near objects to be focused on the retina.

The posterior lens surface is attached to the anterior vitreous face by the hyaloid capsular ligament, a circular ring adhesion. Within this ring is a potential space, the retrolental space (of Berger), an area of nonadhesion between the vitreous and the lens (see Figure 6-12).

LENS DIMENSIONS

The lens is biconvex, with the posterior surface having the steeper curve. The *anterior* radius of curvature measures 8 to 14 μm, and the *posterior* surface radius of curvature measures 5 to 8 μm. The centers of the anterior and posterior surfaces are called the **poles,** and the **lens thickness** is the distance from the anterior to posterior pole. The thickness of the unaccommodated lens is 3.5 to 5 mm and it increases 0.02 mm each year throughout life.[1-3] The **lens diameter** is the nasal-to-temporal measurement and in the infant is 6.5 mm. The diameter reaches 9 mm during the teenage years and does not change significantly,[4-6] although some report a small age-related increase in diameter.[7] The **equator** is the largest circumference of the lens at a location between the two poles.

The refractive power of the unaccommodated lens is approximately 20 diopters (D) and depends on the (1) surface curvatures, (2) refractive index, (3) change in index between the lens and surrounding environment, and (4) length of the optical path. The lens has a gradient refractive index because of changes in optical density throughout the lens; the index increases from the anterior to the center of the lens and decreases toward the posterior surface. The refractive index is a factor of protein concentration within the lens fibers.[8] The variations in index provide additional refractive power.[9,10] The power of the lens increases in accommodation, with the maximum accommodative amplitude, 14 D, reached between ages 8 and 12 years.[11] Accommodative power decreases with age, approaching zero after 50 years.[12]

EMBRYOLOGIC DEVELOPMENT

The structure of the adult lens is determined during embryologic development. The lens vesicle, the first lenslike structure observable in the developing embryo, is composed of a layer of epithelial cells that form a hollow sphere. The cells are positioned so that the apical surface lines the lumen of this sphere. The posterior cells differentiate and elongate, forming the **primary lens fibers.** As these fibers grow and reach the anterior cells (Figure 5-2), the center of the sphere fills. Thus the adult lens has no posterior epithelium because it was used to form these first lens fibers. During the rest of the life of the lens, cell division occurs in the germinative zone of the epithelium just anterior to the lens equator, and the cells thus formed elongate to form secondary lens fibers that are laid down outer to all earlier fibers. With age, the lens continues to grow as it forms new fibers (see Chapter 7).

HISTOLOGY

LENS CAPSULE

The **lens capsule** is a transparent envelope that surrounds the entire lens. The capsule is a basement membrane and with time becomes the thickest in the body.[13] Its thickness varies with location. At the posterior pole, it is thinnest (approximately 3.5 μm) and does not appreciably increase with age; the thickness at the equator increases slightly with age, and on average is 7 μm. The capsule thickness at the anterior pole increases with age from approximately 11 to 15 μm. The annular region surrounding the anterior pole appears to be the thickest. It too increases with age from approximately 13.5 to 16 μm.[14] The capsule consists primarily of collagen; it contains no elastic fibers but is highly elastic because of the lamellar arrangement of the fibers.[4,15] It encloses all lens components and helps to mold the shape of the lens. The capsule would prefer to take a more spherical

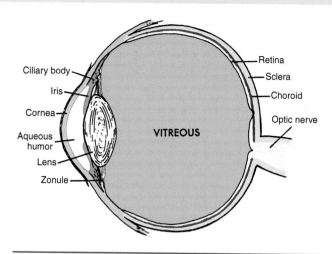

FIGURE 5-1
Diagram showing relationship of the lens and zonule to other ocular structures. (From Paterson CA, Delamere NA: The lens. In Hart WM Jr, editor: *Adler's physiology of the eye*, ed 9, St Louis, 1992, Mosby.)

shape, but this tendency is counteracted by the pull from the zonular fibers. The zonular fibers insert into the capsule, merging with it in an area from the equator to near both poles. This coincides with the annular area mentioned previously. This outer superficial zone of the capsule is called the zonular lamella and consists of zonules interconnected with matrix.[4] The lens capsule provides some barrier function preventing large molecules, such as albumin and hemoglobin,[4] from entering the lens. The anterior lens capsule is produced by the anterior epithelium and thickens with age. The posterior lens capsule may receive some contribution from the basal membrane of lens fibers, but the thickness of the posterior capsule changes minimally throughout life (Figure 5-3).[16-18]

LENS EPITHELIUM

Adjacent to the anterior lens capsule is a layer of cuboidal epithelium—the **anterior lens epithelium** (Figure 5-4). These cells secrete the anterior capsule throughout life and are the site of metabolic transport mechanisms. As noted, no posterior epithelium is present because it was used during embryologic development to form the primary lens fibers. The basal aspect of the epithelial cell is adjacent to the capsule, and the apical portion is oriented inward toward the center of the lens. The lateral membranes of the epithelial cells are joined by desmosomes and gap junctions.[17,19-22] Although zonula occludens were once thought to join the epithelial cells,[23] more recent studies report few, if any, tight junctions.[18]

The band of cells in the *preequatorial* region that lies just anterior to the equator is called the **germinal**

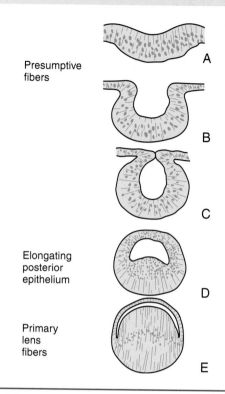

FIGURE 5-2
Development of embryonic nucleus. A, Formation of lens placode, precursor of lens. **B,** Invagination forming lens vesicle. **C,** Hollow lens vesicle lined with epithelium. **D,** Posterior cells elongate, becoming primary lens fibers. **E,** Primary lens fibers fill lumen, forming embryonic nucleus. Curved line formed by cell nuclei is lens bow. Anterior epithelium remains in place.

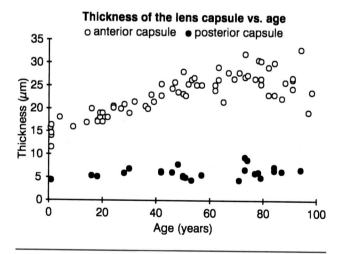

FIGURE 5-3
Thickness of the anterior and posterior lens capsule in relation to age. (From Krag S, Andreassen TT: Mechanical properties of the human posterior lens capsule, *Invest Ophthalmol Vis Sci* 44[2]:691, 2003.)

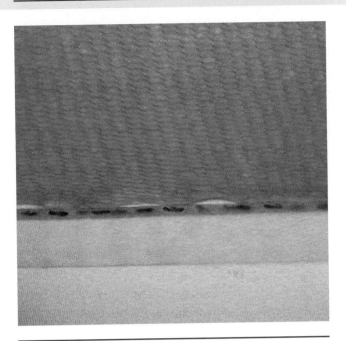

FIGURE 5-4
Light micrograph of anterior lens epithelium and capsule. Honeycomb appearance of lens fibers above epithelium.

zone, the location of cell mitosis. Cell division continues throughout life; as each cell divides, a daughter cell migrates posteriorly towards the equator, withdraws from the cell cycle, and differentiates into a lens fiber. Each newly formed cell elongates; the *basal* aspect stretches toward the *posterior* pole and the *apical* aspect toward the *anterior* pole (Figure 5-5). This process occurs all around the equator, with fibers stretching toward the poles from all aspects of the lens periphery. As the cells in each layer elongate, the cellular nuclei move with the cytoplasm. A line drawn to connect the dots of these nuclei would have an arcuate shape toward the anterior aspect, a configuration called the lens bow (see Figure 5-2). Eventually, as it loses all cellular organelles, the elongated cell becomes a **lens fiber.** The anterior end of the lens fiber (the apical surface) insinuates itself between the epithelial layer and the underlying lens fibers. The new fibers are laid down outer to the older fibers; the more superficial fibers are longer than deeper fibers, and the youngest cells lie directly below the epithelium and the capsule. All fibers formed from mitosis in the germinative zone are called **secondary lens fibers.** Once it loses its nucleus, the mature lens fiber has lost its attachment to the basement membrane.[17]

LENS FIBERS

Lens fiber production continues throughout life, with the new lens fibers being laid down outer to the older fibers; growth results in concentric layers of secondary lens fibers. The structure of the lens is similar to an onion; each layer of fibers approximates a layer of an onion, but then each layer is made up of adjacent fibers. A section through the equator of the lens shows that the fibers cut in cross section are mostly hexagonal in shape and arranged in concentric rings (Figure 5-6). The cross section dimensions of a fiber are approximately 3 by 9 μm.[24] Each fiber has a long crescent shape, with the broad sides parallel to the lens surface and the narrow sides at an angle to the surface and located near the lens poles.

Lens fiber cytoplasm contains a high concentration of proteins, known as crystallins, which account for approximately 40% of the net weight of the fiber. The distribution and concentration of crystallins contribute to the **gradient refractive index.**[25] The crystallin concentration varies from approximately 15% in the cortex to 70% in the nucleus.[26] A cytoskeletal network of microtubules and filaments provides structure and also provides stability by being anchored to the plasma membrane.[18,25] The lateral membranes have numerous and elaborate interdigitations along the fiber length that take various shapes, such as ball-and-socket and tongue-in-groove junctions, and allow for sliding between fibers[4,17,18] (Figure 5-7). The fibers also are joined by desmosomes.

Because the lens has no vascular supply and the fibers lose their cellular organelles as they age, some cell-to-fiber and fiber-to-fiber mechanism of communication is necessary. There is an extensive network of gap junctions throughout the lens along the lateral fiber membranes to account for the facility with which nutrients and ions move within the lens.[17,27] These gap junctions have a different packing arrangement and different protein connexins, forming the channel than do the typical gap junctions.[21] The gap junctions are not evenly distributed throughout the lens, with few near the poles, more toward the equator, and seemingly fewer junctions in deeper layers.[13,21,22] Micropinocytic vesicles at apical and basal aspects of fiber membranes and significant areas of membrane fusion also allow movement of material from fiber to fiber, contributing to communication between fibers in addition to the gap type of junctions described.[13,20,22,28]

EPITHELIUM-FIBER INTERFACE

The border between the apical membrane of the anterior epithelium and the apical membrane of the elongating fiber is known as the **epithelium-fiber interface (EFI).** Nutrients and ions are exchanged across the EFI. It was once assumed that such movement was facilitated by gap junctions, but disagreement now exists on whether gap junctions are present.[19,22,27,28] Gap junctions are usually found on the lateral cell membrane,

FIGURE 5-5

Composite drawing of crystalline lens, cortex, epithelium, capsule, and zonular attachments. **A,** Anterior central lens epithelium, seen in flat section and cross section. Size and shape of these cells can be compared with those of cells in **B,** intermediate zone, and **C,** equatorial zone. At equator, dividing cells are elongating (*arrows*) to form lens cortical cells. As they elongate, cells send processes anteriorly and posteriorly toward sutures, and their nuclei migrate somewhat anterior to equator to form lens bow. At the same time, nuclei become more and more displaced into lens as new cells are formed at equator. Lens capsule (*d*) is thicker anterior and posterior to equator than at equator itself. Anterior and equatorial capsule contains fine filamentous inclusions (*double arrows*); these are not present posteriorly. Lens fibers elongate into flattened hexagons (*e*) in cross section. Zonular fibers (*f*) attach to anterior and posterior capsule and to equatorial capsule, forming pericapsular or zonular lamella of lens (*g*). (From Hogan MJ, Alvarado JA, Weddell JE: *Histology of the human eye*, Philadelphia, 1971, Saunders.)

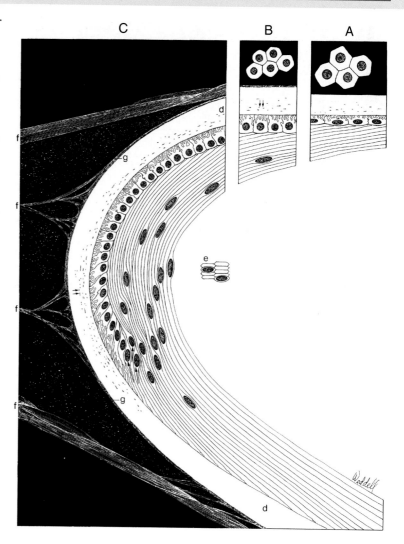

and the EFI involves apical surfaces. Few true gap junctions have been visualized in tissue preparations. Minimal coupling occurs between the epithelium and fibers in the central zone (i.e., near the poles and sutures), but such junctions increase toward the germinative zone.[21] Pinocytosis does occur at this interface, facilitating exchange.[18]

DIVISIONS OF LENS

The **primary lens fibers** from the elongating posterior epithelium form the very center of the lens, the **embryonic nucleus,** and all subsequent lens fibers are laid down outer to this core. Cell mitosis then begins in the preequatorial region of the epithelium, the new cell migrates toward the equator, and then elongates, forming a lens fiber. All such fibers formed are **secondary lens fibers.** The **fetal nucleus** includes the embryonic nucleus and the fibers surrounding it that are formed before birth. The **adult nucleus** is considered to include the embryonic and fetal nuclei

and the fibers formed from birth to sexual maturation. The **lens cortex** contains the fibers formed after sexual maturation (Figure 5-8, *C*). The cortex can be divided into superficial, internal, and deep zones,[13] but these are arbitrary divisions and generally are not clinically significant. Some consider the fibers formed before sexual maturation the "juvenile nucleus," those added before middle age the "adult nucleus," and the remaining fibers the "cortex."[25] The lens cortex has the lowest and the embryonic nucleus has the highest index of refraction.

LENS SUTURES

As the lens fibers reach the poles they meet with the other fibers in their layer, forming a junction known as a **suture.** The anterior suture is formed by the joining of the apical aspects of the fibers, and the posterior suture is formed by the joining of the basal aspects.[4,13] The secondary fibers formed during embryologic development meet in three branches,

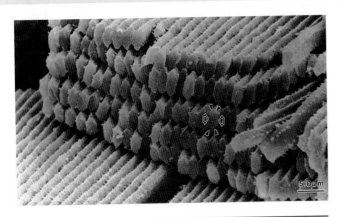

FIGURE 5-6
Scanning electron micrograph shows characteristic hexagonal cross-sectional profiles of lens fiber cells. (From Paterson CA, Delamere NA: The lens. In Hart WM Jr, editor: *Adler's physiology of the eye*, ed 9, St Louis, 1992, Mosby.)

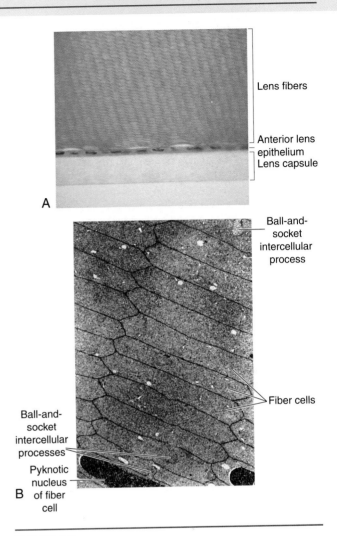

FIGURE 5-7
A, Light micrograph showing lens capsule, anterior lens epithelium, and lens fibers of cortex. **B,** Fiber cells of lens cortex. (Transmission electron microscope; ×6000.) (**B** from Krause WJ, Cutts JH: *Concise text of histology*, Baltimore, 1981, Williams & Wilkins.)

forming **Y sutures.** The **anterior suture** is an *upright-Y* shape and the **posterior suture** an *inverted-Y* shape (see Figure 5-8, *A*).[18] As growth continues and the lens becomes larger, the sutures become asymmetric and dissimilar. The limbs of the anterior and posterior sutures are offset, and the complexity of the sutures contributes to lens transparency.[29] The sutures formed after birth are more stellate shaped; sutures formed through early adulthood have 6 to 9 branches; and 9 to 15 complex branched stars are formed in middle to old age[29] (see Figure 5-8, *B*).

ZONULES (OF ZINN)

The lens is attached to the ciliary body by a group of threadlike fibers, the **zonules (of Zinn),** or the **suspensory ligament of the lens** (Figure 5-9). The fibers belong to a category termed microfibrils. The macromolecular composition that accounts for the remarkable extensibility of the zonules is complex and still undetermined.[15,30] The zonules appear to be formed of extracellular matrix, that includes fibrillin and elastin, both of which have a role in the synthesis of elastic fibers.[31] However, biomolecular analysis indicates that there are no true elastic fibers present in the zonules.[31]

The fibers arise from the basement membrane of the nonpigmented ciliary epithelium in the pars plana and from the valleys between the ciliary processes in the pars plicata.[4] They form two columnlike structures on both sides of a ciliary process and end at the lens capsule (see Figure 3-12). Most fibers attach to the lens capsule at the preequatorial and postequatorial regions; few attach directly at the equator.[32] The zonules are interwoven into the components of the capsule. Those that attach to the lens are known as primary zonules. Secondary zonules join the primary zonules with each other or connect processes to one another or to the pars plana, and "tension" fibers anchor the primary zonules to the ciliary valleys to form a fulcrum.[32]

ACCOMMODATION

When the emmetropic eye is viewing a distant object, the ciliary muscle is relaxed, the diameter of the ciliary ring is relatively large, and the zonules are in a stretched configuration exerting tension on the lens capsule holding the lens in the unaccommodated state, such that the image lies on the retina. When a near object is to be focused on the retina, an increase in the refractive power of the eye must occur. This increase in power is called

FIGURE 5-8
Fetal and adult lenses, showing sutures and arrangement of lens cells. **A,** Fetal nucleus. Anterior γ suture is at *a,* and posterior suture is at *b.* Lens cells are depicted as wide bands. Cells that attach to tips of γ sutures at one pole of lens attach to fork of γ at opposite pole. **B,** Adult lens cortex. Anterior and posterior organization of sutures is more complex. Lens cells that arise from tip of a suture branch insert farther anteriorly or posteriorly into a fork at opposite pole. This arrangement conserves shape of lens. In this drawing, for educational purposes, the suture appears to lie in a single plane, but the reader should remember that the suture extends throughout the thickness of the cortex and nucleus to the level of the γ sutures in the fetal nucleus. **C,** Adult lens, showing nuclear zones, epithelium, and capsule. Thickness of lens capsule in various zones is shown. (From Hogan MJ, Alvarado JA, Weddell JE: *Histology of the human eye,* Philadelphia, 1971, Saunders.)

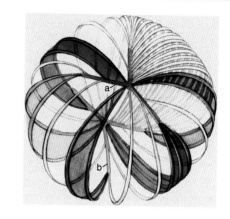

A

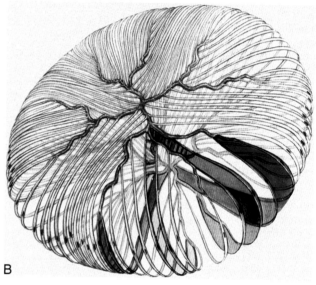

B

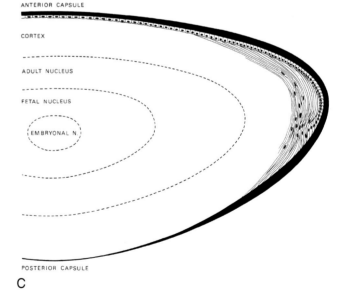

ANTERIOR CAPSULE

CORTEX

ADULT NUCLEUS

FETAL NUCLEUS

EMBRYONAL N.

POSTERIOR CAPSULE

C

accommodation and is accomplished by a change in lens shape brought about by contraction of the ciliary muscle. Von Helmholtz[33] is credited with determining that the following occur during accommodation:
1. Lens thickness increases anterior to posterior.
2. The lens thins along the equator.
3. The anterior lens surface moves forward and thus the anterior chamber becomes shallower.
4. There is no change in the position of the posterior pole.

These factors result in a thickened lens with more sharply curved surfaces and thus increased lens power. The stimulus that initiates the accommodative mechanism is retinal blur.[34] The accommodative mechanism is dependent on cone stimulation with little influence by rods.[35]

When the ciliary muscle contracts, the diameter of the ciliary ring surrounding the lens decreases, reducing the tension that the zonules exert on the lens and allowing the lens capsule to assume its preferred spherical shape. The lens capsule transmits the reduction in the zonular pull to the lens, molding the lens into its accommodated form.

The lens becomes more sharply curved, and because of the thickness variation of the capsule, a bulge is most apparent at the center of the anterior surface.[36,37] The posterior surface increases in curvature only slightly; however, the steepness of the anterior surface does not become greater than that of the posterior surface.[12] As the lens thickens axially, the equatorial diameter decreases, and the anterior lens pole moves toward the cornea. It was previously thought that there was no posterior lens movement, but a small amount of movement of the posterior pole in a posterior direction has been identified.[8,38,39] The curvature of the internal surfaces, seen at the zones of discontinuity and the boundaries of the nuclei, mimics the changes in the surface curvatures and contributes to the increase in the total dioptric power.[8] This thickening of the lens from anterior to posterior occurs in the nuclear region, but the thickness of the lens cortex remains unchanged.[40] The changes occurring in accommodation described in 1855 by Helmholtz have been demonstrated using current technology.[5,41]

The vitreous has a passive role in accommodation, probably serving only as support for the lens.[42] During ciliary muscle contraction, the choroid is pulled forward slightly, perhaps aiding in the correct orientation of the photoreceptors in relation to the entrance pupil. Contraction of the ciliary body in accommodation, by decreasing the circumference of the sclera, may lead to an elongation of the axial length of the eye.[39] The ciliary muscle and trabecular meshwork are both attached to the scleral spur, and accommodation can cause a widening of the intertrabecular spaces, facilitating aqueous outflow and can result in decreased intraocular pressure (IOP).[43]

When the ciliary muscle relaxes, the muscle is moved outward, and the ciliary body is stretched posteriorly by the elastic tissue of Bruch's membrane. The ciliary ring expands, and the tension in the zonules stretches the capsule, restoring the lens to its unaccommodated state.

Clinical Comment: Presbyopia

The ability to focus at near distances decreases with age, and this loss in accommodative ability is called **presbyopia.** *The objective measurement of accommodation nears zero by the age of 50, although subjective measurements of accommodative amplitude may be higher due to the depth of focus.[44] The easiest response to patients when explaining presbyopia is that a "weakness of the muscle" causes this decrease in focusing ability. However, changes in the ciliary body, zonules, lens capsule, and the lens itself all influence the loss of accommodation; yet the precise nature of the impact each has is still unclear. Although ciliary muscle tissue is lost and replaced by connective tissue, this occurs in very old age, not when presbyopia begins.[45] The force of ciliary muscle contraction does not decrease with age[46]; no loss of parasympathetic innervation occurs that would account for decreased muscle contraction and maximal contractile ability of the muscle decreases only slightly if at all with age.[5] The diameter of the unaccommodated ciliary ring decreases in older eyes, thus the circumlental space between ciliary body and lens equator decreases with age, causing a decrease in zonular tension in the unaccommodated eye.[47,48] There is some dispute as to whether the zonule-free area at the anterior lens surface decreases with age. The increase in anterior lens convexity and the increase in anterior lens capsule thickness might cause the appearance of what is called an anterior shift in the anterior zonule insertion on the capsule.[48] There is no apparent increase in zonular length that presumably would accompany such an anterior shift.[49] Some loss of fiber extensibility with age has been measured.[31,49] The lens capsule becomes thicker, less elastic, and more brittle with*

age.[50] Older lens fibers become more resistant to deformity, and thus the ability of the lens to change shape in response to the forces exerted by the capsule diminishes with age.[10,51-54] As the lens continues to grow throughout life, the mass and volume increase, with a forward movement of the center of the lens. The increase in the bulk of the lens and the anterior displacement alter the vector relationship between the lens and the zonules, causing the zonular force to be more tangential to the lens surface and less able to change lens capsule tension.[3,8] As the lens becomes more curved and little change occurs in lens power, greater force will be required to increase the power necessary for near focus.[10,55]

Clinical Comment: Slit-Lamp Appearance of Lens

An optic section through the lens demonstrates the biconvexity of the structure (Figure 5-10). The first bright line is convex forward and is the anterior lens capsule; posterior to this is a dark line, the anterior epithelium. The next bright line is the cortex, then various gray zones (zones of discontinuity) are seen. The anterior Y suture of the fetal nucleus may be evident. The vertical center, the embryonic nucleus, has no anterior or posterior curvature. The posterior inverted-Y suture may be seen in the posterior aspect of the fetal nucleus. Posterior to this, the zones of discontinuity are concave forward, with the final zone being the posterior capsule.[56] The zones of discontinuity are apparent because of changes in light-scattering properties (Table 5-1). A diffuse view of the anterior lens surface illustrates lens shagreen, with the lens surface resembling the surface of an orange, likely caused by the conformation of the capsule to the epithelial cell undulations.[57]

LENS PHYSIOLOGY

The primary function of the lens is the refraction of light, and it is imperative that the transparent lens have minimal light scatter. Transparency is a function of (1) the absence of blood vessels, (2) few cellular organelles in the light path, (3) an orderly arrangement of fibers, and (4) the short distance between components of differing indices relative to the wavelength of light.[58] Since extensive metabolic activity occurs in the anterior epithelium maintaining cell and fiber function, and the preequatorial region has a high level of miotic activity, a significant amount of energy is used by these cells. Because the lens is avascular, most nutrients are obtained from the surrounding aqueous, with a small contribution from the vitreous. Thus the epithelium is rich in transport mechanisms (e.g., $Na^+/K^+/ATPase$ pumps) that maintain electrolyte balance. Anaerobic glycolysis is the source of the energy required for cellular metabolism and cellular replication within the lens.

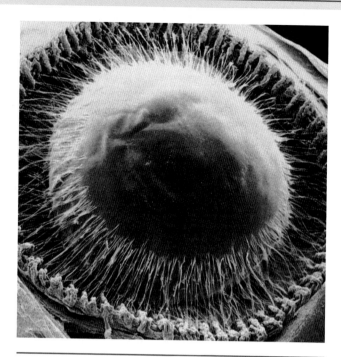

FIGURE 5-9
Scanning electron micrograph of anterior zonular insertion after removal of cornea and iris. Note angle between anterior and posterior zonules and attachment to lens capsule. (From Streeton BW: In Jakobiec JA, editor: *Ocular anatomy, embryology, and teratology*, Hagerstown, Md, 1982, Harper & Row.)

Free radicals are a normal by-product of metabolic processes, but ultraviolet (UV) light absorption can also produce oxidative changes within tissue causing the formation of free radicals. Free radicals disrupt cellular processes and cause cellular damage.

LENS CAPSULE

The lens capsule is first evident in early embryologic development and completely surrounds the early lens fibers. The lens is said to have immune-privilege and protection from infectious viruses and bacteria because the capsule sequesters the lens epithelium and fibers from early in prenatal development. Postnatally, the anterior lens epithelium and the posterior lens fibers continue to secrete and deposit matrix into the inner aspect of the capsule.[59] As the lens itself grows throughout life, the capsule must expand as well, although the molecular mechanisms that regulate this are unknown. The capsule is permeable to water and small solutes and the proteins necessary for lens growth and function. Size and molecular charge may both influence passage through the capsule.[59] A slow turnover of radio-labeled substances has been demonstrated within the capsule matrix (months to years), as compared with basement membranes elsewhere (hours).[59] The capsule acts as a reservoir for the accumulation of

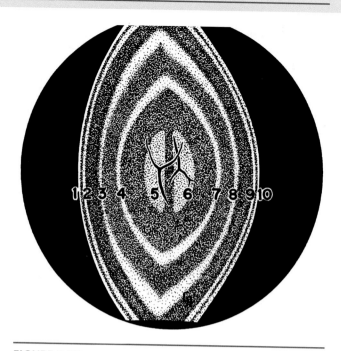

FIGURE 5-10
Optical section of normal adult lens. *1*, Anterior capsule; *2*, anterior line of disjunction (anterior epithelium); *3*, anterior surface of adult nucleus; *4*, anterior surface of fetal nucleus; *5*, inner layer of anterior half of fetal nucleus, containing anterior γ suture; *6*, inner layer of posterior half of fetal nucleus, containing posterior γ suture; *7*, posterior surface of fetal nucleus; *8*, posterior surface of adult nucleus; *9*, posterior line of disjunction; *10*, posterior capsule. (From Phelps CD: In Duane TD, editor: *Clinical ophthalmology*, vol 1, Hagerstown, Md, 1978, Harper & Row.)

molecules and growth factors that promote and regulate lens processes, such as proliferation, migration, and differentiation.[59]

LENS FIBERS

Fiber Components

The lens is 65% to 70% water and 30% to 35% protein; the cortex has a higher water content (73% to 80%) than the nucleus (68%).[60,61] The refractive index of the cortex is 1.38, and 1.41 is the index of the nucleus. An outer fiber can be 1 cm in length in the adult from suture to suture in the adult.[62] Soluble lens proteins are known as crystallins, and insoluble proteins include those forming the cell membrane and the cytoskeleton.

The proteins manufactured during lens development must be durable because they need to last a lifetime. Eighty percent to 90% of the proteins within the lens are **water soluble crystallins;** this concentration is three times higher than in typical cells.[62] Lens crystallins are from the alpha family or the beta/gamma super family. Interaction among crystallins, particularly the alpha crystallins, produce a phenomenon that contributes to lens transparency, and gives the lens a significantly higher index of refraction than surrounding fluids.[63] Alpha crystallins are molecular chaperones and, as such, they stabilize beta and gamma proteins, preventing them from undergoing chemical changes and forming aggregates. When crystallins aggregate they undergo a change in density, become water *insoluble*, and when of sufficient size cause light scatter.[64] Alpha crystallins also appear to be important in maintaining certain functions of lens cells and fibers. The beta/gamma crystallins are more diverse and their functions are unclear.[63,64]

Actin is an insoluble protein and an important component in the scaffolding of the lens fiber, its cytoskeleton. Microtubules are part of the cytoskeleton and help to stabilize the fiber membrane and may have a role in transporting vesicles to the ends of the elongating fibers.[62] Numerous actin microfilaments, just inside the cell membrane, are linked to the adhesive junctions between lens fibers. Actin also helps to maintain crystallin organization.[66] Lens fiber membranes have the highest cholesterol content of human cells and a high concentration of sphingomyelin. The function of sphingomyelin is unclear since it can cause rigidity in membranes and lens fibers must exhibit flexibility.[62]

Formation of Lens Fibers

Lens fiber formation is a complex and multistep process and various molecules influence the mechanism. Growth factors, present in the aqueous and the vitreous, accumulate in the lens capsule. The concentration and the distribution of specific factors along the lens surface direct cellular processes.[65] Growth factors that influence proliferation and migration are concentrated along the anterior surface; other growth factors that influence differentiation are concentrated at the equator.[66] Biomolecules that regulate interactions among actin filaments, adhering junction integrins, and extracellular matrix increase fiber mass.[67] Significant protein synthesis must occur to form crystallins, aquaporin channel proteins, and gap junction components as the fibers elongate.[67] As the fiber cell elongates, the cell membrane permeability increases, causing K^+ and Cl^- accumulation in the cytoplasm, driving water entrance and cell volume increase.[68]

As the cell elongates, the apical aspect slides along the apical aspect of the anterior epithelium, and the basal aspect slides along the posterior capsule. Once the elongating end reaches the end of an elongating fiber from the opposite side of the lens, they join, forming a suture. The basal end detaches from the capsule and once this detachment occurs, the membrane-bound organelles (nucleus, endoplasmic reticulum, mitochondria) degrade in an apoptosis-like process; the loss of organelles is complete within a few hours.[67,69,70]

Fiber Junctions

The membranes of adjacent fibers interdigitate, forming interlocking junctions along their long lateral sides. These junctures help to stabilize the fibers so that as the lens changes shape in accommodation, the lateral membranes slide against each other and remain close together. Adhesion complexes joining the lateral membrane also enable close contact between fibers during lens shape change and decrease extracellular space, minimizing spacing between fibers and decreasing light scatter.

Although mature lens fibers lack cellular organelles, they still require nutrients. The fibers deep within the lens are far from the aqueous and vitreous, and fiber-to-fiber transport is important. An intracellular network of gap junctions facilitates movement of ions and small molecules between fibers.[71] The lens has a higher concentration of gap junctions than other cells in the body; the lens gap junctions contain; some channel proteins that are unique to the lens.[13,62]

LENS METABOLISM

The lens obtains glucose from the aqueous humor and because of the low oxygen concentration in the neighborhood of the lens, 70% of ATP production is via anaerobic metabolism. Aerobic glycolysis and the Krebs cycle are limited to the epithelium or superficial fibers that still have mitochondria. The thickness of the lens cortex, in which newer fibers are present and which still contains organelles, is approximately 100 microns.[62] ATP activity is higher in the epithelial cells and the newer fibers of the cortex near the equator and is lower near the poles. There is no such activity in the lens nucleus, and the fibers in the nucleus are not capable of protein synthesis.[69]

IONIC CURRENT

An ionic current has been identified flowing out of the lens at the equator and into the lens at the poles (Figure 5-11).[24,69] It is likely that ATPase activity contributes to this current because the distribution of ATPase pumps is coincident with this pattern.[71] The Na^+K^+/ATPase activity generates an electrochemical gradient with the interior of the lens more negative than its surrounding environment. This circulating ionic flow might help circulate solutes to the deep lens fibers and transport wastes out of the fibers and out of the lens.[68] The fluid would follow the same pathway as the ionic current, facilitating water and metabolite (glucose, ascorbate, and amino acids) movement into the deeper fibers.[24] Water and solutes enter the lens through extracellular spaces at the anterior and posterior polar regions,

Anterior pole

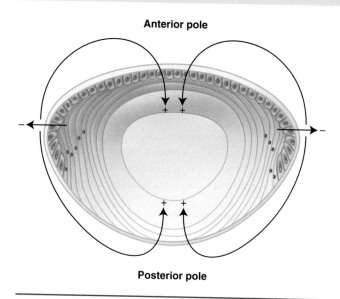

Posterior pole

FIGURE 5-11
Schematic of the ionic current in the lens.

cross fiber membranes to the lens interior, and then flow through fibers back to the surface at the equator, matching the distribution of the ionic pumps and channels.[68]

REGULATION OF FLUID VOLUME

Cl^- flux appears to be the important factor in regulating fluid volume.[68] The $Na^+K^+/2Cl^-$ and $K^+/2Cl^-$ cotransporters and Cl^- channels maintain ion concentration gradients at a level that keeps water in equilibrium across the cell and fiber membranes.[24,68] The membranes of the epithelium and the fibers are highly permeable and aquaporins are numerous, enhancing water movement into and out of the lens.[72]

ULTRAVIOLET RADIATION (UVR)

The cornea absorbs wavelengths below 300 nm, the lens absorbs wavelengths between 300 and 400 nm, and wavelengths greater than 400 nm are transmitted to the retina. The lens absorbs almost all UVR to which it is exposed, and any resulting unstable free radicals cause molecular changes.[73] The first active tissue of the lens that encounters UVR is the lens epithelium, which is susceptible to damage from free radicals. Morphologic changes apparent in the epithelial layer may lead to irreversible changes throughout the lens, although the mechanism by which this progresses has not been defined.[74]

UVR absorbed by lens fibers causes oxidative damage, leading to degradation and modification of lens

proteins. An association exists between ocular exposure and increased risk of lens opacity.[75,76] UVR absorption also increases chromophore concentration; yellow pigments accumulate in the center of the lens.[73] The yellowing may progress to a dark-brown hue, which is called **lens brunescence.**[25]

OXIDATIVE STRESS

Free radicals are generated both by UVR absorption and by cellular metabolic processes. Oxidative stress results when the rate of free radical production is greater than the rate of their degradation. Oxidative stress can impair the structure and function of connexins (gap junction proteins), can modify lens crystallins, and can cause aggregation of proteins, all of which contribute to cataract development.[77] **Glutathione** is a reducing agent that detoxifies free radicals, thus preventing such damage. It is found in high concentration within the lens and the aqueous humor and is transported into the lens from the aqueous. It can be synthesized and regenerated by the lens epithelial cells and young lens fibers.[68] The deeper fibers rely on diffusion of glutathione from superficial fibers.[78] Glutathione also has a role in maintaining membrane transport mechanisms.[78]

Ascorbic acid also provides some protection to lens epithelium against UV-induced damage to deoxyribonucleic acid (DNA) and is present in relatively high levels in the aqueous humor.[79]

AGING CHANGES IN CRYSTALLINE LENS

The lens grows throughout life. The majority of the increase in thickness occurs between ages 8 and 40, accompanied by an increase in surface curvatures, a forward movement of the center of the lens, and a decrease in anterior chamber depth.[2,35,53,80] Other physical changes that accompany age were described in the section about presbyopia. Changes occur in lens physiology as mature lens fibers lose all cellular organelles. A coincident decrease in the transport of ions, nutrients, and antioxidants may lead to damage contributing to cataract formation.[81] With age there is an increase in fiber membrane permeability and the ionic pumps may not be able to compensate, disrupting ion balance. Circulation within the lens changes and restriction of the flow of water and of glutathione occurs at the cortex/nucleus border. Significant changes in aquaporins occur, causing a disruption of water flow.[82]

The amount of water soluble alpha crystallins decreases with age, and by age 45 there are no alpha crystallins evident in the lens nucleus. Since the alpha crystallins help to prevent other crystallins from forming aggregates, water insoluble aggregates increase with age.[77] Some components of the cytoskeleton disassemble.[83] Levels of UVR filters in the lens decrease approximately 12% per decade, allowing increased UVR damage.[63]

Clinical manifestations of aging are presbyopia and cataract formation. Both processes affect vision and are a significant concern to the patient and to the clinician, particularly because few preventive measures are available. Recommendations to patients should include the use of UVR-absorbing lenses when outdoors; the incidence of cataract is higher in those exposed to greater levels of sunlight.[73]

Clinical Comment: The Lens Paradox

Because the lens continues to grow, it would seem that its refractive power should change, yet it remains constant. With age the radii of curvature decrease; the anterior radius of curvature decreases to approximately 8.25 μm and the posterior radius to about 7 μm by 80 years of age.[55] As the lens surface becomes more steeply curved, refractive power should increase. However, the lens thickness increases primarily in the width of the lens cortex, and as the lens becomes more optically homogenous, there is less of an affect from the gradient nature of the index of refraction; these changes apparently compensate for the increased surface curvatures, and the power of the lens remains stable.[84-87]

CATARACTS

Clinical Comment: Clinical Cataract

Although any lens opacity is accurately called a cataract, the clinician should be aware of the impact that the word "cataract" may have on a patient. Cataracts are the greatest cause of blindness worldwide. The etiology of cataract formation is complex, and cataract development is often the result of multiple factors that influence lens metabolism. Risk factors include aging, disease, genetics, nutritional or metabolic deficiencies, trauma, congenital factors, and environmental stress (e.g., radiation), with age being the major contributor.[88]

*Cataracts are named according to location or cause and can be graded based on severity (Figure 5-12). An opacity located in the embryonic, fetal, or adult nucleus is called a **nuclear cataract** (Figure 5-13). The center opacification accompanying the onset of a nuclear cataract can increase refractive power, and in the hyperopic patient this myopic shift causes a temporary improvement in vision. **Brunescence** accompanies nuclear cataracts caused by increased chromophore concentration. The increase in yellow coloration results in the absorption of wavelengths in the blue end of the spectrum, which may actually provide some protection for the macula.*

*A **cortical cataract**, located in the cortex, has a spokelike shape; thicker in the periphery and tapering toward the lens center, it follows the shape of the fiber (Figure 5-14). Cortical cataracts generally progress slowly; with time the spoke width expands as the opacity spreads to adjacent fibers.[89,90] Fluid accumulates and membrane rupture in the equatorial area can occur.[91] Cortical cataracts affect vision only when they spread into the center of the lens and cause light scatter in the pupillary region.*

Table 5-1   Zones of Discontinuity

Zones of Discontinuity	Correlative Lens Morphology
Anterior capsular zone	Anterior lens capsule
Anterior subcapsular zone	Anterior lens epithelium, elongating fibers, and outermost cortical fibers
Anterior zone of disjunction	Anterior segments of cortical fibers formed after sexual maturation, complex sutures
Anterior zone of the adult nucleus	Anterior half of the adult nucleus consisting of secondary fibers formed after birth to sexual maturation
Anterior zone of the fetal nucleus	Anterior half of the fetal nucleus consisting of secondary fibers formed before birth
	Location of upright Y suture
Zone of the embryonic nucleus	Embryonic nucleus consisting of primary lens fibers formed during first 2 months of embryonic development
Posterior zone of the fetal nucleus	Posterior half of the fetal nucleus consisting of secondary fibers formed before birth
	Location of inverted Y suture
Posterior zone of the adult nucleus	Posterior half of the adult nucleus consisting of secondary fibers formed after birth to sexual maturation
Posterior subcapsular zone	Posterior segments of elongating fibers and the outermost cortical fibers, complex sutures
Posterior capsular zone	Posterior lens capsule

Adapted from Kuszak JR, Deutsch TA, Brown HG: Anatomy of aged and senile cataractous lenses. In Albert DM, Jakobiec FA, editors: *Principles and practice of ophthalmology: basic sciences*, Philadelphia, 1994, Saunders.

*A **posterior subcapsular cataract** is a disturbance located just beneath the posterior capsule (Figure 5-15). This type of cataract impacts vision early and significantly given its location along the visual axis and near the nodal point of the eye. A significant risk factor for posterior subcapsular cataracts is long-term, high-dose steroid use.*

Clinical Comment: Cataract Surgery

The decision for cataract removal is determined by the effect the cataract has on the patient's everyday life. When a person is not able to perform the usual daily activities because of reduced vision caused by the opacity, the lens should be removed. Cataract extraction is a relatively safe surgical procedure usually done under local anesthesia. A small incision is made to allow entrance of surgical instruments into the anterior chamber. The anterior lens capsule is opened and the lens epithelium and all fibers are removed, with the lens capsule remaining intact. An intraocular lens (IOL) can then be inserted into the lens capsule to replace the power of the missing lens. Multifocal IOLs that correct for presbyopia may be an option.

The Physiology of Cataract Formation

Numerous mechanisms are presumed causative for cataracts, including fluid and ion imbalance, oxidative damage, protein modification, and metabolic disruption.[66] A disturbance in fluid regulation can be caused by ionic pump dysfunction and/or membrane permeability increase that allows water accumulation. If Na^+/K^+ ATPase pump activity decreases significantly, a rise in Na^+ in the cytoplasm is accompanied by an influx of water, the lens fibers swell and transparency diminishes.[69] An increased level of cytoplasmic Ca^{++} is also associated with a loss of transparency.[69] Water accumulation between fibers can form vacuoles causing a disruption of fiber arrangement and increased light scatter. UVR and oxidative damage as a result of free radical accumulation affects cellular function, damages lens DNA, causes protein modification, and high-molecular-weight crystallin aggregations, any of which can increase light scatter.[25] Alpha crystallins, as molecular chaperones, help to stabilize beta/gamma crystallin configuration but by age 40 have disappeared from the lens nucleus, although the normal lens usually remains fairly transparent for years past that age.[92] But as the concentration of alpha crystallins is reduced, aggregates accumulate and with time form light-scattering opacities.

Glutathione and ascorbate maintain a reducing environment providing some protection from free radical damage and preventing protein modification. Reduced levels of glutathione allow oxidative damage to membranes and proteins.[77] A decrease in glutathione

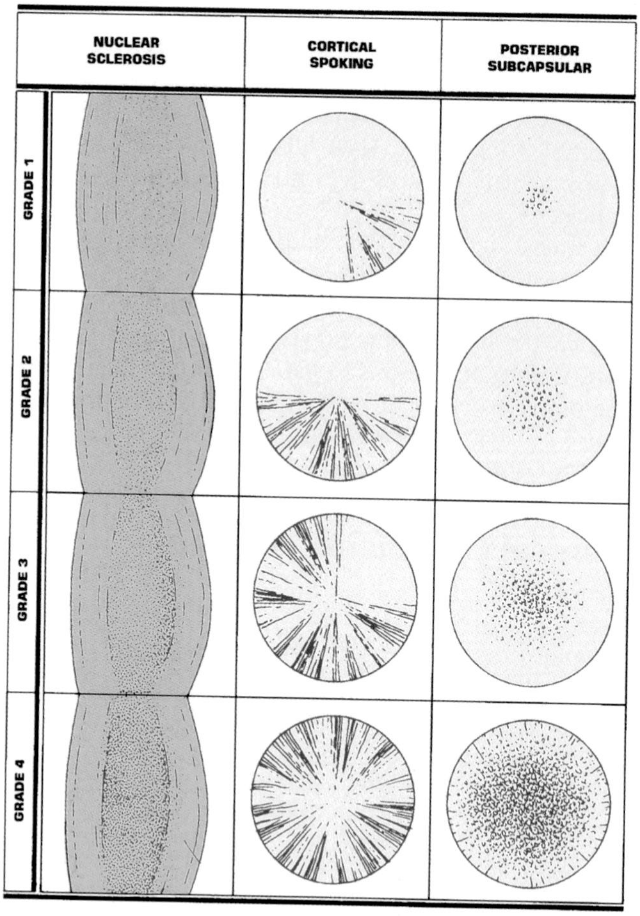

FIGURE 5-12
Grading system for age-related cataracts. Nuclear sclerotic changes are shown in cross section, with anterior surface to the left. Cortical and posterior subcapsular changes are seen in retroillumination. (From Fingeret M, Casser L, Woodcome HT: *Atlas of primary eyecare procedures*, Norwalk, Conn, 1992, Appleton & Lange.)

concentration is associated with cataract development.[92,93] A barrier, speculated to develop in middle age and located at the interface of the cortex and nucleus, seems to impede the flow of small molecules from the cortex into the nucleus and might account for the reduction in glutathione in the nucleus.[91] A modification of the connexins in gap junctions causes a disruption in communication between fibers and might be one cause of this barrier.[94,95] Changes occur in aquaporin channel proteins in the innermost nuclear regions of the lens as early as age 5 and by middle age (age 40 to 50), half of such channels are lost in the region of the speculated barrier.[82] These changes can lead to the occlusion of the water channels and contribute to the barrier function.

A **diabetic cataract** results from elevated glucose levels and can develop rapidly. With increased blood glucose, excess glucose present in the aqueous enters

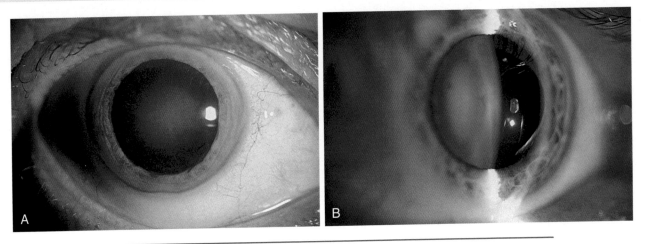

FIGURE 5-13
Nuclear cataract seen with **A,** diffuse illumination, and **B,** optic section. (From Kanski JJ, Nischal KK: *Ophthalmology: clinical signs and differential diagnosis,* St Louis, 2000, Mosby.)

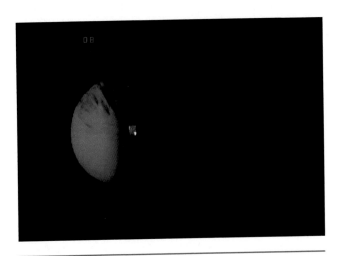

FIGURE 5-14
Spokes of a cortical cataract visible against the red reflex. (Courtesy Pacific University Family Vision Center, Forest Grove, Ore.)

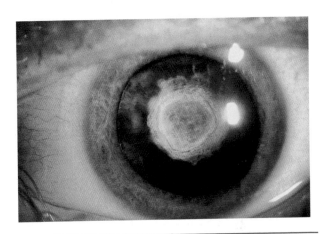

FIGURE 5-15
Posterior subcapsular cataract. (From Kanski JJ, Nischal KK: *Ophthalmology: clinical signs and differential diagnosis,* St Louis, 2000, Mosby.)

the lens. As this excess glucose is metabolized, sorbitol accumulates faster than it is converted to fructose. Sorbitol concentration increases within the lens fiber, because sorbitol does not readily pass through the fiber membrane, and thus water is drawn into the fiber. The fibers swell, the lens loses transparency, and the fibers may eventually rupture.

Age-Related *Cortical* Cataract

High lifetime exposure to UVR is associated with increased incidence of cortical cataracts; the paradox is that the most severe damage in cortical cataracts occurs near the equator initially, the area most protected from sunlight by the iris. Cortical cataracts are associated with increased membrane permeability and ion transporters, pumps, and exchangers are not able to maintain the

homeostatic concentration.[71] An increased concentration of Ca^{++} in the fiber cytoplasm also drives fluid accumulation.[69] Affected regions of the fiber show disruption of structure and can include membrane rupture. The changes first occur in the center of the elongated fiber (that is at the equatorial region), with the apical and basal ends remaining transparent. Generally the tapered fiber ends, located at the sutures in the optical axis, are only affected very late in the life of the cortical cataract.

Age-Related *Nuclear* Cataract

Age-related nuclear cataracts are associated with a decline of glutathione, making the fibers susceptible to oxidative damage. Levels can be significantly reduced in the nucleus while levels in the cortex remain within the normal range.[78,94] Oxidative protein modification increases significantly after age 50, contributing to the damage seen in *senile nuclear sclerosis*.[92] The color changes that often accompany nuclear cataracts are usually seen as various hues of yellow or brown; this pigmentation is primarily protein-bound.[91]

Posterior Subcapsular Cataract (PSC)

The opacity in the posterior subcapsular region is formed by epithelial-like cells that migrate from the equatorial region. These cells accumulate at the posterior pole forming an opacity.[96] It is speculated that radiation damage is one causative factor as patients undergoing radiation therapy for cancer treatments also develop PSCs and/or cortical cataracts.[62] There are some sutural congenital cataracts that occur at this location, but they are caused by swelling of the basal ends of cortical fibers.[62]

Steroid-Induced Cataract

Steroid-induced cataracts are also located in the posterior subcapsular region. Dosage and the duration of steroid use appear to be controlling factors, although individuals may have varying levels of susceptibility. Children develop such cataracts at a faster rate than do adults. Reversal of the cataract can occur but this is rare.[5,37,66] The opacity appears to be formed of undifferentiated epithelial cells at the interface of the posterior cortex and capsule. These misplaced cells (which should only be present in the lens epithelium) display aberrant behavior. The undifferentiated cells may have migrated from the preequatorial area, influenced by a change in the concentration of growth factors.[66] The growth factors governing mitosis, migration, and differentiation are obtained from aqueous and reside in the lens capsule. If steroids influence production of these growth factors that are present in the aqueous, and the concentration and location in the capsule is altered, cellular processes can be affected.[66]

REFERENCES

1. Patterson CA, Delamere NA: The lens. In Hart WM, editor: *Adler's physiology of the eye*, ed 9, St Louis, 1992, Mosby, p 348.
2. Dubbelman M, van der Heijde GL, Weeber HA: The thickness of the aging human lens obtained from corrected Scheimpflug images, *Optom Vis Sci* 78(6):411, 2001.
3. Koretz JE, Strenk SA, Strenk LM, et al: Scheimpflug and high resolution magnetic resonance imaging of the anterior segment: a comparative study, *J Opt Soc Am A Opt Image Sci Vis* 21:346–354, 2004.
4. Hogan MJ, Alvarado JA, Weddell JE: *Histology of the human eye*, Philadelphia, 1971, Saunders, p 638.
5. Strenk SA, Semmlow JL, Strenk LM, et al: Age-related changes in ciliary muscle and lens: a magnetic resonance imaging study, *Invest Ophthalmol Vis Sci* 40:1162, 1999.
6. Jones CE, Atchison DA, Pope JM: Changes in lens dimensions and refractive index with age and accommodation, *Optom Vis Sci* 84:990–995, 2007.
7. Rosen AM, Denham DB, Fernandez V, et al: in vitro dimensions and curvatures of human lenses, *Vision Res* 46:1002–1009, 2006.
8. Glasser A, Kaufman PL: Accommodation and presbyopia. In Kaufman PL, Alm A, editors: *Adler's physiology of the eye*, ed 10, St Louis, 2003, Mosby, p 197.
9. Smith G, Pierscionek BK: The optical structure of the lens and its contribution to the refractive status of the eye, *Ophthalmic Physiol Opt* 18(1):21, 1998.
10. Pierscionek BK: Refractive index contours in the human lens, *Exp Eye Res* 64:887, 1997.
11. Borish IM: *Clinical refraction*, ed 3, Chicago, 1975, Professional Press, p 169.
12. Koretz JF, Handelman GH, Brown NP: Analysis of human crystalline lens curvature as a function of accommodative state and age, *Vision Res* 24:1141, 1984.
13. Kuszak JR, Brown HG: Embryology and anatomy of the lens. In Albert DM, Jakobiec FA, editors: *Principles and practice of ophthalmology*, Philadelphia, 1994, Saunders, p 82.
14. Barraquer RI, Michael R, Abreu R, et al: Human lens capsule thickness as a function of age and location along the sagittal lens perimeter, *Invest Ophthalmol Vis Sci* 47:2053–2060, 2006.
15. Alexander RA, Garner A: Elastic and precursor fibres in the normal human eye, *Exp Eye Res* 36:305, 1983.
16. Krag S, Olsen T, Andreassen TT: Biomechanical characteristics of the human anterior lens capsule in relation to age, *Invest Ophthalmol Vis Sci* 38(2):357, 1997.
17. Kuwabara T: The maturation of the lens cell: a morphologic study, *Exp Eye Res* 20:427, 1975.
18. Kuszak JR, Peterson KL, Brown HG: Electron microscopic observations of the crystalline lens, *Microsc Res Tech* 33:441, 1996.
19. Bassnett S, Kuszak JR, Reinisch L, et al: Intercellular communication between epithelial and fiber cells of the eye lens, *J Cell Sci* 107:799, 1994.
20. Rae J: Physiology of the lens. In Albert DM, Jakobiec FA, editors: *Principles and practice of ophthalmology*, Philadelphia, 1994, Saunders, p 123.
21. Kuszak JR, Novak LA, Brown HG: An ultrastructural analysis of the epithelial-fiber interface (EFI) in primate lenses, *Exp Eye Res* 61:579, 1995.
22. Lo WK, Harding CV: Structure and distribution of gap junctions in lens epithelium and fiber cells, *Cell Tissue Res* 244(2):253, 1986.
23. Lo WK, Harding CV: Tight junctions in the lens epithelia of human and frog: freeze-fracture and protein tracer studies, *Invest Ophthalmol Vis Sci* 24(4):396, 1983.
24. Mathias RT, Kistler J, Donaldson P: The lens circulation, *J Membr Biol* 216:1–16, 2007.
25. Vavvas D, Azar NF, Azar DT: Mechanisms of disease: cataracts, *Ophthalmol Clin North Am* 15:49, 2002.
26. Clark JI: Development and maintenance of lens transparency. In Albert DM, Jakobiec FA, editors: *Principles and practice of ophthalmology*, Philadelphia, 1994, Saunders, p 114.
27. Mathias RT, Rae JL: Transport properties of the lens, *Am J Physiol* 249(3):181, 1985.
28. Dahm R, van Marle J, Prescott AR, et al: Gap junctions containing alpha8-connexin (MP70) in the adult mammalian lens epithelium suggests a re-evaluation of its role in the lens, *Exp Eye Res* 69:45, 1999.
29. Kuszak JR, Peterson KL, Sivak JG, et al: The interrelationship of lens anatomy and optical quality. II. Primate lenses, *Exp Eye Res* 59(5):521, 1994.
30. Streeten BW, Licari PA: The zonules and the elastic microfibrillar system in the ciliary body, *Invest Ophthalmol Vis Sci* 24(6):667, 1983.
31. Bourge JL, Robert AM, Renard G: Zonular fibers, multimolecular composition as related to function (elasticity) and pathology, *Pathol Biol (Paris)* 55:347–359, 2007.

32. Rohen JW: Scanning electron microscopic studies of the zonular apparatus in human and monkey eyes, *Invest Ophthalmol Vis Sci* 18:133, 1979.

33. Von Helmholtz HH: Treatise on physiologic optics, Mineola, NY, 1962, Dover (Translated by JPC Southhall), p 143.

34. Von Noorden G: *Burien and von Noorden's binocular vision and ocular motility*, ed 5, St Louis, 1996, Mosby, p 85.

35. Johnson CA: Effects of luminance and stimulus distance on accommodation and visual resolution, *J Opt Soc Am* 66:138–142, 1976.

36. Garner LF, Smith G: Changes in equivalent and gradient refractive index of the crystalline lens with accommodation, *Optom Vis Sci* 74(2):114, 1997.

37. Garner LF, Yap MK: Changes in ocular dimensions and refraction with accommodation, *Ophthalmic Physiol Opt* 17(1):12, 1997.

38. Drexler W, Baumgartner A, Findl O, et al: Biometric investigation of changes in the anterior eye segment during accommodation, *Vision Res* 37:2789, 1997.

39. Drexler W, Findl O, Schmetterer L, et al: Eye elongation during accommodation in humans: differences between emmetropes and myopes, *Invest Ophthalmol Vis Sci* 39(11):2140, 1998.

40. Koretz JF, Bertasso AM, Neider MW, et al: Slit-lamp studies of the rhesus monkey eye. II. Changes in crystalline lens shape, thickness and position during accommodation and aging, *Exp Eye Res* 45:317, 1987.

41. Ludwig K, Wegscheider E, Hoops JP, et al: in vivo imaging of the human zonular apparatus with high-resolution ultrasound biomicroscopy, *Graefes Arch Clin Exp Ophthalmol* 237:361–371, 1999.

42. Fisher RF: The vitreous and lens in accommodation, *Trans Ophthalmol Soc U K* 102:318, 1982.

43. Mauger RR, Likens CP, Applebaum M: Effects of accommodation and repeated applanation tonometry on intraocular pressure, *Am J Optom Physiol Opt* 6(1):28, 1984.

44. Hamasaki D, Ong J, Marg E: The amplitude of accommodation in presbyopia, *Am J Optom Arch Am Acad Optom* 33:3–14, 1956.

45. Pardue MT, Sivak JG: Age-related changes in human ciliary muscle, *Optom Vis Sci* 77:204, 2000.

46. Hermans EA, Dubbelman M, van der Heijde GL, et al: Change in the accommodative force on the lens of the human eye with age, *Vision Res* 48:119–126, 2008.

47. Strenk SA, Strenk LM, Guo S: Magnetic resonance imaging of aging, accommodating, phakic, and pseudophakic ciliary muscle diameters, *J Cataract Refract Surg* 32:1792–1798, 2006.

48. Sakabe I, Oshika T, Lim SJ, et al: Anterior shift of zonular insertion onto the anterior surface of human crystalline lens with age, *Ophthalmology* 105(2):295, 1998.

49. Assia EI, Apple DJ, Morgan RC, et al: The relationship between stretching capability of the anterior capsule and zonules, *Invest Ophthalmol Vis Sci* 32:2835–2839, 1991.

50. Fisher RF: The influence of age on some ocular basement membranes, *Eye* 1:184–189, 1987.

51. Krag S, Andreassen TT: Mechanical properties of the human posterior lens capsule, *Invest Ophthalmol Vis Sci* 44:691, 2003.

52. Seland JH: Ultrastructural changes in the normal human lens capsule from birth to old age, *Acta Ophthalmol* 52:688, 1974.

53. Glasser A, Campbell MC: Biometric, optical and physical changes in the isolated human crystalline lens with age in relation to presbyopia, *Vision Res* 39:1991, 1999.

54. Beers AP, van der Heijde GL: Age-related changes in the accommodation mechanism, *Optom Vis Sci* 73(4):235, 1996.

55. Brown N: The change in lens curvature with age, *Exp Eye Res* 19:175, 1974.

56. Brandreth RH: *Clinical slit lamp biomicroscopy*, Berkeley, Calif, 1978, Brandreth.

57. Sasaki K, Kojirna M, Hara T: in vivo observation of the crystalline lens capsule, *Ophthalmic Res* 20(3):154, 1988.

58. Trokel S: The physical basis for transparency of the crystalline lens, *Invest Ophthalmol* 1:493, 1962.

59. Danysh BP, Duncan MK: The lens capsule, *Exp Eye Res* 88:151–164, 2009.

60. Hejtmancik JF: Congenital cataracts and their molecular genetics, *Semin Cell Dev Biol* 19:134–149, 2008.

61. Chong HNV: *Clinical ocular physiology*, Butterworth Heinemann, Linacre House, Oxford, UK, 1996, Jordan Hill, p 41.

62. Beebe DC: The lens. In Kaufman PL, Alm A, editors: *Adler's physiology of the eye*, ed 10, St Louis, 2003, Mosby, p 117.

63. Truscott RJ: Presbyopia. Emerging from a blur towards an understanding of the molecular basis for this most common eye condition, *Exp Eye Res* 88:241–247, 2009.

64. Takemoto L, Sorensen CM: Protein-protein interactions and lens transparency, *Exp Eye Res* 87:496–501, 2008.

65. Zelenka PS, Arpitha P: Coordinating cell proliferation and migration in the lens and cornea, *Sem Cell Develop Bio* 19:113–124, 2008.

66. Jobling AI, Augusteyn RC: What induces steroid cataracts? A review of steroid-induced posterior subcapsular cataracts, *Clin Exp Optom* 85:61–75, 2002.

67. Rao PV, Maddala R: The role of the lens actin cytoskeleton in fiber cell elongation and differentiation, *Sem Cell Dev Bio* 17:698–711, 2006.

68. Donaldson PJ, Chee KS, Lim JC, et al: Regulation of lens volume: Implication for lens transparency, *Exp Eye Res* 88:144–150, 2009.

69. Delamere NA, Tamiya S: Lens Na$^+$, K$^+$-ATPase. In Tombran-Tink J, Barnstable CJ, editors: *Ophthalmology research: ocular transporters in ophthalmic diseases and drug delivery*, Totowa, NJ, 2008, Humana Press, pp 111–123.

70. Bassnett S, Beebe DC: Coincident loss of mitochondria and nuclei during lens fiber cell differentiation, *Dev Dyn* 194:85–92, 1992.

71. Delamere NA, Tamiya S: Lens ion transport: from basic concepts to regulation of Na$^+$, K-ATPase activity, *Exp Eye Res* 88:140–143, 2009.

72. Zampighi GA: The lens. In Fischbarg J, editor: *The biology of the eye*, Amsterdam, 2006, Elsevier, pp 149–179.

73. Young RW: The family of sunlight-related eye diseases, *Optom Vis Sci* 71(2):125, 1994.

74. Hightower KR, Reddan JR, McCready JP, et al: Lens epithelium: a primary target of UVB irradiation, *Exp Eye Res* 59:557, 1994.

75. Hightower KR: The role of the lens epithelium in development of UV cataract, *Curr Eye Res* 14:71, 1995.

76. West SK, Duncan DD, Muñoz B, et al: Sunlight exposure and risk of lens opacities in a population-based study, *Arch Ophthalmol* 116:1666, 1998.

77. Berthoud VM, Beyer EC: Oxidative stress, lens gap junctions, and cataracts, *Antioxid Redox Signal* 11:339–353, 2009.

78. Reddy VN: Glutathione and its function in the lens—an overview, *Exp Eye Res* 50:771–778, 1990.

79. Reddy VN, Giblin FJ, Lin LR, et al: The effect of aqueous humor ascorbate on ultraviolet-B-induced DNA damage in lens epithelium, *Invest Ophthalmol Vis Sci* 39(2):344, 1998.

80. Alió JL, Schimchak P, Negri HP, et al: Crystalline lens optical dysfunction through aging, *Ophthalmology* 112:2022–2029, 2005.

81. Moffat BA, Landman KA, Truscott RJ, et al: Age-related changes in the kinetics of water transport in normal human lenses, *Exp Eye Res* 69(6):663, 1999.

82. Korlimbinis A, Berry Y, Thibault D, et al: Protein aging: truncation of aquaporin 0 in human lens regions is a continuous age-dependent process, *Exp Eye Res* 88:966–973, 2009.

83. Friedrich MG, Truscott RJ: Membrane association of proteins in the aging human lens: Profound changes take place in the fifth decade of life, *Invest Ophthalmol Vis Sci* 50:4786–4793, 2009.

84. Pierscionek BK: Age-related response of human lenses to stretching forces, *Exp Eye Res* 60:325, 1995.

85. Moffat BA, Atchison DA, Pope JM: Age-related changes in refractive index distribution and power of the human lens as measured by magnetic resonance micro-imaging in vitro, *Vis Res* 42:1683, 2002.

86. Dubbelman M, van der Heijde GL: The shape of the aging human lens: curvature, equivalent refractive index and the lens paradox, *Vision Res* 41:1867, 2001.

87. Charman WN: The eye in focus: accommodation and presbyopia, *Clin Exp Optom* 91:207–225, 2008.

88. Cruickshanks KJ, Klein BE, Klein R: Ultraviolet light exposure and lens opacities: the Beaver Dam Eye Study, *Am J Public Health* 82(12):1658, 1992.

89. Brown NP, Harris ML, Shun-Shin GA, et al: Is cortical spoke cataract due to lens fibre breaks? The relationship between fibre folds, fibre breaks, waterclefts and spoke cataract, *Eye* 7:672, 1993.

90. Vrensen G, Willekens B: Biomicroscopy and scanning electron microscopy of early opacities in the aging human lens, *Invest Ophthalmol Vis Sci* 31(8):1582, 1990.

91. Truscott RJ: Age-related nuclear cataract-oxidation is the key, *Exp Eye Res* 80:709–725, 2005.

92. Sweeney MH, Truscott RJ: An impediment to glutathione diffusion in older normal human lenses: a possible precondition for nuclear cataract, *Exp Eye Res* 67:587, 1998.

93. Truscott RJ: Age-related nuclear cataract: a lens transport problem, *Ophthalmol Res* 32:185, 2000.

94. Sweeney MH, Truscott RJ: An impediment to glutathione diffusion in older normal human lenses: a possible precondition for nuclear cataract, *Exp Eye Res* 67:587–595, 1998.

95. Moffat BA, Landman KA, Truscott RJ, et al: Age-related changes in the kinetics of water transport in normal human lenses, *Exp Eye Res* 69:663–669, 1999.

96. Streeten BW, Eshaghian J: Human posterior subcapsular cataract. A gross and flat preparation study, *Arch Ophthalmol* 96:1653–1658, 1978.

The aqueous and vitreous are contained in three chambers within the eye. The anterior and posterior chambers contain aqueous humor, and the vitreous chamber contains the vitreous gel. A description of each chamber will be followed by an explanation of the formation, composition, and function of the aqueous and the vitreous.

ANTERIOR CHAMBER

The anterior chamber is bounded anteriorly by the corneal endothelium; peripherally by the trabecular meshwork, a portion of the ciliary body, and the iris root; and posteriorly by the anterior iris surface and the pupillary area of the anterior lens (Figure 6-1). The center of the anterior chamber is deeper than the periphery. The anterior chamber angle is formed at the periphery of the chamber, where the corneoscleral and uveal coats meet. The aqueous humor exits the anterior chamber through the structures located in this angle.

ANTERIOR CHAMBER ANGLE STRUCTURES

The structures through which aqueous exits, collectively called the filtration apparatus, consist of the trabecular meshwork and Schlemm's canal. These structures and the scleral spur occupy the excavated area located at the internal corneoscleral junction known as the **internal scleral sulcus.**

Scleral Spur

The **scleral spur** lies at the posterior edge of the internal scleral sulcus (see Chapter 2). The posterior portion of the scleral spur is the attachment site for the tendon of the longitudinal ciliary muscle fibers, whereas many of the trabecular meshwork sheets attach to the spur's anterior aspect, such that the collagen of the spur is continuous with that of the trabeculae[1] (Figure 6-2).

Trabecular Meshwork

The **trabecular meshwork** encircles the circumference of the anterior chamber, occupying most of the inner aspect of the internal scleral sulcus. In cross section it

has a triangular shape, with its *apex* at the termination of Descemet's membrane (Schwalbe's line) and its *base* at the scleral spur (Figure 6-3). The inner face borders the anterior chamber, and the outer side lies against corneal stroma, sclera, and Schlemm's canal. The meshwork is composed of flattened perforated sheets, with three to five sheets at the apex. These sheets branch into 15 to 20 sheets as they extend posteriorly from Schwalbe's line to the scleral spur.[2] The trabecular meshwork is an open latticework, the branches of which interlace. The intertrabecular spaces between the sheets are connected through pores, or openings within the sheets (historically called the "spaces of Fontana").[3] The openings are of varying sizes and become smaller near Schlemm's canal. No apertures directly join the meshwork with the canal.[2] A small aspect of the meshwork at the most anterior location is adjacent to connective tissue of the limbus and differs in structure from the filtering portion. Some believe that this is a niche where cells reside that have properties similar to stem cells. These cells may be capable of replacing the endothelial cells of the trabecular meshwork after injury.[4]

The meshwork can be separated into two anatomic divisions. The **corneoscleral meshwork** is the outer region; its sheets attach to the scleral spur. The inner sheets, which lie inner to the spur and attach to the ciliary stroma and longitudinal muscle fibers, make up the **uveal meshwork;** some of these sheets may attach to the iris root.[3,5] The two portions differ slightly in structure; the corneoscleral meshwork is sheetlike, and the uveal meshwork is cordlike[2] (Figure 6-4). The pores in the uveal meshwork are the largest, and pore size diminishes in the sheets closer to the canal. Projections from the surface layer of the iris, known as iris processes, connect to the trabeculae, usually projecting no farther forward than the midpoint of the meshwork.[2]

The meshwork trabeculae consist of an inner core of collagen and elastic fibers[6] embedded in ground substance and covered by basement membrane and endothelium.[7] The endothelial cells are a continuation of the corneal endothelium.[5,8] The endothelial cells contain the cellular organelles for protein synthesis and apparently are capable of replacing the connective tissue components. These cells also contain lysosomes, which give them the capacity for phagocytosis.[5] Gap junctions and short areas of tight junctions join the endothelial

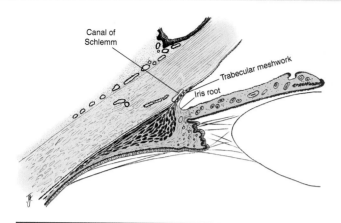

FIGURE 6-1

Periphery of the anterior segment. Structures of the anterior chamber angle are labeled.

cells; no zonula occludens are found.[9] Cytoplasmic projections connect cells of neighboring sheets.[5,9,10]

At the scleral spur, the trabecular sheets lose their endothelial covering, but the collagenous and elastic fibers continue into the connective tissue of the spur and ciliary body.[2,5] Some connective tissue fibers of the ciliary muscle pass forward and merge with the inner sheets of the meshwork.[11]

Canal of Schlemm

The **canal of Schlemm** is a circular vessel and is considered to be a venous channel, although it normally contains aqueous humor rather than blood. It is outer to the trabecular meshwork and anterior to the scleral spur. The external wall of the canal lies against the limbal sclera, and the internal wall lies against the juxtacanalicular connective tissue and the scleral spur (see Figure 6-2). Thin tissue septa may bridge the lumen, dividing it into several channels.[2,3]

The lumen is lined with endothelial cells, many of which are joined by zonula occludens.[2,9,12] The endothelial cells have an incomplete basement membrane.[2,3,7] The continuous endothelial lining with cells joined by tight junctions make the canal similar to blood vessels, whereas the discontinuous basement membrane make it similar to lymph channels.[13] The tight junctions of the inner wall restrict flow into the canal between the lateral walls of the cells. Pores and pinocytic vesicles in the cell membrane may be an avenue for passage of aqueous humor.[2,3,14-16]

Juxtacanalicular Connective Tissue

The region separating the endothelial cell lining of the canal from the trabecular meshwork is called the **juxtacanalicular tissue**[5,11] or the **cribriform layer**.[5,15,17] It consists of endothelial cells and fibroblasts embedded in a matrix of collagen, elastic-like fibers, and ground

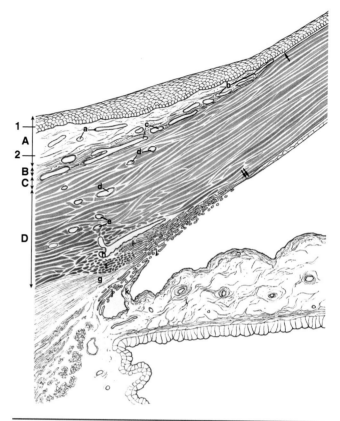

FIGURE 6-2

Drawing of the limbus. Limbal conjunctiva (*A*) is formed by an epithelium (*1*) and a loose connective tissue stroma (*2*). Tenon's capsule (*B*) forms a thin, poorly defined connective tissue layer over episclera (*C*). Limbal stroma occupies the area (*D*) and is composed of scleral and corneal tissues, which merge in this region. Conjunctival stromal vessels are seen at *a*; they form peripheral corneal arcades (*b*), which extend anteriorly to termination of Bowman's layer (*arrow*). Episcleral vessels (*c*) are cut in different planes. Vessels forming intrascleral plexus (*d*) and deep scleral plexus (*e*) are shown within limbal stroma. Scleral spur, with its coarse, dense collagen fibers, is shown at *f*. Anterior part of longitudinal portion of ciliary muscle (*g*) merges with scleral spur and trabecular meshwork. Lumen of Schlemm's canal (*h*) and loose tissues of its wall are clearly seen. Sheets of trabecular meshwork (*i*) are outer to cords of uveal meshwork (*j*). An iris process (*k*) arises from iris surface and joins trabecular meshwork at level of anterior portion of scleral spur. Descemet's membrane terminates (*double arrows*) within anterior portion of the triangle, outlining aqueous outflow system. (From Hogan MJ, Alvarado JA, Weddell JE: *Histology of the human eye,* Philadelphia, 1971, Saunders.)

substance.[15,18-20] The cells of this region have processes occasionally joined by adhering and gap junctions. The cells also form similar connections with the endothelium of the inner wall of Schlemm's canal.[21] There are micronsized spaces within the juxtacanalicular tissue that appear to lack extracellular matrix (although these may be presumed spaces whose material is yet to be observed)[22]

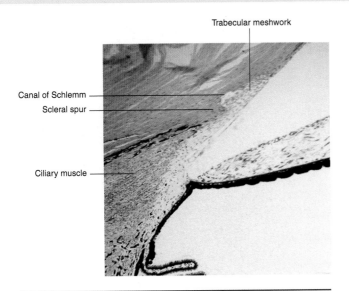

Trabecular meshwork

Canal of Schlemm —

Scleral spur —

Ciliary muscle —

FIGURE 6-3
Light micrograph of transverse section through anterior chamber angle showing trabecular meshwork, scleral spur, and Schlemm's canal.

and may provide a tortuous pathway for fluid to move toward the inner wall of the canal. The endothelium of Schlemm's canal is anchored to the juxtacanalicular tissue by a network of elastic-containing fibrils that is also connected to the scleral spur and the tendon of the ciliary muscle.[19] This connective network might help in modulating aqueous outflow.[21]

Clinical Comment: Gonioscopy

The condition of the anterior chamber angle structures is clinically important because this angle is the location of exit for aqueous humor. It must be able to flow freely and unimpeded out of the anterior chamber. If its exit is blocked, pressure within the eye will increase, and ocular tissue damage will occur. The width of the angle can be estimated and graded using biomicroscopy to determine whether the angle appears wide enough to provide easy access to the trabecular meshwork.

If the angle does not appear to be wide enough or if there is concern that aqueous exit is inadequate, a view of the chamber angle structures might be necessary. A direct view of the angle cannot be achieved because the limbus is opaque, and light directed obliquely through the cornea into the angle does not exit because of total internal reflection. Therefore a clinical procedure, gonioscopy, is performed that uses a special lens, a goniolens (Figure 6-5). A goniolens can overcome total internal reflection and contains mirrors in which the examiner views the angle. The image the examiner sees is as if he or she is facing the angle and sighting along the anterior surface of the iris. If all structures can be seen, they appear in the following order, beginning at the inferior aspect: iris root, ciliary body, scleral spur, trabecular meshwork, and Schwalbe's line (Figure 6-6). (The iris root may or may

not be visible.) Schlemm's canal lies behind the trabecular meshwork in this view and appears as a thin red line within the meshwork if blood is backed up in the canal. Such pooling of blood occurs if the examiner exerts pressure on the goniolens, thereby compressing the episcleral veins and causing the episcleral venous pressure to exceed intraocular pressure.[23]

In a wide-open anterior chamber angle, the entire trabecular meshwork can be seen. As peripheral iris tissue approaches the meshwork, the angle becomes narrower, and access to the trabecular openings may be diminished. In certain conditions, cellular debris or pigment accumulates within the meshwork, interfering with aqueous drainage; such an occurrence would be evident with gonioscopy.

FUNCTION OF THE FILTRATION APPARATUS

The primary function of Schlemm's canal and the trabecular meshwork is to provide an exit for the aqueous humor. In addition, with the movement of aqueous through these structures, nutrients can diffuse into surrounding tissue, thereby supplying nutrients to the nearby deep limbal and scleral tissue.[8]

POSTERIOR CHAMBER

The **posterior chamber** is an annular area located behind the iris and bounded by the posterior iris surface, the equatorial zone of the lens, the anterior face of the vitreous, and the ciliary body. The ciliary processes that secrete the aqueous humor project into the posterior chamber. The zonule fibers arise from the internal limiting membrane of the nonpigmented epithelium of the ciliary body, pass through the posterior chamber, and insert into the lens capsule.[1] The posterior chamber contains two regions: The area occupied by the zonules is the **canal of Hannover,** and the *retrozonular space,* the area from the most posterior zonules to the vitreal face, is the **canal of Petit**[2] (Figure 6-7). The canal of Petit might be better described as a potential space.

AQUEOUS DYNAMICS

The aqueous humor provides necessary metabolites, primarily oxygen and glucose, to the avascular cornea and lens. It is produced in the pars plicata of the ciliary body and is secreted into the posterior chamber through the epithelium covering the ciliary processes. It passes between the iris and lens, entering the anterior chamber through the pupil (Figure 6-8). In the anterior chamber, the aqueous circulates in *convection currents,* moving down along the cooler cornea and up along the warmer iris and exiting through the periphery of the chamber.

FIGURE 6-4

Drawing of aqueous outflow apparatus and adjacent tissues. Schlemm's canal (*a*) is divided into two portions. An internal collector channel (of Sondermann) (*b*) opens into posterior part of canal. Sheets of corneoscleral meshwork (*c*) extend from corneolimbus (*e*) anteriorly to scleral spur (*d*). Ropelike components of uveal meshwork (*f*) occupy inner portion of trabecular meshwork; they arise in ciliary body (CB) near the angle recess and end just posterior to termination of Descemet's membrane (*g*). An iris process (*h*) extends from iris root to merge with uveal meshwork at approximately the level of anterior part of scleral spur. Longitudinal ciliary muscle (*i*) is attached to scleral spur, but a portion of muscle joins corneoscleral meshwork (*arrows*). Descemet's membrane terminates within deep corneolimbus. Corneal endothelium becomes continuous with trabecular endothelium at *j*. A broad transition zone (*double-headed arrows*) begins near termination of Descemet's membrane and ends where uveal meshwork joins deep corneolimbus. (From Hogan MJ, Alvarado JA, Weddell JE: *Histology of the human eye*, Philadelphia, 1971, Saunders.)

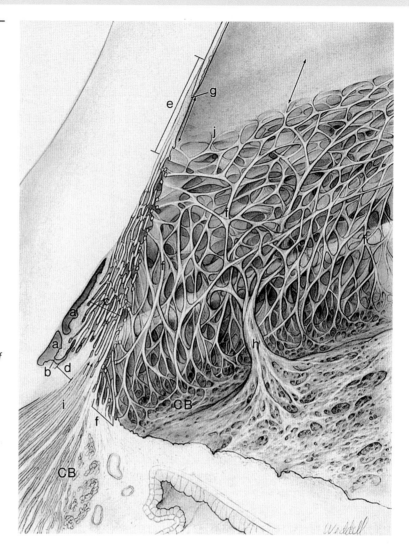

There are two avenues by which aqueous exits the anterior chamber. It can pass through the spaces within the uveal meshwork; this pathway is called the *unconventional outflow* and accounts for a relatively small amount (variously reported in the literature as 5% to 35% of the total outflow[24-26]). The fluid then passes into the connective tissue spaces surrounding the ciliary muscle bundles,[27] moves into the suprachoroidal space, and is absorbed into and through the sclera.[28] Alternately, the fluid is absorbed into the anterior ciliary veins and vortex veins. Additional veins recently identified may represent suprachoroidal collector channels designed to accommodate this uveoscleral flow.[24] There is some evidence that lymphatic channels exist in the ciliary stroma, which might provide an additional avenue for aqueous exit.[29]

The remainder of the aqueous follows the *conventional outflow* pathway and moves through the meshwork and into the narrower pores of the corneoscleral meshwork and through the juxtacanalicular tissue and the endothelial lining into Schlemm's canal.[18] In histologic sections, many of the endothelial cells lining the inner wall of the canal have been found to contain giant vacuoles,[7,12,16,30-32] some of which exhibit openings into the lumen.[10,33,34] The vacuoles apparently open and close intermittently, creating transient, transcellular, unidirectional channels that provide a means for transporting large molecules, such as proteins, across the endothelium. Flow occurs only into the canal.[14,15,35] An indentation forms in the basal surface of the endothelial cell, gradually enlarges, and eventually opens onto the apical surface (Figure 6-9). Then the cytoplasm in the basal aspect of the cell moves to occlude the opening.[35] The number of pores throughout the endothelium is uncertain because some may be artifacts caused by tissue preparation.[36] Smaller pinocytic vesicles also provide a transport system for substances. However, the greatest volume of aqueous humor diffuses passively into Schlemm's canal. Recent speculation suggests that the tight intercellular junctions may respond to changing physiologic conditions (i.e., effects of pharmacologic agents) by modifying their permeability and increasing the ease by which aqueous flows into the canal.[9,12] The

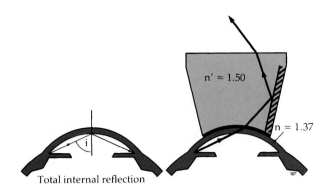

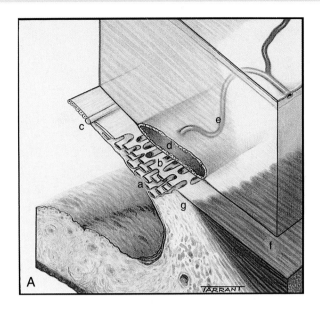

FIGURE 6-5
Optical principles of gonioscopy: *n* and *n'*, refractive index. (From Kanski JJ: *Clinical ophthalmology: a systematic approach*, ed 5, Oxford, UK, 2003, Butterworth-Heinemann.)

endothelial cells of the trabecular meshwork may actually release cellular factors that can increase the permeability of the inner wall of Schlemm's canal.[37]

The internal wall of Schlemm's canal contains a number of evaginations, or blind pouches, that extend into the juxtacanalicular tissue toward the trabecular meshwork. These **internal collector channels (of Sondermann)**[38] can be fairly long and branching, and serve to increase the surface area of the canal[2] (Figure 6-10). Their endothelium is always separated from the trabecular space by a sheet of connective tissue.

The endothelial cells lining the external wall of Schlemm's canal are joined by *zonula occludens* and contain no vacuoles. Approximately 25 to 35 **external collector channels** are distributed around the outer wall of Schlemm's canal and branch from it to empty into either the **deep scleral plexus** or the **intrascleral plexus** of veins,[5,39,40] which in turn drain into the episcleral and conjunctival veins.[2] **Aqueous veins (of Ascher),** that pass from the outer wall of the canal directly to the episcleral veins, provide another route from the canal.[41]

FACTORS AFFECTING INTRAOCULAR PRESSURE

The aqueous carries nutrients to the lens and cornea and carries waste products away, and a constant volume of aqueous helps to maintain the intraocular pressure (IOP) within the eye. IOP must be kept at a level that is not detrimental to ocular tissue and is maintained within a fairly small range by the complex equilibrium between the rate of production and the rate of exit. Homeostatic mechanisms normally preserve this balance, but small variations in either the production or the exit can cause significant changes in IOP. Production remains fairly constant; most cases of increased IOP are caused by decreased aqueous outflow.

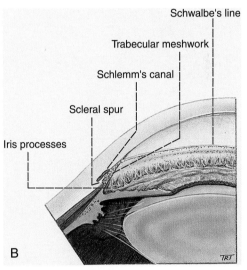

FIGURE 6-6
A, Anatomy of outflow channels: *a,* uveal meshwork; *b,* corneoscleral meshwork; *c,* Schwalbe's line; *d,* Schlemm's canal; *e,* collector channels; *f,* longitudinal muscle of ciliary body; *g,* scleral spur. **B,** Anatomy of anterior chamber angle structures. (From Kanski JJ: *Clinical ophthalmology: a systematic approach*, ed 3, Oxford, UK, 1995, Butterworth-Heinemann.)

The outflow can be impeded at various sites along the pathway. Aqueous that exits through the ciliary body (the unconventional outflow) passes into the ciliary body from the anterior chamber either through the uveoscleral meshwork or directly into the ciliary body. There is no continuous layer of epithelium covering the ciliary body as it borders the anterior chamber and thus the tissue offers little resistance to aqueous passage. The uveoscleral outflow is believed to be a fairly constant amount not affected by IOP.[26,42] Figure 6-11 shows the affect that IOP has on flow through the two outflow pathways.

Canal of Petit

Canal of Hannover

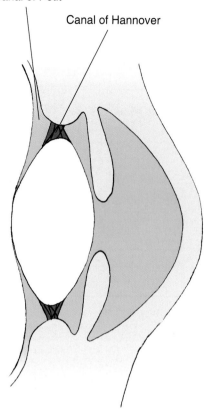

FIGURE 6-7
Regions of the posterior chamber.

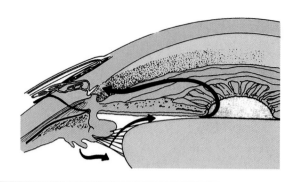

FIGURE 6-8
Normal flow of aqueous humor. Aqueous is formed in ciliary processes, moves out around crystalline lens and through pupil, and flows out of anterior chamber through trabecular meshwork into Schlemm's canal and then to episcleral veins. (From Bartlett JD, Jaanus SD: *Clinical ocular pharmacology*, ed 2, Boston, 1989, Butterworth-Heinemann.)

Canal of Schlemm

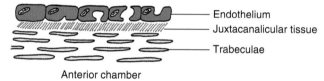

Endothelium
Juxtacanalicular tissue
Trabeculae

Anterior chamber

FIGURE 6-9
Formation of giant vacuoles in endothelial cells lining Schlemm's canal. (Modified from Bartlett JD, Jaanus SD: *Clinical ocular pharmacology*, ed 2, Boston, 1989, Butterworth-Heinemann.)

FIGURE 6-10
Drawing of Schlemm's canal, an internal collector channel, and adjacent tissues. Lumen of canal *(sc)* is lined by endothelium *(e)*. Endothelium of inner wall is very irregular, with many folds and outpouchings. Giant vacuoles *(gv)* are seen in endothelial cells along inner wall. External wall of canal *(ew)* is shown. Internal wall *(iw)* lies between endothelium and nearest trabecular space *(ts)*. Internal collector channel *(icc)* arises near posterior canal wall and extends into trabecular meshwork, where it is lost. As with Schlemm's canal, it is surrounded by a wall *(a)* that separates its lumen from adjacent trabecular spaces. Corneoscleral trabecular sheets *(cst)* branch frequently, and their endothelial cells often form bridges between adjacent sheets. (From Hogan MJ, Alvarado JA, Weddell JE: *Histology of the human eye*, Philadelphia, 1971, Saunders.)

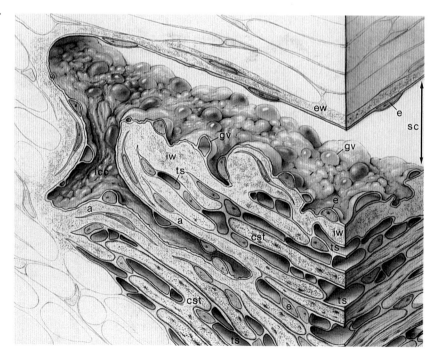

There is greater variability in the amount exiting via the conventional pathway. Resistance in this outflow pathway is a major factor in the rate of aqueous exit and influences intraocular pressure. There is normally little resistance to aqueous passage through the sheets of the trabecular meshwork unless pigment or debris has accumulated within the pores. When Schlemm's canal is wide open it also provides little to no resistance to outflow; likewise the external collector channels and aqueous veins normally provide negligible resistance.[22] The location of the highest resistance to aqueous movement seems to be in the region of the juxtacanalicular tissue (JCT) and (according to some) the endothelium of the inner wall of Schlemm's canal.[13,21,22,43] Plaquelike material that accumulates in the extracellular matrix of the juxtacanalicular area either directly or indirectly increases resistance in the outflow pathway.[13] In the normal eye, the cells of the trabecular meshwork and the cells within the JCT are speculated to have some self-regulating ability that can influence changes in resistance and thus IOP.[21,44,45] Sustained resistance to outflow usually results in elevated IOP.

Because of the elastic-like network of fibers joining the scleral spur, the ciliary muscle, and the meshwork, ciliary muscle contraction can alter the geometry of the trabeculum by widening the spaces between the sheets, resulting in a decrease in outflow resistance.[11,43] Elastic fibers of the spur are continuous with elastic fibers in the JCT, and fibers from the JCT connect with the endothelium of Schlemm's canal. Interaction among these fibers during accommodation can increase the lumen diameter.[21]

It is important that the amount of aqueous formed (flow in) is equal to the amount that exits the eye (flow out) and can be represented as $F_{in} = F_{out}$. This represents a balance between the factors affecting production and those involved in exit. As discussed in Chapter 3, aqueous production (F_{in}) is dependent on molecules moving out of the ciliary body capillaries and through the ciliary stroma and epithelium. Movement out of the blood vessels occurs because the pressure within the capillaries is greater than the pressure within the eye (IOP), and can be represented as ($P_{CB\ caps}$ – IOP).[42] The ease with which the molecules pass through tissue is called facility and will be represented as (C_{in}). (Facility is the reciprocal of resistance, as resistance increases, facility decreases.) The final factor in aqueous production is the rate at which energy-utilizing pumps actively move material toward secretion into the posterior chamber and is designated as (S). Thus $F_{in} = (P_{CB\ caps} - IOP)\ C_{in} + S$.[42] S is generally considered to be a constant; the other factors might fluctuate.

Flow out (F_{out}) includes both conventional and unconventional outflow. Flow from Schlemm's canal and into the episcleral veins is represented as (IOP – P_{ev})[42] and the ease with which the aqueous moves through the trabecular meshwork and into Schlemm's canal is

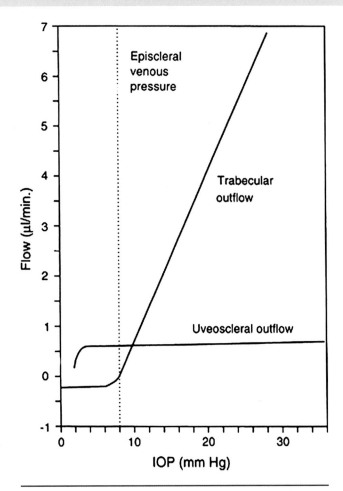

FIGURE 6-11
From Alm showing affect of IOP on outflow.

the facility, represented by (C_{out}). The small amount that exits through the uveoscleral meshwork is represented by (U) and is generally fairly constant.

$$F_{in} = F_{out} = (P_{CB\ caps} - IOP)\ C_{in} + S = (IOP - P_{ev})\ C_{out} + U^{42}$$

Although this equation is an over-simplification, it does give an indication of the factors to be considered and their interdependence. It represents the steady state of homeostasis, and in the normal eye, only small fluctuations occur throughout the day.[46] The amount of aqueous produced usually does not change appreciably and so when the steady state is disrupted, it is usually the flow out that is compromised and an elevation of IOP can follow. If aqueous exit is compromised, it is usually because of an in increase in resistance to aqueous exit (thus a decrease in facility); the major location of the increased resistance is likely to be the juxtacanalicular tissue between the last trabecular sheet and the inner wall of Schlemm's canal.

Small fluctuations in IOP might have some small effect on the egress of aqueous from the ciliary processes, but this is usually negligible.

Clinical Comment: Measurement of IOP

INTRAOCULAR PRESSURE can be estimated clinically with a tonometer. The commonest instruments used are the noncontact tonometer and the Goldmann applanation tonometer. IOP is measured in millimeters of mercury (mm Hg) and a reading between 10 and 20 is considered normal. Readings in the low to mid 20s may be suspect and IOP measurements in the upper 20s or higher require monitoring. The noncontact tonometer (also called the air-puff tonometer) detects the force necessary to applanate the cornea by a rapid pulse of air. When performing Goldmann applanation tonometry a topical anesthetic must be instilled so that a prism/probe can contact the cornea. As the practitioner changes the force exerted by the probe, causing applanation of a given area of the corneal surface, the force required gives an estimate of the pressure within the eye. IOP is only one of the clinical findings that aids in the diagnosis of glaucoma, the appearance of the optic nerve head and the nerve fiber layer are assessed and the visual field is examined for defects.

Clinical Comment: Glaucoma

GLAUCOMA is a complex disease process that is not completely understood. Many patients with glaucoma have higher than normal IOP. Increased IOP can contribute to damage of the retinal nerve fiber layer, either directly by mechanical pressure or indirectly through impeding blood perfusion. In normotensive glaucoma, retinal nerve fibers are damaged but IOP measurements are normal or even low. In these cases, the likely cause is a decrease of perfusion pressure in the retinal tissue resulting in loss of metabolites and cell death. Nerve fiber loss is most evident at the optic disc and can cause enlargement and deepening of the physiologic cup.

Deposits of pigment or debris on the trabecular sheets and cords can restrict aqueous flow through the trabecular spaces. Proliferation of the juxtacanalicular tissue increases with age and has been found to cause a decrease in outflow.[5] Some histologic preparations of ocular tissue from glaucomatous eyes give evidence for a decrease in outflow. A reduction in the cross-sectional diameter of Schlemm's canal and fewer pores in the endothelial lining of the canal were found in glaucomatous eyes when compared with normal eyes.[47,48] Other studies show an increase in the fibrillar component of the matrix in the juxtacanalicular tissue in glaucomatous eyes.[43]

Drugs that Effect IOP

Glaucoma treatment consists of attempts to reduce pressure using drugs that either decrease aqueous production or increase aqueous outflow. One of the earliest treatment plans prescribed a cholinergic agonist that caused the iris sphincter and ciliary muscle to contract, thus changing the configuration of the trabecular sheets to facilitate outflow, perhaps by allowing more separation between the sheets.[11,49,50] Pilocarpine was commonly used; however, compliance was often poor because of the uncomfortable side effects—miosis and ciliary spasm.

Drugs that inhibit production act on the ciliary epithelia, either by interfering with neural pathways or by inhibiting intracellular enzymes that maintain the ionic transport mechanisms important in the formation of aqueous.[51] Although the role of sympathetic innervation in aqueous production is unclear, beta-blockers and alpha-adrenergic agonists do decrease aqueous production, perhaps by interfering with ciliary epithelial function. There is some speculation that drugs that have vasoconstrictive action can decrease aqueous production by decreasing blood flow in the ciliary vessels, causing a reduction in oxygen availability to the tissue.[51] During the 1970s and 1980s, beta-blockers were the preferred method of treatment.[52]

Carbonic anhydrase inhibitors are also common in glaucoma treatment but are not well tolerated in many patients. They inhibit key enzymes necessary for ionic transport across the epithelial layers. Currently the most effective drugs used in glaucoma treatment are prostaglandins; they are well tolerated and compliance is good because instillation may only be necessary once a day. Prostaglandins enhance outflow through the uveoscleral pathway, although the exact mechanism has not been fully defined. They are found to relax ciliary muscle tone and to remodel the extracellular matrix within the connective tissue between muscle bundles, increasing the spacing between bundles and increasing tissue permeability for increased aqueous flow.[25,26,45,53-55] Certain prostaglandin analogues may also increase trabecular meshwork outflow.[56]

Clinical Comment: Surgical Treatment

Surgical procedures in the treatment of glaucoma are often the last resort when nerve fiber layer damage continues even with vigorous pharmacologic treatment. In trabeculoplasty, small laser holes are made in the trabecular meshwork to increase fluid movement. In trabeculectomy, a wedge of meshwork is removed and often a scleral flap is formed so that aqueous can percolate through the trabecular opening and accumulate beneath the flap to be absorbed into episcleral tissue. A recent surgical procedure, endoscopic cyclophotocoagulation, reduces aqueous production by applying a laser to damage tissue of the ciliary processes.

AGING CHANGES IN THE ANTERIOR CHAMBER

With age, the anterior chamber angle width narrows and the anterior chamber volume decreases, probably secondary to lens growth. This narrowing is more significant in women and may be related to the higher incidence of angle-closure glaucoma in elderly women.[57]

Other age-related changes include a decrease in aqueous production, a reduction in uveoscleral outflow reduction, a decrease in the density and size of giant vacuoles, an accumulation of extracellular matrix plaques in the juxtacanalicular tissue, and an increase in the outflow resistance in the vicinity of the juxtacanalicular tissue and the inner wall of Schlemm's canal.[22,58,59] An increase in the amount of connective tissue in the ciliary muscle may be the cause of the reduction in uveoscleral outflow.[26] However, no age-related increase in IOP is seen in healthy individuals with pressures below 22 mm Hg.[58]

VITREOUS CHAMBER

The **vitreous chamber** is filled with the gel-like vitreous body and occupies the largest portion of the globe. It is bounded on the front by the posterior surface of the lens and the retrozonular portion of the posterior chamber. Peripherally and posteriorly, it is bounded by the pars plana of the ciliary body, the retina, and the optic disc. All surfaces that interface with the vitreous are basement membranes. The center of the anterior surface contains the **patellar fossa,** an indentation in which the lens sits. The vitreous makes up about 80% of the entire volume of the eye.

VITREAL ATTACHMENTS

The vitreous forms several attachments to surrounding structures. The strongest of these is the vitreous base, located at the ora serrata. The other attachments (in order of decreasing strength) are to the posterior lens, to the optic disc, at the macula, and to retinal vessels.

The **vitreous base,** the most extensive adhesion, extends 1.5 to 2 mm anterior to the ora serrata, 1 to 3 mm posterior to it, and several millimeters into the vitreous[2,60] (Figure 6-12). The vitreal fibers that form the base are embedded firmly in the basement membrane of the nonpigmented epithelium of the ciliary body and the internal limiting membrane of the peripheral retina.[39,61]

The **hyaloideocapsular ligament (of Weiger),** or **retrolental ligament,** forms an annular attachment 1 to 2 mm wide and 8 to 9 mm in diameter between the posterior surface of the lens and the anterior face of the vitreous.[60] This is a firm attachment site in young persons, but the strength of the bond diminishes after age 35.[62] Within the ring formed by this ligament is a potential space, the **retrolental space (of Berger),** which is present because the lens and vitreous are juxtaposed but not joined.[2]

The peripapillary adhesion around the edge of the optic disc also diminishes with age. The annular ring of attachment at the macula is 3 to 4 mm in diameter.[2]

The attachment of the vitreous to retinal blood vessels consists of fine strands that extend through the internal

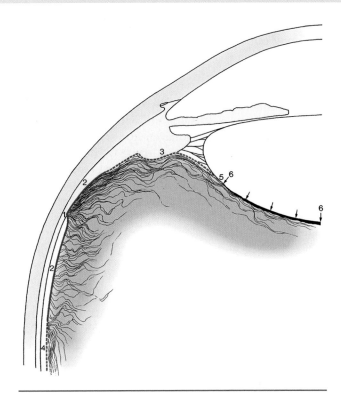

FIGURE 6-12
Vitreous relationships in the anterior eye. Ora serrata (*1*) is termination of retina. Vitreous base (*2*) extends forward approximately 2 mm over ciliary body and posteriorly approximately 4 mm over peripheral retina. Collagen in this region is oriented at a right angle to surface of retina and ciliary body, but anteriorly over pars plana, it is more parallel to inner surface of ciliary body. Posterior hyaloid (*4*) is continuous with retina and anterior hyaloid (*3*) with zonules and lens. Also depicted are hyaloideocapsular ligament (*5*) and space of Berger (*6*). (From Hogan MJ, Alvarado JA, Weddell JE: *Histology of the human eye*, Philadelphia, 1971, Saunders.)

limiting membrane to branch and surround the larger retinal vessels.[61,63] These strands may account for hemorrhages that occur when there is vitreal traction on the retina. The nature of the attachment between the vitreous and the retinal internal limiting membrane throughout the rest of the retina remains uncertain. It is unlikely that fibrils from the posterior vitreous insert into the internal limiting membrane.[64-66] But rather the vitreoretinal interface contains a "molecular glue" linking the outer part of the cortex and the inner part of the limiting membrane.[2,67,68] This area contains extracellular matrix—molecules, including laminin and fibronectin, that have been identified as having adhesive properties.[62]

VITREOUS ZONES

The vitreous can be divided into zones that differ in relative density. The outermost zone is the vitreous cortex, the center zone is occupied by Cloquet's canal, and the intermediate zone is inner to the cortex and surrounds the center canal.

Vitreous Cortex

The **vitreous cortex,** also called the **hyaloid surface,** is the outer zone.[69] It is 100 μm wide,[2] and it is composed of tightly packed collagen fibrils, some of which run parallel and some perpendicular to the retinal surface.[70,71] The anterior cortex lies anterior to the base and is adjacent to the ciliary body, posterior chamber, and lens. The posterior cortex extends posterior to the base and is in contact with the retina. It contains transvitreal channels that appear as holes—the *prepapillary hole,* the *premacular hole,* and *prevascular fissures.* The prepapillary hole can sometimes be seen clinically when the posterior vitreous detaches from the retina.[60] The premacular hole, a weak area, may be a region of decreased density rather than an actual hole.[60,71] The prevascular fissures provide the avenue by which fine fibers enter the retina and encircle retinal vessels.[61]

Intermediate Zone

The **intermediate zone** contains fine fibers that are continuous and unbranched and that run anteroposteriorly.[60,70,72] These fibers arise at the region of the vitreous base and insert into the posterior cortex.[73] The peripheral fibers parallel the cortex, whereas the more central fibers parallel Cloquet's canal. Membranelike condensations, called vitreous tracts, may be differentiated as areas that have differing fiber densities (Figure 6-13).[71]

Cloquet's Canal

Cloquet's canal, also called the **hyaloid channel** or the **retrolental tract,** is located in the center of the vitreous body.[2] It has an S shape, rotated 90 degrees with the center dip downward, and is the former site of the hyaloid artery system, which was formed during embryologic development (see Chapter 7). Cloquet's canal arises at the retrolental space. Its anterior face is approximately 4 to 5 mm in diameter.[2] It terminates at the **area of Martegiani,** a funnel-shaped space at the optic nerve head that extends forward into the vitreous to become continuous with the canal.[2,60]

COMPOSITION OF VITREOUS

The highly transparent vitreous is a dilute solution of salts, soluble proteins, and hyaluronic acid contained within a meshwork of the insoluble protein, collagen. Vitreous is 98.5% to 99.7% water and has been described as having connective tissue status and being an extracellular matrix.[71,74] Because of its high water content, study

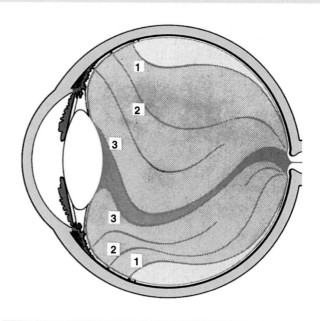

FIGURE 6-13

Eisner's interpretation[71] of vitreous structures (according to slit-lamp examinations of eyes obtained at autopsy). Vitreous body is divided into three zones: Externally, as far as retina extends, there is a relatively thick vitreous cortex (light orange). It has holes at characteristic locations: in front of papilla, in region of fovea centralis, in front of vessels, and in front of anomalies of ora serrata region (enclosed ora bays, meridional folds, zonular traction tufts). Intermediate zone (medium orange) contains vitreal tracts, membranelles that form funnels packed into one another and that diverge from region of papilla anteriorly. Central channel (dark orange) is space delimited by hyaloid tract. It is closed off anteriorly by a retrolental section of anterior vitreous membrane. It contains no typical tracts but only irregularly arranged vitreous fibers, part of which are residua of Cloquet's canal. Outermost vitreous tract, the preretinal tract (*1*), separates intermediary substance from vitreous cortex. Innermost tract, the hyaloid tract (*3*), inserts at the edge of the lens. Between these tracts extends the median tract (*2*) to median ligament of pars plana and the coronary tract to coronary ligament. (From Sebag J: The vitreous. In Hart WM Jr, editor: *Adler's physiology of the eye,* ed 9, St Louis, 1992, Mosby.)

of the vitreous is difficult. Attempts at tissue fixation often have dehydrating effects that introduce artifacts. Recent investigations suggest that the epithelium of the pars plana has a significant role in the production and secretion of several connective tissue macromolecules of the vitreous body.[74]

Collagen

The collagen content of the vitreous is highest in the vitreous base, next highest in the posterior cortex, next in the anterior cortex, and lowest in the center.[60] A fine meshwork of uniform collagen fibrils, each 8 to 16 nm in diameter, is evident on electron microscopy and fills the vitreous body.[69,75-77] The individual fibrils cannot be seen with the slit lamp, but the pattern of variations in their density and regularity can be seen. The density of this collagen fibril network differs throughout the vitreous.[44]

Hyaluronic Acid (hyaluronan)

The second major vitreal component, **hyaluronic acid (HA)**, a glycosaminoglycan, is a long unbranched molecule coiled into a twisted network.[72] This hydrophilic macromolecule is located in specific sites within the collagen fibril network and is believed to maintain the wide spacing between fibrils.[60] The concentration of HA is highest in the posterior cortex and decreases centrally and anteriorly.[68,78] The gel structure is a result of the interaction of collagen and HA. HA stabilizes the network formed by the collagen strands.

Hyalocytes

Vitreous cells, or **hyalocytes,** are located in a single, widely spaced layer in the cortex near the vitreal surface and parallel to it.[60,72] Various functions have been attributed to these cells. Some investigators have determined that these cells synthesize HA.[79-81] Others have found evidence that hyalocytes synthesize glycoproteins for the collagen fibrils.[60,82] Still others indicate that hyalocytes have phagocytic properties.[72,81,83] Apparently, hyalocytes can have different appearances depending on their activity at a given time.[60] Cells located in the vitreous base are fibroblast-like when anterior to the ora serrata and macrophage-like when posterior to it.[64]

Fibroblasts present in the vitreous are located in the vitreous base near the ciliary body and near the optic disc. Although composing less than 10% of the cell population, fibroblasts may have been mistaken for hyalocytes in the past. It is believed that fibroblasts synthesize the collagen fibrils that run anteroposteriorly and are active in pathologic conditions.[60]

Other cells that have been identified as macrophages likely originate in the nearby retinal blood vessels.[2,71]

VITREAL FUNCTION

The vitreous body provides physical support holding the retina in place next to the choroid, the blood supply for the outer retina. (Neural retina and choroid are only connected to each other at the disc and the ora serrata.) The vitreous is a storage area for metabolites for the retina and lens and provides an avenue for the movement of these substances within the eye.[41] The vitreous, because of its viscoelastic properties, acts as a "shock absorber," protecting the fragile retinal tissue during rapid eye movements and strenuous physical activity.[2,71] The vitreous transmits and refracts light, aiding in focusing the rays on the retina. Minimal light scattering occurs in the vitreous because of its extremely low concentration of particles and the interfibrillar spacing ensured by the HA-collagen complex.

AGE-RELATED VITREAL CHANGES

In the infant the vitreous is a very homogeneous, gel-like body. With maturation, changes occur in which the gel volume decreases and the liquid volume increases; this is called vitreous liquefaction or vitreous synersis.[60] By age 40 years, the vitreous is 80% gel and 20% liquid, and by 70 or 80 years it is 50% liquid,[70] with most of the liquefaction occurring in the central vitreous.[71] Both HA and collagen may be detrimentally affected by free radicals that cause conformational changes in the HA molecule and breakdown in collagen cross-links. Subsequent displacement of collagen from the HA-collagen network influences the change from gel to liquid.[46,84,85] As the dissolution of the HA-collagen complex occurs, the macromolecule moves out of the collagen network, causing the fibrils to coalesce into fibers and then into bands.[85,86] The redistribution of collagen leaves spaces adjacent to these bundles, allowing pooling of liquid vitreous; these pockets are called lacunae.[68,86,87]

Clinical Comment: Peripheral Retinal Traction

With aging, the vitreous base adhesion extends further posteriorly, and the border approaches the equator.[88,89] These changes can increase traction on peripheral retina and might contribute to the development of retinal tears and detachment.

Clinical Comment: Posterior Vitreal Detachment

As the HA is displaced from the collagen network and as the fibrils coalesce into bundles, the bundles can contract and apply traction to the vitreous and thus to the posterior retina. One of the most common abnormalities that occurs at the posterior retinal-vitreous interface is a **posterior vitreal detachment** caused by this traction. The vitreous usually detaches from the retinal internal limiting membrane at the peripapillary ring, forming a retrocortical space. If glial tissue is torn away with the vitreous, a circular condensation, Weiss' ring (senile annular ring), may be visible within the vitreous.[90] If liquid vitreous seeps into the retrocortical space through the prepapillary and premacular areas, a synersis, or collapse, of the vitreous can follow because of the volume displacement.[86,91]

PHYSIOLOGY OF THE VITREOUS

The vitreous was thought to merely passively interact and support surrounding tissues but a new understanding of the dynamic vitreous is developing. The cells in the cortex reamin largely quiescent because factors present in the vitreous prevent cell migration and proliferation. The interaction between HA and collagen fibrils contributes to the viscoelastic properties of the vitreous[92,93] and influences the physical properties, i.e., the balance between gel and liquid, of the vitreous state.[60] Most of the water in the vitreous is bound in the widely-spaced network of collagen and HA. A disruption in the HA-collagen complex can cause the collagen fibrils to aggregate into bundles, which may become large enough to be visible clinically, and reported by a patient as floaters.

While there is little metabolic activity within the vitreous and a slow degradation occurs with age, an intact vitreous gel may be quite important to ocular health; age-related degeneration of the vitreous gel and liquefaction accompanies several age-related ocular diseases, such as nuclear sclerotic cataract and neovascular diabetic retinopathy.[94] Studies suggest a correlation between vitreous degeneration and the development of nuclear sclerotic cataract (NSC), inferring that an intact vitreous provides some protection against lens nuclear changes. A much higher incidence of NSC after vitrectomy was found in patients over 50 than in those younger.[95,96] It may be that the younger lens is more resistant to cataractous changes or that the presence of anterior vitreous that is still adherent to posterior lens (it was not removed in the vitrectomy because of the stronger adhesion) provides some protection against NSC.

Nuclear sclerotic cataract is the result of oxidative changes within the lens nucleus. The vitreous has a high concentration of ascorbate (up to 40 times higher than blood plasma) and might have a role in the regulation of intraocular molecular oxygen.[94] As oxygen diffuses into the vitreous from the retinal vessels, it is likely to be consumed by ascorbate before it reaches the lens and anterior segment, providing some protection from oxidative stress. The lens might therefore be exposed to a greater concentration of oxygen after vitrectomy. Vitreous *gel* has a higher concentration of ascorbate and consumes oxygen at a faster rate than *liquid* vitreous.[97] Vitreous loss due to liquefaction or vitrectomy can be linked to disease processes in which excessive oxygen causes oxidative stress and tissue damage.

Another hypothesis suggests that some might benefit from vitreous liquefaction or surgical removal of the vitreous. Vitreous loss that results in increased intraocular molecular oxygen may benefit ischemic retinal disease by lowering vascular endothelial growth factor (VEGF) and thus reduce neovascularization.[94] The importance of the vitreous and a better understanding of its relationship with neighboring tissues will become more evident as studies continue.

REFERENCES

1. Fine BS, Yanoff M: The vitreous body. In Fine BS, Yanoff M, editors: *Ocular histology*, ed 2, Hagerstown, Md, 1979, Harper & Row, p 131.
2. Hogan MJ, Alvarado JA, Weddell JE: *Histology of the human eye*, Philadelphia, 1971, Saunders.
3. Warwick R: *Eugene Wolff's anatomy of the eye and orbit*, ed 7, Philadelphia, 1976, Saunders.
4. Kelley MJ, Rose AY, Keller KE, et al: Stem cells in the trabecular meshwork: present and future promises, *Exp Eye Res* 88:747–751, 2009.
5. Lütjen-Drecoll E, Rohen JW: Functional morphology of the trabecular meshwork. In Tasman W, Jaeger EA, editors: *Duane's foundations of clinical ophthalmology*, vol 1, Philadelphia, 1994, Lippincott, p 1.
6. Alexander RA, Garner A: Elastic and precursor fibres in the normal human eye, *Exp Eye Res* 36:305, 1983.
7. Gong H, Ruberti J, Overby D, et al: A new view of the human trabecular meshwork using quick-freeze, deep-etch electron microscopy, *Exp Eye Res* 75:347, 2002.
8. Fine BS: Structure of the trabecular meshwork and the canal of Schlemm, *Trans Am Acad Ophthalmol Otolaryngol* 70:777, 1966.
9. Bhatt K, Gong F, Freddo TF: Freeze-fracture studies of interendothelial junctions in the angle of the human eye, *Invest Ophthalmol Vis Sci* 36(7):1379, 1995.
10. Raviola G, Raviola E: Paracellular route of aqueous in the trabecular meshwork and canal of Schlemm. A freeze-fracture study of the endothelial junctions in the sclerocorneal angle of the macaque monkey eye, *Invest Ophthalmol Vis Sci* 21:52, 1981.
11. Kaufman PL: Enhancing trabecular outflow by disrupting the actin cytoskeleton, increasing uveoscleral outflow with prostaglandins, and understanding the pathophysiology of presbyopia interrogating Mother Nature: asking why, asking how, recognizing the signs, following the trail, *Exp Eye Res* 86:3–17, 2008.
12. Ye W, Gong H, Sit A, et al: Interendothelial junctions in normal human Schlemm's canal respond to changes in pressure, *Invest Ophthalmol Vis Sci* 38(12):2460, 1997.
13. Johnson M: What controls aqueous humour outflow resistance? *Exp Eye Res* 82:545–557, 2006.
14. Bill A: Scanning electron microscopic studies of the canal of Schlemm, *Exp Eye Res* 10:214, 1970.
15. Epstein DL, Rohen JW: Morphology of the trabecular meshwork and inner-wall endothelium after cationized ferritin perfusion in the monkey eye, *Invest Ophthalmol Vis Sci* 32:160, 1991.
16. Ethier CR, Coloma FM, Sit AJ, et al: Two pore types in the inner-wall endothelium of Schlemm's canal, *Invest Ophthalmol Vis Sci* 39(11):2041, 1998.
17. Lütjen-Drecoll E, Futa R, Rohen JW: Ultrahistochemical studies on tangential sections of the trabecular meshwork in normal and glaucomatous eyes, *Invest Ophthalmol Vis Sci* 21:563, 1981.
18. Inomata H, Bill A, Smelser GK: Aqueous humor pathways through the trabecular meshwork and into Schlemm's canal in the cynomolgus monkey (Macaca irus), *Am J Ophthalmol* 73:760, 1972.
19. Rohen JW, Futa R, Lütjen-Drecoll E: The fine structure of the cribriform network in normal and glaucomatous eyes as seen in tangential sections, *Invest Ophthalmol Vis Sci* 21:574, 1981.
20. Umihira J, Nagata S, Nohara M, et al: Localization of elastin in the normal and glaucomatous human trabecular meshwork, *Invest Ophthalmol Vis Sci* 35(2):486, 1994.

21. Acott TS, Kelley MJ: Extracellular matrix in the trabecular meshwork, *Exp Eye Res* 86:543–561, 2008.
22. Overby DR, Stamer WD, Johnson M: The changing paradigm of outflow resistance generation: towards synergistic models of the JCT and inner wall endothelium, *Exp Eye Res* 88:656–670, 2009.
23. Kanski JJ: *Clinical ophthalmology*, ed 3, Oxford, UK, 1994, Butterworth-Heinemann.
24. Krohn J, Bertelsen T: Corrosion casts of the suprachoroidal space and uveoscleral drainage routes in the human eye, *Acta Ophthalmol Scand* 75:32, 1997.
25. Nilsson SF: The uveoscleral outflow routes, *Eye* 11:149, 1997.
26. Alm A, Nilsson SF: Uveoscleral outflow—a review, *Exp Eye Res* 88:760–768, 2009.
27. Bill A: Some aspects of aqueous humour drainage, *Eye* 7:14, 1993.
28. Krohn J, Bertelsen T: Light microscopy of uveoscleral drainage routes after gelatine injections into the suprachoroidal space, *Acta Ophthalmol Scand* 76(5):521, 1998:(abstract).
29. Gupta N, Patel M, Ly T, et al: Evidence of a new uveolymphatic outflow pathway in human and sheep; implications for aqueous drainage and glaucoma, *Invest Ophthalmol Vis Sci* 49, 2008.
30. Holmberg AS: The fine structure of the inner wall of Schlemm's canal, *Arch Ophthalmol* 62:956, 1959.
31. Speakman JS: Drainage channels in the trabecular wall of Schlemm's canal, *Br J Ophthalmol* 44:513, 1960.
32. Parc CE, Johnson DH, Brilakis HS: Giant vacuoles are found preferentially near collector channels, *Invest Ophthalmol Vis Sci* 41:2984, 2000.
33. Feeney L: Outflow studies using an electron dense tracer, *Trans Am Acad Ophthalmol Otolaryngol* 70:791, 1966.
34. Anderson DR: Scanning electron microscopy of primate trabecular meshwork, *Am J Ophthalmol* 71:90, 1971.
35. Tripathi ERC: Mechanism of the aqueous outflow across the trabecular wall of Schlemm's canal, *Exp Eye Res* 11:116, 1971.
36. Sit AJ, Coloma FM, Ethier CR, et al: Factors affecting the pores of the inner wall endothelium of Schlemm's canal, *Invest Ophthalmol Vis Sci* 38(8):1517, 1997.
37. Alvarado JA, Alvarado RG, Yeh RF, et al: A new insight into the cellular regulation of aqueous outflow: how trabecular meshwork endothelial cells drive a mechanism that regulates the permeability of Schlemm's canal endothelial cells, *Br J Ophthalmol* 89:1500–1505, 2005.
38. Sondermann R: The formation, morphology and function of Schlemm's canal, *Acta Ophthalmol* 11:280, 1933.
39. Dvorak-Theobold G: Schlemm's canal: its anastomosis and anatomic relations, *Trans Am Ophthalmol Soc* 32:574, 1934.
40. Ashton N: Anatomical study of Schlemm's canal and aqueous veins by means of neoprene casts. Part I. Aqueous veins, *Br J Ophthalmol* 35:291, 1951.
41. Ascher KW: Aqueous veins: preliminary notes, *Am J Ophthalmol* 25:31, 1942.
42. Gabfelt BT, Kaufman PL: Aqueous humor hydrodynamics. In Kaufman PL, Alm A, editors: *Adler's physiology of the eye*, ed 10, St Louis, 2003, Mosby, p 293.
43. Tamm ER: The trabecular meshwork outflow pathways: structural and functional aspects, *Exp Eye Res* 88:648–655, 2009.
44. Selbach JM, Gottanka J, Wittmann M, et al: Efferent and afferent innervation of primate trabecular meshwork and scleral spur, *Invest Ophthalmol Vis Sci* 41(8):2184, 2000.
45. Faralli JA, Schwinn MK, Gonzalez JM Jr, et al: Functional properties of fibronectin in the trabecular meshwork, *Exp Eye Res* 88:689–693, 2009.
46. Lund-Andersen H, Sander B: The vitreous. In Kaufman PL, Alm A, editors: *Adler's physiology of the eye*, ed 10, St Louis, 2003, Mosby, p 293.
47. Johnson S, Chan D, Read AT, et al: The pore density in the inner wall endothelium of Schlemm's canal of glaucomatous eyes, *Invest Ophthalmol Vis Sci* 43(9):2950, 2002.
48. Allingham RR, de Kater AW, Ethier CR: Schlemm's canal and primary open angle glaucoma: correlation between Schlemm's canal dimensions and outflow facility, *Exp Eye Res* 62(1):101, 1996:(abstract).
49. Rohen J, Unger HH: Studies on the morphology and pathology of the trabecular meshwork in the human eye, *Am J Ophthalmol* 46:802, 1958.
50. Grierson I, Lee WR, Abraham S: Effects of pilocarpine on the morphology of human outflow apparatus, *Br J Ophthalmol* 62:302, 1978.
51. Keil JW, Reithamer HA: Relationship between ciliary blood flow and aqueous production: does it play a role in glaucoma therapy? *J Glaucoma* 15:172–181, 2006.
52. Zimmerman TJ: Topical ophthalmic beta blockers: a comparative review, *J Ocul Pharmacol* 9:373–384, 1993.
53. Alm A: Uveoscleral outflow, *Eye* 14:488, 2000.
54. Lütjen-Drecoll E, Gabelt AT, Tian B, et al: Outflow of aqueous humor, *J Glaucoma* 10(Suppl 1):42, 2001.
55. Cracknell KPB, Grierson I: Prostaglandin analogues in the anterior eye: their pressure lowering action and side effects, *Exp Eye Res* 88:786–791, 2009.
56. Toris CB, Gabelt BT, Kaufman PL: Update on the mechanism of action of topical prostaglandins for intraocular pressure reduction, *Surv Ophthalmol* 53(Suppl1):S107–S120, 2008.
57. Chen HB, Kashiwagi K, Yamabayashi S, et al: Anterior chamber angle biometry: quadrant variation, age change and sex difference, *Curr Eye Res* 17(2):120, 1998:(abstract).
58. Toris CB, Yablonski ME, Wang YL, et al: Aqueous humor dynamics in the aging human eye, *Am J Ophthalmol* 127:407, 1999.
59. Boldea RC, Roy S, Mermoud A: Ageing of Schlemm's canal in nonglaucomatous subjects, *Int Ophthalmol* 24:67, 2001.
60. Sebag J: The vitreous. In Hart WM Jr, editor: *Adler's physiology of the eye*, ed 9, St Louis, 1992, Mosby, p 268.
61. Mutlu F, Leopold IH: Structure of the human retinal vascular system, *Arch Ophthalmol* 71:93, 1964.
62. Lund-Andersen H, Sebag J, Sander B, et al: The vitreous. In Fischbarg J, editor: *The biology of the eye*, Amsterdam, 2006, Elsevier, pp 181–194.
63. Wolter JR: Pores in the internal limiting membrane of the human retina, *Arch Ophthalmol* 42:971, 1964.
64. Gaertner J: Vitreous electron microscopic studies on the fine structure of the normal and pathologically changed vitreoretinal limiting membrane, *Surv Ophthalmol* 9:219, 1964.
65. Matsumato B, Blanks JC, Ryan SJ: Topographic variations in rabbit and primate internal limiting membrane, *Invest Ophthalmol Vis Sci* 25:71, 1984.
66. Malecaze F, Caratero C, Caratero A, et al: Some ultrastructural aspects of the vitreoretinal juncture, *Ophthalmologica* 191:22, 1985.
67. Russell SR, Shepherd JD, Hageman GS: Distribution of glycoconjugates in the human retinal internal limiting membrane, *Invest Ophthalmol Vis Sci* 32(7):1986, 1991.
68. La Goff MM, Bishop PN: Adult vitreous structure and postnatal changes, *Eye* 22:1214–1222, 2008.
69. Schwarz W: Electron microscopic observations on the human vitreous body. In Smelser GK, editor: *Structure of the eye*, New York, 1961, Academic Press, p 283.
70. Balazs EA: Functional anatomy of the vitreous. In Tasman W, Jaeger EA, editors: *Duane's foundations of clinical ophthalmology*, vol 1, Philadelphia, 1994, Lippincott.
71. Eisner G: Clinical anatomy of the vitreous. In Tasman W, Jaeger EA, editors: *Duane's foundations of clinical ophthalmology*, vol 1, Philadelphia, 1994, Lippincott.

72. Balazs EA, Toth LZ, Eckl EA, et al: Studies on the structure of the vitreous body. XII. Cytological and histochemical studies on the cortical tissue layer, *Exp Eye Res* 3:57, 1964.

73. Sebag J, Balazs EA: Morphology and ultrastructure of human vitreous fibers, *Invest Ophthalmol Vis Sci* 30:1867, 1989.

74. Bishop PN, Takanosu M, Le Goff M, et al: The role of the posterior ciliary body in the biosynthesis of vitreous humour, *Eye* 16:454, 2002.

75. Pirie A, Schmidt G, Waters JW: Ox vitreous humor. I. The residual protein, *Br J Ophthalmol* 32:321, 1948.

76. Matoltsy AG: A study on the structural protein of the vitreous body (vitrosin), *J Gen Physiol* 36:29, 1952.

77. Gross J, Matoltsy AG, Cohen C: Vitrosin: a member of the collagen class, *J Biophys Biochem Cytol* 1:215, 1955.

78. Bembridge BA, Crawford CN, Pirie A: Phase-contrast microscopy of the animal vitreous body, *Br J Ophthalmol* 36:131, 1952.

79. Osterlin SE: The synthesis of hyaluronic acid in the vitreous. IV. Regeneration in the owl monkey, *Exp Eye Res* 7:524, 1968.

80. Hultsch E, Balazs EA: In vitro synthesis of glycosaminoglycans and glycoproteins by cells of the vitreous, *Invest Ophthalmol Vis Sci* 14(Suppl):43, 1973.

81. Freeman MI, Jacobson B, Balazs EA: The chemical composition of vitreous hyalocyte granules, *Exp Eye Res* 29:479, 1979.

82. Ayad S, Weiss JB: A new look at vitreous-humor collagen, *Biochem J* 218:835, 1984.

83. Szirmai JA, Balazs EA: Studies on the structure of the vitreous body. Cells in the cortical layer, *Arch Ophthalmol* 59:34, 1958.

84. Armand G, Chakrabarti B: Conformational differences between hyaluronates of gel and liquid human vitreous: fractionation and circular dichroism studies, *Curr Eye Res* 6:445, 1987.

85. Ponsioen TL, Deemter M, Bank RA, et al: Mature enzymatic collagen cross-links, hydroxylysylpyridinoline and lysylpyridinoline, in the aging human vitreous, *Invest Ophthalmol Vis Sci* 50:1041–1046, 2009.

86. Sebag J: Age-related differences in the human vitreoretinal interface, *Arch Ophthalmol* 109(7):966, 1991.

87. Kishi S, Shimizu K: Posterior precortical vitreous pocket, *Arch Ophthalmol* 108:979, 1990.

88. Teng CC, Che HH: Vitreous changes and the mechanism of retinal detachment, *Am J Ophthalmol* 44:335, 1957.

89. Wang J, McLeod D, Henson DB, et al: Age-dependent changes in the basal retinovitreous adhesion, *Invest Ophthalmol Vis Sci* 44(5):1793, 2003.

90. Spalton DJ, Hitchings RA, Hunter PA: *Atlas of clinical ophthalmology*, Philadelphia, 1984, Lippincott, p 124.

91. Lindner B: Acute posterior vitreous detachment and its retinal complications, *Acta Ophthalmol Suppl* 87:1, 1966.

92. Weber H, Landwehr G: A new method for the determination of the mechanical properties of the vitreous, *Ophthalmic Res* 14:326, 1982.

93. Weber H, Landwehr G, Kilp H, et al: The mechanical properties of the vitreous of pig and human donor eyes, *Ophthalmic Res* 14:335, 1982.

94. Holekamp NM: The vitreous gel: more than meets the eye, *Am J Ophthalmol* 149:32–36, 2010.

95. Harocopos GJ, Shui Y, McKinnon M, et al: Importance of vitreous liquefaction in age-related cataract, *Invest Ophthalmol Vis Sci* 45:77–85, 2004.

96. Melberg NS, Thomas MA: Nuclear sclerotic cataract after vitrectomy in patients younger than 50 years of age, *Ophthalmology* 102:1466–1471, 1995.

97. Shui B, Holekamp NM, Kramer BC, et al: The gel state of the vitreous and ascorbate-dependent oxygen consumption: relationship to the etiology of nuclear cataracts, *Arch Ophthtalmol* 127:475–482, 2009.

7 *Ocular Embryology*

This chapter follows the chapters describing the globe and orbit because the study of embryology can be difficult if the adult structure, organization, and function of the eye are not known. Although studying the development of a structure after studying the structure itself might seem backward, in my experience this has proved to be a useful sequence for the student. In this chapter, the development of each structure is described separately, but the reader must keep in mind that these events are occurring simultaneously.

With the explosion of information from improved technology and human genome study, new information is reported daily about the processes that control cellular development, structure, and function. A number of growth factors have been identified that bind to receptor sites on target cells to control normal development by modulating proliferation, migration, and differentiation.[1] These processes are at the basis of structure development. Cells from germ layers *migrate* to a specific location and then *proliferate*, forming the population of cells that will *differentiate* into the specific cell type necessary.

DEVELOPMENT OF OCULAR STRUCTURES

By the third week of embryonic development, the three primary germ layers—ectoderm, mesoderm, and endoderm—have formed the embryonic plate.[2] (Of these three, only ectoderm and mesoderm will take part in the developing ocular structures.) A thickening in the ectoderm, visible on the dorsal surface of the embryo, forms the **neural plate,** which will give rise to the central nervous system, including ocular structures. A groove forms down the center of this plate at approximately day 18 of gestation, and the ridges bordering the groove grow into **neural folds.** As the groove expands, these folds grow toward one another and fuse to form the **neural tube** along the dorsal aspect of the embryo. Just before fusing, an area of cells on the crest of each of the neural folds separates from the ectoderm; these are **neural crest cells.** They form islands of cells within the mesoderm, which now surrounds the neural tube. The neural tube is formed on or near day 22.[2] The tissue of the neural tube is now called **neural ectoderm** and the surface layer is now called **surface ectoderm.** Neural and surface ectoderm differ in anatomic location and in differentiation potentials (Box 7-1). Figure 7-1 illustrates these events.

OPTIC PITS

Indentations form in the inner surface of the neural tube on both sides of the forebrain region even before the tube is completely closed. These indentations are the **optic pits**. On approximately day 25, after the neural tube has closed, the optic pits expand forming lateral sac-shaped extensions, the **optic vesicles**.[3] The cavity within the optic vesicle is continuous with the lumen of the neural tube. The surface of each vesicle expands until it comes in contact with surface ectoderm then

---

▲ **BOX 7-1**

Embryologic Derivation of Ocular Structures

Surface ectoderm gives rise to:
- Lens
- Corneal epithelium
- Conjunctival epithelium
- Epithelium of eyelids and cilia, meibomian glands, and glands of Zeis and Moll
- Epithelium lining nasolacrimal system

Neural ectoderm gives rise to:
- Retinal pigment epithelium
- Neural retina
- Optic nerve fibers
- Neuroglia
- Epithelium of ciliary body
- Epithelium of iris
- Iris sphincter and dilator muscles

Neural crest gives rise to:
- Corneal stroma (which gives rise to Bowman's layer)
- Corneal endothelium (which gives rise to Descemet's membrane)
- Most (or all) of sclera
- Trabecular structures
- Uveal pigment cells
- Uveal connective tissue
- Ciliary muscle
- Meninges of optic nerve
- Vascular pericytes

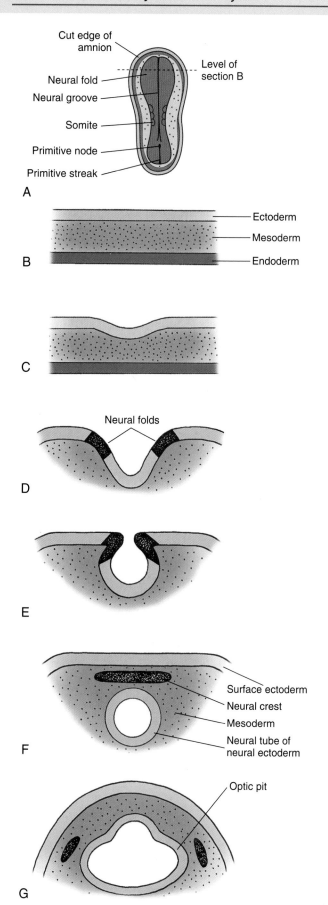

gradually becomes separated from it by cells of neural crest origin and mesoderm.[4]

Neural crest cells and mesoderm collectively make up the **mesenchyme,** from which the connective tissue of the globe and orbit develop. Although most orbital connective tissue is derived from neural crest, determining whether a structure is of neural crest or mesodermal origin sometimes is difficult because mesodermal cells and neural crest cells appear similar cytologically.[5] If the origin is uncertain, mesenchyme is cited as the germ layer.

As the optic vesicle evaginates, the tissue joining the vesicle to the neural tube constricts, forming the optic stalk (Figure 7-2). The cells lining the inner surface of this entire formation are ciliated, and the outer surface is covered by a thin basal lamina.[3] The cavity of the optic stalk, as well as that of the optic vesicle, is continuous with the space that will become the third ventricle.

While the wall of the optic vesicle is in contact with surface ectoderm, it thickens and flattens to form the retinal disc.[5] The lower wall of the optic vesicle and optic stalk begins to buckle and move inward toward the upper and posterior walls. This invagination forms a cleft, variously called the **optic fissure,** embryonic fissure, or fetal fissure. (It has also been called the "choroidal fissure," but this name will be avoided because it may imply that the choroid is involved in the fissure, which it is not.) The inferior wall continues to move inward, pulling the anterior wall of the optic vesicle with it and placing the retinal disc in the approximate location of the future retina. The edges of the fissure grow toward one another and begin to fuse at 5 weeks; fusion starts at the center and proceeds anteriorly toward the rim of the optic cup and posteriorly along the optic stalk. Closure is complete at 7 weeks, forming the two layers of the optic cup and optic stalk[6] (Figure 7-3). Mesenchyme enters the fissure and moves into the cavity of the developing optic cup.

FIGURE 7-1

Formation of neural tube. A, Dorsal surface of embryo as seen from above. **B,** Horizontal section through three-layered embryonic disc. **C,** Neural groove forms in neural plate area of ectoderm. **D,** Neural groove invaginates, and neural folds are formed. **E,** Neural folds continue to grow toward each other. **F,** Neural crest cells separate from ectoderm of neural folds as the folds fuse; neural tube is formed (of neural ectoderm); and surface ectoderm is again continuous. **G,** Evaginations in area of forebrain form the optic pits.

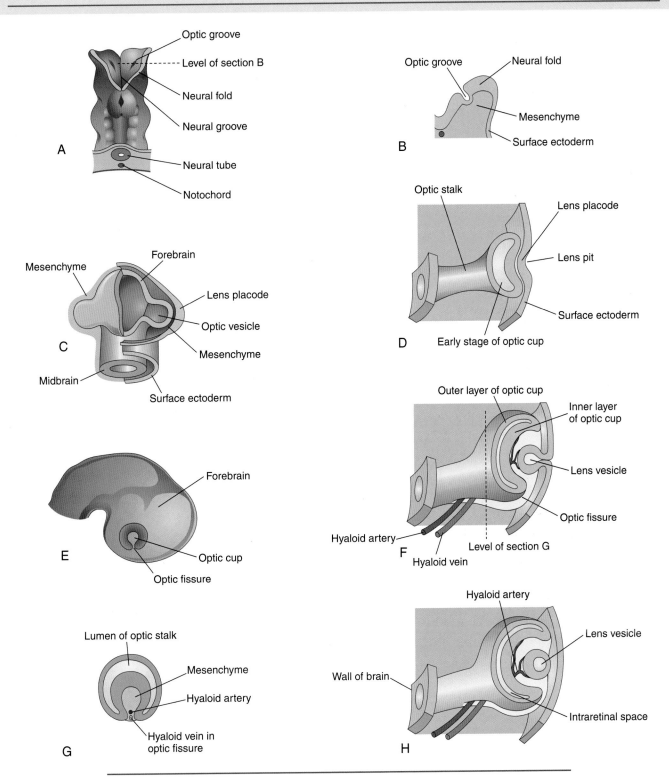

FIGURE 7-2
Early eye development. **A,** Dorsal view of cranial end of 22-day embryo showing first indication of eye development. **B,** Transverse section through neural fold showing an optic groove. **C,** Forebrain and its covering layers of mesenchyme and surface ectoderm from approximately 28-day-old embryo. **D, F,** and **H,** Sections of developing eye, illustrating successive stages in development of the optic cup and lens vesicle. **E,** Lateral view of brain of approximately 32-day-old embryo showing external appearance of optic cup. **G,** Transverse section through optic stalk showing optic fissure and its contents. (From Moore KL: *Before we are born: essentials of embryology and birth defects*, ed 5, Philadelphia, 1998, Saunders.)

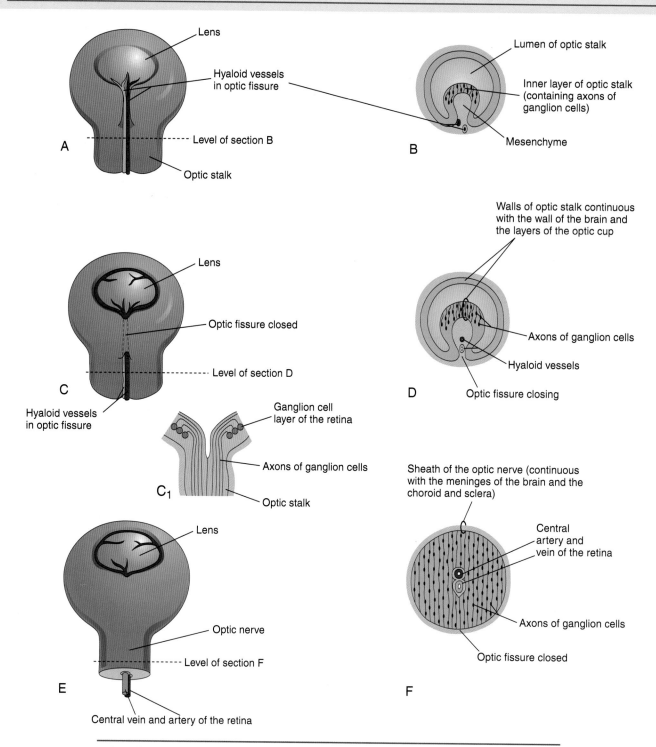

FIGURE 7-3

Closure of optic fissure and formation of optic nerve. **A, C, and E,** Views of inferior surface of optic cup and stalk showing progressive stages in closure of optic fissure. Longitudinal section of portion of optic cup and optic stalk **(C)** showing axons of ganglion cells of retina growing through optic stalk to brain. **B, D, and F,** Transverse sections through optic stalk showing successive stages in closure of optic fissure and formation of optic nerve. Optic fissure normally closes during sixth week. Defects of closure of optic fissure results in defect in iris known as coloboma of the iris. Note that lumen of optic stalk is obliterated gradually as axons of ganglion cells accumulate in the inner layer of the stalk. Formation of optic nerve occurs between sixth and eighth weeks. (From Moore KL: *Before we are born: essentials of embryology and birth defects*, ed 5, Philadelphia, 1998, Saunders.)

OPTIC CUP, LENS, AND HYALOID VESSELS

Optic Cup

The **optic cup** at this stage of development is composed of two layers of cells (both neuroectodermal in origin) that are continuous with each other at the rim of the cup. The cells of the inner and outer layers of the optic cup are positioned apex to apex and are separated by the *intraretinal space* (see Figure 7-2, *H*), which, as the two layers approach each other, finally will become only a potential space. The **outer layer** of the optic cup will become the retinal pigment epithelium (RPE), the outer pigmented epithelium of the ciliary body, and the anterior iris epithelium. The **inner layer** will become the neural retina, the inner nonpigmented ciliary body epithelium, and the posterior iris epithelium.

Mesenchyme proliferates and migrates around the optic cup, and once the cells reach their destination, they proliferate and differentiate, contributing to the connective tissue of the eye and orbit. Neural crest cells will form corneal stroma and endothelium, uveal stroma and melanocytes, ciliary muscle, much of the sclera, the connective tissue and meningeal sheaths of the optic nerve, and the connective tissue of the lids, conjunctiva, and orbit. Vascular endothelium and striated muscle cells are formed by mesoderm.[1]

Clinical Comment: Coloboma

*Incomplete closure of the optic fissure may affect the developing optic cup or stalk and the adult derivations of these structures, resulting in an inferior nasal defect in the optic disc, retina, ciliary body, or iris. This defect is called a **coloboma** and can vary from a slight notch to a large wedgelike defect. A large iris coloboma produces a keyhole-shaped pupil, although the remainder of the iris develops normally (Figure 7-4, A). When the coloboma is unilateral, the affected iris may have denser pigmentation than the opposite normal iris.[7] Colobomas affecting the sensory retina and RPE also involve the choroid because its differentiation depends on an intact RPE layer.[8] Bare sclera is seen in the area affected, with retinal vessels passing over the defect (Figure 7-4, B).*

Induction

During embryologic development, formation and growth of structures depend on tissue differentiation and interactions among these tissues. Some structures will not develop unless they are near another developing area at a specific time. In some cases the two structures must actually come in contact; in others the structures must just be in proximity to each other, allowing biochemical signals to pass between them.[9] The influence that one developing structure has on another is termed **induction.** It is likely that the mechanism of induction is not a single event but a series of separate steps that presumably occur on a biochemical level.[10]

Lens

Induction occurs between the developing optic cup and the developing lens, apparently through a reciprocal relationship.[11] As the surface ectoderm comes in contact with the optic vesicle, the invagination of the optic cup begins (approximately day 27), and the surface ectoderm adjacent to the vesicle begins to thicken, forming the **lens plate (lens placode)** (Figures 7-5 and 7-6, *A*). This thickening is caused by an elongation of the ectodermal cells and by a regional increase in cell division.[5] If the area of contact between the optic vesicle and surface ectoderm is less than normal, a perfectly formed but microphthalmic eye can result.[12] Some investigators believe that transformation of the lens plate into the lens vesicle might be independent of direct contact with the optic vesicle.[13] In addition to signals from the developing optic vesicle, complete lens differentiation might also depend on factors that inhibit lens formation in the ectoderm adjacent to the lens plate.[14]

Cell division ceases in the center of the lens plate, forming a pit, and cell division accelerates in the periphery such that the lens plate invaginates rapidly.[15] As invagination continues, the lens vesicle is formed and then separates from the surface ectoderm at approximately day 33.[3,9] The **lens vesicle** is a hollow sphere composed of a single layer of cells, the apical surface of the cell lines the lumen, and the basal aspect is covered by a thin basal lamina; with the addition of more material, the basal lamina will become the lens capsule (Figure 7-6, *B* and *C*).

Once the lens vesicle is formed, the posterior epithelial cells adjacent to the future vitreous cavity elongate to fill in the lumen within the lens vesicle (Figure 7-6, *D, E*). In chick embryos if the lens is turned 180 degrees the epithelium that was once at the anterior of the lens vesicle is now adjacent to the developing optic cup and this is the epithelium that elongates filling in the lumen.[16] The developing retina secretes biochemical mediators and is apparently the inducing factor for this elongation.[15] The orientation of the lens is also influenced by the developing vitreous.[12,17] The posterior epithelial cells become the *primary lens fibers* and form the **embryonic nucleus** at the center of the lens. This nucleus has no sutures. The fact that the posterior epithelium was used to form the embryonic nucleus accounts for the lack of an epithelial layer beneath the posterior lens capsule in the fully formed lens. The anterior epithelial cells remain in place, and the cells near the equator begin to undergo mitosis. Each new cell elongates anteriorly and posteriorly, forming *secondary lens fibers* that are laid down around the embryonic nucleus.

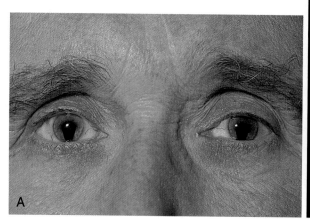
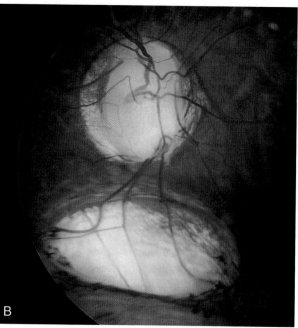

FIGURE 7-4
A, Iris coloboma (OU); pupil has keyhole appearance. **B,** Coloboma of retina. Retinal tissue and choroidal tissue are absent, retinal vessels course across the intact sclera. (**A** from Kanski JJ, Nischal KK: *Ophthalmology; clinical signs and differential diagnosis*, St Louis, 1999, Mosby; **B** courtesy Pacific University Family Vision Center, Forest Grove, Ore.)

The first layer of secondary fibers is completed by week 7.[9] Secondary lens fibers continue to form and each layer surrounds the previous layer. The ends of the fibers meet in an *upright* Y-suture immediately posterior to the anterior epithelium and in an *inverted* Y-suture immediately anterior to the posterior capsule. These sutures are visible during the third month.[18] The **fetal nucleus** contains the Y-sutures and all fibers formed before birth. If a line were drawn to connect the cellular nuclei within a lens fiber layer, an arcuate shape would be revealed. This configuration is called the *lens bow* (Figure 7-7).

Mitosis, cell elongation, and lens fiber formation continue throughout development and throughout life. The lens is initially spherical in shape but becomes more ellipsoid with additional fibers.[16] The lens capsule is evident at 5 weeks, evolving from the basement membrane of the invaginating surface ectoderm and from secretions of the lens epithelium.[18]

Clinical Comment: Congenital Cataract

The spectrum of lens opacities that can result from problems during lens development range from pinpoint densities having no effect on vision to significant opacities causing extensive loss of vision.[19] If the tissue near the developing lens fails to induce the lens fibers to elongate and pack together in an orderly way, the lens fibers will be misaligned, forming a cataract of the primary fibers. Interference with secondary lens fibers can lead to sutural cataracts.[20]

Viral infection affecting the mother during the first trimester often causes congenital malformations, including a cataract. The developing lens is vulnerable to the rubella virus (German measles) between the fourth and seventh week of development, when the primary fibers are forming. After this period the virus cannot penetrate the lens capsule and thus will not affect the lens. The cataract usually is present at birth but may develop weeks to months later because the virus can persist within the lens for up to 3 years. The opacity may be dense and opaque or it may be diffuse; the cataract may affect the nucleus only or may involve most of the lens.[21]

Hyaloid Arterial System

A branch of the internal carotid artery enters the optic cup through the fetal fissure to become the **hyaloid artery** during week 5.[1] This vessel produces a highly branching network that fills the vitreous cavity and forms the *posterior vascular tunic of the lens (posterior tunica vasculosa lentis)*, a vascular network covering the posterior lens (Figure 7-8). By the end of the second month, the hyaloid vasculature is fully formed.[1]

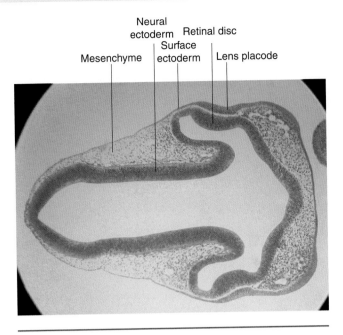

FIGURE 7-5
Light micrograph of 6-mm pig embryo showing thickening of lens placode.

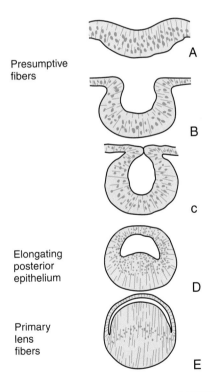

FIGURE 7-6
A, Formation of lens placode. B, Invagination forming lens vesicle. C to E, Development of embryonic nucleus. C, Hollow lens vesicle is lined with epithelium. D, Posterior cells elongate, becoming primary lens fibers. E, Primary lens fibers fill lumen, forming embryonic nucleus. Curved line formed by cell nuclei is called the lens bow. Anterior epithelium remains in place.

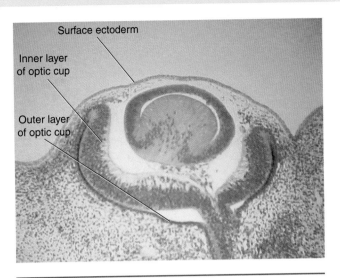

FIGURE 7-7
Light micrograph of 15-mm pig embryo showing lens vesicle filling with primary lens fibers; lens bow configuration is evident.

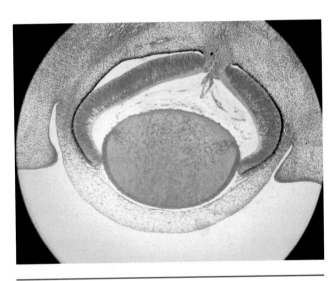

FIGURE 7-8
Light micrograph of 25-mm pig embryo showing the hyaloid arterial system filling future vitreal cavity. Vessels are evident extending through the optic stalk and the vascular network attached to posterior lens is evident. Early layers of corneal epithelium, stroma, and endothelium are present.

Branches near the lens equator anastomose with the **annular vessel** at the margin of the optic cup. The annular vessel sends loops forward onto the anterior surface of the lens to form the *anterior vascular tunic of the lens (anterior tunica vasculosa lentis)* during the seventh week[1,22,23] (Figure 7-9). These vascular networks carry nutrients to the developing lens until production of the aqueous humor occurs. These vessels drain into a network located in the region that will become the ciliary body.[3] The vessels of the hyaloid system cannot

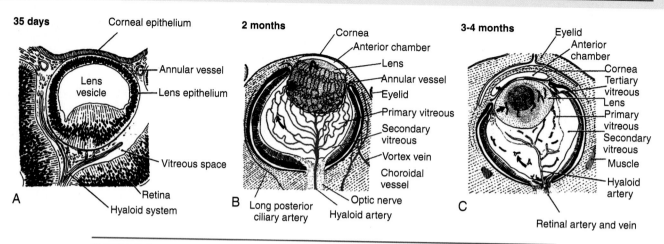

FIGURE 7-9

Schema of main features in vitreous development and regression of hyaloid system, shown in drawings of sagittal sections. **A,** At 5 weeks, hyaloid vessels and branches occupy much of space between lens and neural ectoderm. **B,** By 2 months, vascular primary vitreous reaches its greatest extent. An avascular secondary vitreous of more finely fibrillar composition forms a narrow zone between peripheral branches of hyaloid system and retina. **C,** During fourth month, vessels of hyaloid system atrophy progressively. Zonular fibers (tertiary vitreous) begin to stretch from growing ciliary region toward lens capsule. Vessels through center of optic nerve connect with hyaloid vessels and send small loops into retina. (From Cook CS, Ozanics V, Jakobiec FA: Prenatal development of the eye and its adnexa. In Tasman W, Jaeger EA, editors: *Duane's foundations of clinical ophthalmology,* vol 1, Philadelphia, 1994, Lippincott.)

be identified as arterial or venous on the basis of their histologic makeup.[22]

Glial cells on the surface of the optic cup form a cone-like mass of tissue around the base of the hyaloid artery. These cells proliferate, forming a glial mantle around the arterial system. The hyaloid vasculature reaches its peak development during the third month[1] and begins to atrophy during the fourth month, at the same time that the retinal vasculature is developing.[1,24] By the seventh month, no blood flow is present in the hyaloid vasculature, which normally should be completely reabsorbed by birth.[3] The extent of the degeneration of the glial tissue mass defines the extent of the adult physiologic optic cup.[25]

Clinical Comment: Bergmeister's Papilla and Mittendorf's Dot

*Remnants of the hyaloid system often are seen clinically during examination of a patient's ocular health. Glial tissue that persists on the nerve head is called **Bergmeister's papilla** (Figure 7-10, A), and a pinpoint remnant of the hyaloid artery on the posterior surface of the lens is called **Mittendorf's dot.** Rarely, a remnant of the entire hyaloid artery will be seen coursing through the vitreous from its attachment at the disc to the posterior lens (Figure 7-10, B).*

Retinal Pigment Epithelium

Apposition of the two layers of the optic cup is essential for development of the **retinal pigment epithelium,**[12] the first retinal layer to differentiate.[25] Cellular structures and melanosomes begin to appear in the outer layer of the optic cup, and pigmentation of the retinal epithelium occurs at approximately week 3 or 4; this is the earliest pigmentation evident in the embryo[3,4,26] (see Figure 7-8). After week 6, the RPE is one cell thick. The cells are cuboidal to columnar in shape, and the base of each cell is external toward the developing choroid and the apex internal toward the inner layer of the optic cup.[27,28]

Neural Retina

Between weeks 4 to 6, the cells of the inner layer of the optic cup (in the area that will become the neural retina) proliferate, and two zones are evident.[1] The cells accumulate in the outer region, the **proliferative zone** or **germinating zone.** The inner **marginal zone (of His)** is anuclear. A thin lamina—the basement membrane of the inner layer of the optic cup and the precursor of the internal limiting membrane—separates the marginal zone from the vitreal cavity.[18] At approximately week 7, cell migration occurs, forming the inner and outer neuroblastic layers, between which lies the **transient fiber layer of Chievitz,** a nucleus-free area.[27,29] The formation of

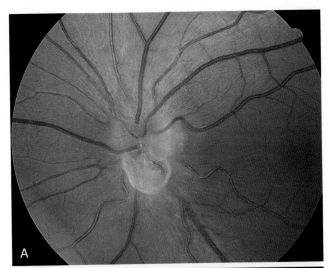

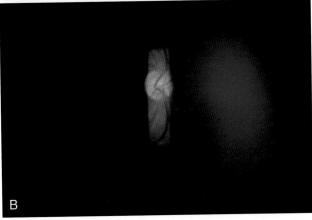

FIGURE 7-10
A, Raised glial tissue on optic disc; Bergmeister's papilla.
B, Persistent hyaloid artery seen extending from optic disc into vitreous. (**A** From Kanski JJ, Nischal KK: *Ophthalmology: clinical signs and differential diagnosis*, St Louis, 1999, Mosby.) (**B** Courtesy Edward B. Mallett, O.D., Pacific University Family Vision Center, Forest Grove, Ore.)

these two neuroblastic layers is complete during the third month. Differentiation of the neural retinal cells begins in the central retina and proceeds to the periphery.[1]

Ganglion cells and amacrine cells differentiate in the vitread portion of the **inner neuroblastic layer.**[30] The ganglion cells migrate, forming a layer close to the basement membrane, and almost immediately send out their axonal processes, which become evident by week 8.[18] Biomolecular agents guide axonal growth toward termination in the lateral geniculate nucleus.[31,32] Müller cells, located rather centrally in the inner neuroblastic layer, develop at the same time. The bodies of the Müller and amacrine cells remain in the inner neuroblastic layer but move slightly sclerad.[30]

Bipolar cells migrate from the **outer neuroblastic layer** and settle near the Müller and amacrine cells; the horizontal cells follow.[1] The fiber layer of Chievitz

is gradually obliterated by this move of the prospective bipolar and horizontal cells.[18] The photoreceptor cells remain in the outer neuroblastic layer. By week 12 the photoreceptors are aligned along the outer side of the inner layer of the optic cup and adhering junctions appear between them. These junctions form the precursor of the external limiting membrane. The photoreceptor cells are the last cells of neural retina to differentiate; this occurs during the fifth month.[1] Cones differentiate first and rods begin to differentiate during the seventh month. The early inner segment produces a protuberance that becomes embedded in the RPE and continues to grow, forming the cilium and outer segment by week 24 or 25.[18,33]

The horizontal, bipolar, amacrine, and Müller cells are developing in the inner nuclear layer, and the inner and outer plexiform layers are filling with neuronal processes.[3] The fibers of the Müller cells appear and extend to the basal lamina, forming the primitive internal limiting membrane, and external processes extend between the rods and cones.[3,27] The Müller cell provides a scaffolding for cell development and appears to be involved with guiding the direction of axonal fiber growth.[34] (The developing interplexiform neuron has not yet been identified.) Figures 7-11 and 7-12 show the development of the neural retina.

Synaptic complexes begin to appear at about the same time as the plexiform layers, with the inner plexiform layer preceding the outer layer.[27,35] Cone pedicles develop earlier than rod spherules, and photoreceptor synapses with bipolar cells are established before the outer segments are completed.[27]

By month 5 the ganglion cell layer is well established.[36] Because retinal development is more advanced centrally than peripherally, the ganglion axons from the periphery must take an arched route above and below the macular area to reach the nerve head.[33,37] This line of deviation at the horizontal temporal meridian is termed the **horizontal raphe.**[3] During the fifth month a reduction of retinal cells by apoptosis begins. By month 6 there is no further mitosis, and retinal growth continues because of cell differentiation, growth, and maturation.[38]

During the sixth month cones begin to differentiate, and a dense accumulation of nuclei in the macular area makes this region thicker than the rest of the retina;[25] up to nine rows of ganglion cells are evident.[36] Foveal development consists of three stages: (1) displacement of inner retinal components to form the depression; (2) migration of photoreceptors toward the center, which increases cone packing; and (3) maturation of the photoreceptors.[39] During the seventh month the ganglion cells and the cells of the inner nuclear layer begin to move to the periphery of the macula. By birth, however, there still is a single layer of ganglion cells and a thin inner nuclear layer across the now-depressed foveal area (Figure 7-13). By 4 months postpartum, both these layers are displaced to the sloping walls of the fovea, leaving the cones of the

**Retina
2½ months**

**Retina
4½ months**

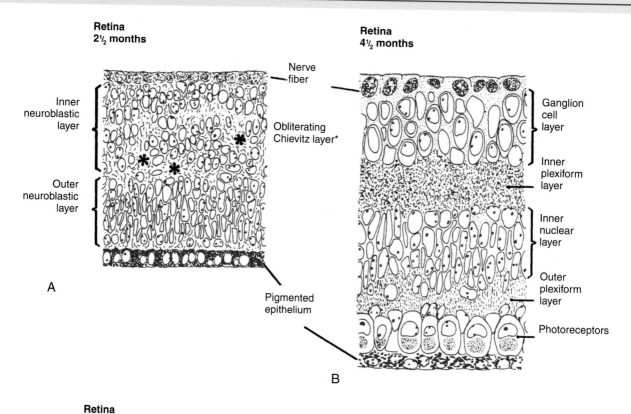

Inner
neuroblastic
layer

Outer
neuroblastic
layer

Nerve
fiber

Obliterating
Chievitz layer*

Pigmented
epithelium

Ganglion
cell
layer

Inner
plexiform
layer

Inner
nuclear
layer

Outer
plexiform
layer

Photoreceptors

A

B

**Retina
5½ months**

Newborn

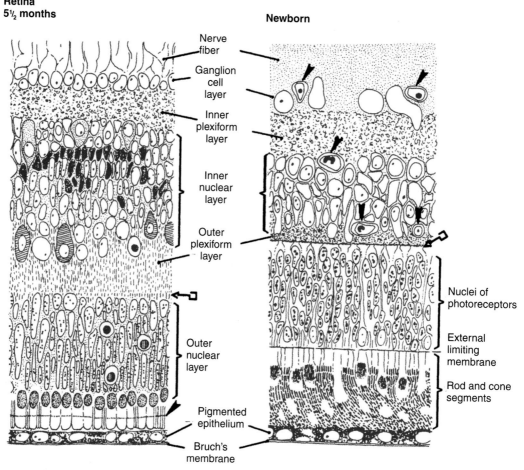

Nerve
fiber

Ganglion
cell
layer

Inner
plexiform
layer

Inner
nuclear
layer

Outer
plexiform
layer

Outer
nuclear
layer

Pigmented
epithelium

Bruch's
membrane

Nuclei of
photoreceptors

External
limiting
membrane

Rod and cone
segments

C

D

FIGURE 7-11

Developing retina. Region of posterior pole is represented in sagittal section in each diagram. **A,** At 2.5 months, transient fiber layer of Chievitz, which separated inner from outer neuroblastic layers of primitive retina, is being obliterated slowly by shifting of nuclear elements and realignment of their processes. Uppermost cells, lying vitread, are differentiating into ganglion cells. Those below the uneven transient layer of Chievitz (*asterisks*) are immature but are destined to differentiate into amacrine and Müller cells. Future inner plexiform layer will be located between shifted nuclei of Müller and amacrine cells and those of ganglion cells. Outer neuroblastic layer contains photoreceptor, bipolar, and horizontal cell elements. **B,** At midterm (4.5 months), retinal lamination essentially is complete. Ganglion cells have multilayered arrangement. Inner plexiform layer, composed of fibers of bipolar, ganglion, and amacrine cells supported by müllerian fibers, has established sites of primitive conventional and ribbon synapses. In the inner nuclear layer the still undifferentiated cellular components are recognizable by shape and position. In the outer nuclear layer, large cone nuclei are aligned adjacent to pigment epithelium, and smaller rod nuclei are positioned more vitread. Outer plexiform layer has primitive lamellar synapses between bipolar cell dendrites and cone pedicles (not indicated). Photoreceptor outer segments are not yet present. **C,** At 5.5 months, ganglion cells have thinned out to one to two layers (except in macular area). Cellular components of inner nuclear layer include amacrine cells with large, pale nuclei in innermost (vitread) zone of this layer and pleomorphic, dark-staining Müller cell nuclei. Both these types originally came from inner neuroblastic layer. Also included are smaller bipolar cells and large, pale-staining horizontal cells in an irregular arrangement sclerad. These two cell types, together with photoreceptors, are derived from outer neuroblastic layer. Outer plexiform layer has a linear arrangement of synapses between bipolar cells and rod spherules (key symbol). Outer nuclear layer consists of six to seven layers of nuclei; outermost layers are cones aligned to external limiting membrane. Growing photoreceptor outer segments project into space between pigment epithelium and external limiting membrane (*arrowhead*). Cell death is represented by round, dark-centered symbols. **D,** Newborn retina has adult configuration, with vascularization (*arrowheads*) reaching outer limits of inner nuclear layer. Outer plexiform layer is thinner than that in adult, but line of synapses is well established (key symbol). Rod and cone inner and outer segments are fully developed, and tips of outer segments contact pigment epithelium. (From Cook CS, Ozanics V, Jakobiec FA: Prenatal development of the eye and its adnexa. In Tasman W, Jaeger EA, editors: *Duane's foundations of clinical ophthalmology*, vol 1, Philadelphia, 1994, Lippincott.)

outer nuclear layer as the only neural cell bodies in the center of the depression.[4,6] The foveal depression continues to deepen until about age 15 months as cells continue to move toward the macular periphery.[39]

The **foveola,** the retinal area of sharpest visual acuity, is the last to reach maturity.[39] Before birth the rod-free area is large compared with that in the adult, but it becomes narrower with migration of the cones centrally, increasing cone density. When examining an area with a diameter of 100 µm at the center of the rod-free zone, the cone population is 18 in the 1-week-old infant. The cone population increases to 42 by age 4 to 5 years, which is the same count as seen in the adult.[39] The cone inner fibers elongate and adopt an oblique orientation (forming *Henle's fiber layer*) in order to synapse with the cells of the inner nuclear layer, which have been displaced to the sloping walls. During the first few years, the outer segment continues to develop and the inner fiber lengthens.

Clinical Comment: Ocular Albinism

Melanocytes that derive their pigment from neural crest (i.e., those located in the choroid, skin, and hair) show a variance that is related to race. Melanocytes that are neuroectodermal in derivation (i.e., retinal pigment, iris, and ciliary body epithelia) are densely pigmented in all races.[36] Melanin production is gene regulated, and in an individual with albinism either or both types of melanocytes can be affected. Because normal development of sensory retina is influenced by a melanin-related agent produced in the RPE, when pigment is absent from this layer, as occurs in ocular albinism, a number of retinal abnormalities are present at birth in addition to the absence of pigmentation. The macula is underdeveloped and the fovea may be absent. The number of rods may be decreased.[40] Abnormal optic nerve projection to the lateral geniculate nucleus occurs, with more crossed fibers than normal, often resulting in binocular problems.[40]

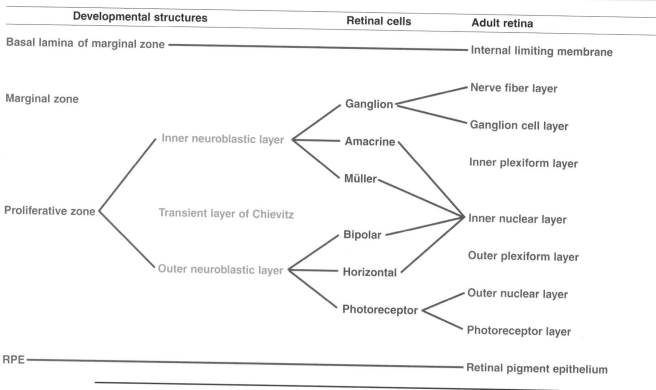

FIGURE 7-12
Flow chart of retinal development.

Retinal Vessels

The fetal fissure along the optic stalk closes around the hyaloid artery, and the portions of the vessel within the stalk become the **central retinal artery.**[3] A branch of the primitive maxillary vein located within the optic stalk is the likely precursor of the **central retinal vein.**[26] Early in the fourth month of development, primitive retinal vessels emerge from the hyaloid artery near the optic disc and enter the developing nerve fiber layer. Signals from biomolecular agents called guidance molecules guide the growth and pathway of neurons and likely also guide the growth of these retinal vessels.[41,42] The vessels of the retina continue to develop, gradually forming the arterioles, venules, and capillary beds, but all vessel structure is not completed until approximately 3 months after birth, with the vessels to the nasal periphery completed before those to the temporal periphery.[3]

Clinical Comment: Retinopathy of Prematurity

*Premature infants who are exposed to a high concentration of oxygen can develop **retinopathy of prematurity** (also called **retrolental fibroplasia**). The immature retinal blood vessels respond to the high concentration of oxygen with vasoconstriction and cease to develop. On removal of the oxygen, vasoproliferation occurs; however, the new vessel growth is composed of "leaky" vessels with poorly formed endothelial tight junctions. Potential serious complications include neovascular invasion of the vitreous and development of vitreoretinal adhesions, which may be followed by hemorrhage and retinal detachment.[43]*

CORNEA

Induction by the developing anterior epithelium of the lens signals multiple steps in corneal development, at about the time the lens vesicle separates from the surface ectoderm (day 33).[12,17,44] One or two layers of epithelial cells from surface ectoderm become aligned and will form the corneal epithelium. During the sixth week, zonula occludens are evident.[1] The first component of the anchoring system is the basal lamina, which is evident by week 9, and hemidesmosomes are present by week 13.[45] By the fifth or sixth month, all the cellular layers of the corneal epithelium are present.[46] **Corneal endothelium,** formed from the first wave of mesenchyme that migrates into the space between the corneal epithelium and the lens, is one to two cells thick by week 6.[3] At 4 months the endothelium is a single row of flattened cells with a basal lamina, the first evidence of **Descemet's membrane.**[3,47] By the middle of the fourth month, tight junctions are apparent in

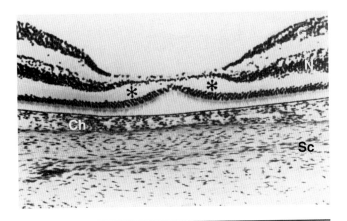

FIGURE 7-13
Fovea of *Macaca mulatta* just before birth (159 days; term at 162 to 165 days). One interrupted row of ganglion cells and one to two layers of bipolar cells still extend across foveal depression. Wide, well-developed horizontal outer plexiform layer of Henle (*asterisks*) and elongated cone inner and outer segments are present. Parafoveal area has large accumulation of cells in ganglion (*G*) and inner nuclear layer (*N*) characteristic of mature macula. *Ch,* Choroid; *Sc,* sclera. (×95.) (From Cook CS, Ozanics V, Jakobiec FA: Prenatal development of the eye and its adnexa. In Tasman W, Jaeger EA, editors: *Duane's foundations of clinical ophthalmology,* vol 1, Philadelphia, 1994, Lippincott.)

the endothelium, coinciding with the beginning of aqueous formation.[48] The material comprising Descemet's membrane before birth has a banded appearance, whereas the tissue secreted by the endothelium after birth (which has a more posterior position) has a homogeneous, unbanded appearance.[49,50]

By week 8, a second wave of mesenchyme proliferates, migrates between the developing epithelium and endothelium, and gives rise to the fibroblasts, collagen, and ground substance of the **stroma.**[3,51] A third wave of mesenchyme migrates into the area between the developing endothelium and lens, giving rise to the pupillary membrane. These three waves of mesenchyme, as well as that giving rise to the sclera, are of neural crest origin (see Box 7-1).[3]

At 3 months all layers of the cornea are present (Figure 7-14) except **Bowman's layer,** which appears during the fourth month[45] and is presumably formed by fibroblasts of the anterior stroma and secretions of the epithelial cells;[52,53] whatever the stage, Bowman's layer is always acellular.[49] Fibroblast arrangement and subsequent production of collagen fibrils begins in posterior corneal stroma and proceeds anteriorly. Rapid growth of the corneal stroma causes an increase in curvature relative to the rest of the globe.[5] At birth the cornea is circular and steep (55D); the curvature decreases to 44D at age 6 months[1].

SCLERA

The sclera first develops anteriorly from condensations in the mesenchyme near the limbus. Growth continues posteriorly until the sclera reaches the optic nerve, and by the end of the third month the sclera has surrounded the developing choroid.[26] During the fourth month connective tissue fibers cross the posterior scleral foramen, running through the optic nerve fibers and producing the first connective tissue strands of the **lamina cribrosa.**[3] By the fifth month, the sclera (including the scleral spur) is well differentiated.[4]

UVEA

Choroid

The mesenchyme that forms the **choriocapillaris** must be in contact with the developing pigment epithelium to differentiate.[4,6] The vessels appear during the second month, and the diaphragm-covered fenestrations are evident by week 12.[28] Bruch's membrane develops during month 4. During the fifth month the layers of the large and medium vessels are evident, as are the vessels that will become vortex veins.[54] The short posterior ciliary arteries also are evident and begin to anastomose to form the circle of Zinn.[3]

At midterm in fetal development the elastic sheet of **Bruch's membrane** is present, the basement membrane of the RPE is developing, and the collagenous layers are thickening. The basement membrane of the choriocapillaris is the last component to appear.[3] By term the choroidal stroma is pigmented.[28]

Ciliary Body

The region of the outer layer of the optic cup, which will become the **outer pigmented epithelium** of the ciliary body, begins to form ridges late in the third month.[55] The **inner nonpigmented epithelium,** from the inner optic cup layer, grows and folds with it. These folds, almost 70 in number, become the ciliary processes. Zonula occludens are evident in the nonpigmented epithelium during the third month.[1] Neural crest cells differentiate into stromal elements; the fenestrations in the capillaries in the processes are visible in week 14.[3,55] During the fourth month the major arterial circle of the iris is formed by the anastomosing long ciliary arteries and replaces the annular vessel.[56] Gap junctions and desmosomes appear, joining the apices of the two epithelial layers during the fourth month. The **ciliary muscle** begins to develop from neural crest[44] during the fifth month. However, the annular muscle (of Müller) remains incomplete at birth.[3,4] Aqueous humor production begins at 4 to 6 months of gestation.[55]

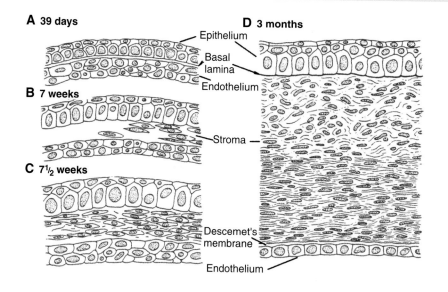

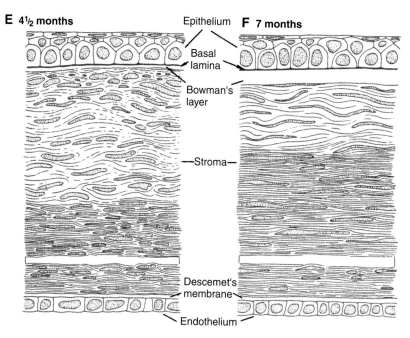

FIGURE 7-14

Developing cornea, central region. A, At 39 days, two-layered epithelium rests on a basal lamina. It is separated from two- to three-layered "endothelium" by narrow cellular space. **B,** At 7 weeks, mesenchyme from periphery migrates into space between epithelium and endothelium, the precursor of future corneal stroma. **C,** Mesenchyme (fibroblasts) is arranged in four or five incomplete layers by 7½ weeks, and a few collagen fibrils appear among them. **D,** By 3 months, epithelium has two or three layers of cells, and stroma has approximately 25 to 30 layers of fibroblasts (keratoblasts), which are more regularly arranged in its posterior half. Thin, uneven Descemet's membrane is between most posterior keratoblasts and monolayered endothelium. **E,** By midterm (4.5 months), some "wing cells" are forming above basal epithelial cells, and an indefinite, acellular Bowman's layer emerges beneath basal lamina. In almost one third of anterior portion of multilayered stroma, keratoblasts are strewn in a disorganized formation. Descemet's membrane is well developed. **F,** At 7 months, adult structure of cornea is established. A few mostly superficial keratoblasts still are randomly oriented with respect to corneal surface. Collagenous lamellae in rest of stroma are in parallel array, and only a few spaces in the matrix lack collagen fibrils. Breaks near bottom of **E** and **F** indicate that central portion of stroma is not represented. (From Cook CS, Ozanics V, Jakobiec FA: Prenatal development of the eye and its adnexa. In Tasman W, Jaeger EA, editors: *Duane's foundations of clinical ophthalmology,* vol 1, Philadelphia, 1994, Lippincott.)

Iris

By the end of the third month, the lip of the optic cup begins to elongate and grows between the lens and the developing cornea. The outer layer of the optic cup becomes the **anterior iris epithelium** and the inner layer forms the **posterior iris epithelium;** these layers remain separated from each other for a time by the marginal sinus. The proliferation of myofilaments in the basal aspect of the anterior epithelium adjoining the stroma transforms the layer into *myoepithelium.*[57] The group of cells that will become the iris sphincter breaks away from the pupillary zone of this epithelial layer during the fifth month and develops into smooth muscle within the iris stroma.[6,57] During the sixth gestational month the fibers of the dilator muscle continue to develop within the epithelial layer, and both muscles are completed by birth. That the sphincter and dilator come from *neural ectoderm* is unusual because most muscle tissue is derived from mesenchyme. Pigmentation in the anterior and posterior epithelium begins to appear at approximately week 10 and is complete during the seventh month. The marginal sinus disappears and the two epithelial layers are joined at their apices by intercellular junctions.[3]

Mesenchymal cells line up, leaving large gaps between them, to form the anterior border layer. The stromal components are of neural crest origin and are said to migrate from the second wave of mesenchyme.[1,58] A sparse distribution of collagen fibers begins to accumulate to form the iris stroma.[3] Stromal melanocytes continue to produce more pigment, and the color of the iris can continue to darken for the first 6 postnatal months, with some stromal organization not complete until age 7 years.[1]

PUPILLARY MEMBRANE

As the lens thickens, its anterior vascular tunic disconnects from the annular vessel, and its constituents are incorporated into the iris stroma; remnants contribute to the minor circle of the iris.[3] During the third month, the **pupillary membrane** forms between the lens epithelium and the corneal endothelium to replace the vascular tunic. This transitory membrane contains components from the third wave of mesenchyme and branches from the major circle of the iris.[1,59] (The pupillary membrane can be seen in Figure 7-15 just anterior to the lens.) Three or four arcades of thin-walled blood vessels separated by a thin mesodermal membrane are completed by the end of the fifth month.[59] The vessels of the pupillary membrane cannot be identified as arterial or venous on the basis of their histologic makeup.[22]

During gestational month 6, the central vessels atrophy and become bloodless. The more peripheral vessels contribute to the minor circle of the iris, and by

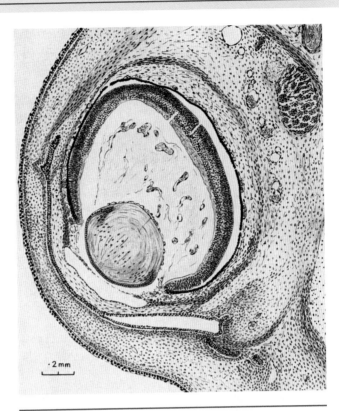

FIGURE 7-15
Section through eye and surrounding structures in 35-mm human embryo (approximately 8 weeks). (From Mann I: *The development of the human eye*, New York, 1964, Grune & Stratton. Copyright 1964, British Medical Association.)

8½ months the central vessels have fragmented and disappeared.[6,59] As reabsorption of the central pupillary membrane occurs, the loops of the midregion form the ridge of the collarette, with other components incorporated into the anterior border layer.[3]

Clinical Comment: Persistent Pupillary Membrane

Remnants of the central portion of the pupillary membrane that do not reabsorb may be seen with a biomicroscope and appear similar to strands of a spider web attached to the surface of the iris. A persistent pupillary membrane may have a variety of presentations, from a single strand of connective tissue (anchored at one or both ends) to several interconnecting strands; pigment cells also might be incorporated. A persistent pupillary membrane is present in 17% to 32% of the population.[59]

ANTERIOR CHAMBER

A mass of cells of neural crest origin and from the first wave of mesenchyme accumulates adjacent to the ciliary body and the iris root in the anterior chamber angle area.[50,60] The method whereby this mass is eliminated to expose the angle remains controversial. The mass may atrophy,[4] the structure may split between the iris and the meshwork, with some tissue contributing to each,[61] or the intercellular spaces may enlarge and the cells reorganize into the surrounding tissue.[62]

The **trabecular meshwork** is visible as a triangular mass of mesenchymal cells during the fourth month; at least part of this tissue is of neural crest origin (see Box 7-1).[63-65] The tissue progressively becomes more organized, and by 9 months the trabecular beams and pores are well developed, with the intratrabecular spaces and pores likely formed by programmed cell death.

Schlemm's canal is derived from the deep scleral plexus.[63,64] During the fourth month, tight junctions are evident in the canal's endothelial lining.[62] During the seventh month, Schlemm's canal is fully formed in some quadrants; during the eighth month, giant vacuoles are seen in the endothelial lining, and the complete circular canal is present during the ninth month.

Once formed, the anterior chamber is lined by a continuous endothelium that covers the trabecular meshwork and the iridocorneal angle.[66] This membrane appears continuous at gestational month 7 but is discontinuous in the region of the meshwork by month 9.[62,67] During the last few weeks before birth, splits occur between cells in the membrane, and the size and number of these splits increase rapidly because of the increase in the size of the anterior ocular structures.[67] The loss of continuity in this membrane over the trabecular meshwork correlates significantly with an increase in the facility of aqueous outflow.[63] Persistence of the uninterrupted endothelial membrane over the meshwork *(Barkan's membrane)* can be a causative factor in congenital glaucoma.[3,8,67]

VITREOUS

The presence of the developing lens is essential for normal accumulation of vitreous.[68] The **primary vitreous** fills the vitreous space early in development (see Figure 7-8) and has both mesenchymal and ectodermal origins. Fibrils derived from the developing lens and from the developing retina and components from the degenerating hyaloid system will form the primary vitreous.[62]

As the **secondary vitreous** develops, apparently produced by neural retina and hyalocytes from the primary vitreous,[1] it encloses the primary vitreous within the region of the atrophying hyaloid vessels, thus forming the funnel-shaped **Cloquet's canal.** This zone, with its apex at the optic disc and its base at the posterior lens, is well formed by the fourth month. It persists in the adult. The secondary vitreous contains a fibril network and primitive hyalocytes.[3] During the third month, a thickening of secondary vitreous in the anterior peripheral area occurs (the marginal bundle of Druault); it forms

attachments at the vitreous base and at the hyaloideo-capsular ligament.[1]

The **zonule fibers** develop in the area between the lens equator and the ciliary body. They have been called *tertiary vitreous* because they do arise in the vitreous and were assumed to be collagenous, but now are believed to be noncollagenous.[1] Questions remain about whether the tertiary vitreous is mesenchymal or epithelial in origin.[3] The fibers forming the zonules pass through the marginal bundle of Druault at right angles. Early zonule fibers appear to be a continuation of a thickening of the internal limiting membrane of the ciliary body, formed by the ciliary epithelium; the fibers run from a zone near the ora serrata and from the valleys between the processes to the lens capsule.[5] The zonules are well formed during the seventh month.

OPTIC NERVE

The optic stalk, the precursor of the **optic nerve,** joins the optic vesicle to the forebrain. As the optic fissure develops along the inferior stalk invagination, a two-layered optic stalk is created. The outer layer of the optic stalk becomes the neuroglial sheath that surrounds the optic nerve; it also gives rise to the glial components of the lamina cribrosa.[3] Programmed cell death occurs in the cells of the inner layer, providing an avenue for passage of the axons from ganglion cells entering the optic stalk; other cells of the inner wall become the glial cells of the optic nerve. As apoptosis occurs in the ganglion cell population, the number of axons in the optic nerve decreases from 2.6 million during the second month to 1.1 million in the eighth month[1]. This decrease makes room for the increase in glial and connective tissue processes that enter the optic nerve.

A band of glial tissue forms around the optic disc, at the junction of the inner and outer layers of the optic cup, thus separating the potential intraretinal space from the fibers of the optic nerve; this tissue will become the *intermediary tissue of Kuhnt.*[1] Ganglion cell axons fill the lumen of the optic nerve (Figure 7-16) and grow toward their termination in the lateral geniculate nucleus. Myelination of the axon begins during the fifth month of gestation once the fiber reaches the lateral geniculate nucleus. Myelination reaches the chiasm during the sixth month, and the lamina cribrosa 1 to 3 months after birth.[3,69] Normally no myelin continues into the retina past the lamina cribrosa.

Clinical Comment: Emmetropization

The globe continues to grow after birth, and the eye will become emmetropic as long as there is coordination between the length of the eye and the power of the refractive components. Although this growth is under genetic control, visual experience that provides feedback for normal growth may influence this process.[1]

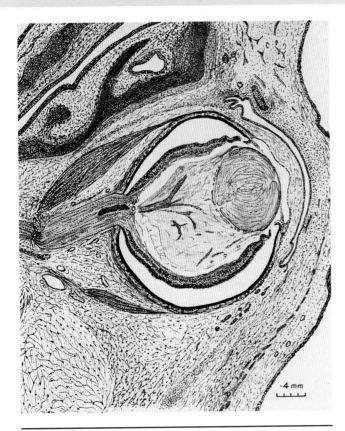

FIGURE 7-16
Section through eye and orbit of 48-mm human embryo (approximately 9.5 weeks). (From Mann I: *The development of the human eye*, New York, 1964, Grune & Stratton. Copyright 1964, British Medical Association.)

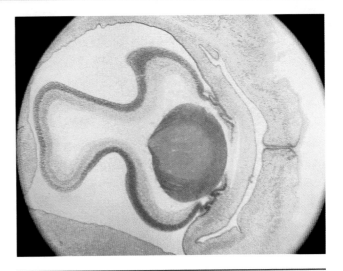

FIGURE 7-17
Light micrograph of eye of 2½-month human embryo; fused eyelids are seen. The mushroom-shape to the inner layer of the optic cup is an artifact.

DEVELOPMENT OF OCULAR ADNEXA

EYELIDS

Early in the second gestational month, folds of surface ectoderm filled with mesenchyme begin to grow toward one another anterior to the developing cornea; these folds will become the **eyelids.** Early formation of these folds can be seen in Figure 7-8. The upper fold is from the frontonasal process, and the lower fold is from the maxillary process.[1] The eyelid margins meet and fuse during the third month of development and remain fused until the lid structures have developed (Figure 7-17).[25] Two layers of epithelium cover the anterior surface to become epidermis and one layer lines the inner surface to become conjunctiva.[70] The tarsal plates are the first structures evident and then epithelial buds from the margins of the eyelid folds grow into the developing tarsal plates to form meibomian glands.[1] The epithelial layers of the skin and conjunctiva, the hair follicles and cilia, and the meibomian glands, Zeis glands, and glands of Moll all develop from surface ectoderm; the

tarsal plates, the orbicularis, the levator, and the tarsal muscle of Müller develop from mesenchyme.[3] The fusion of the eyelids isolates the developing eye from the amniotic fluid[71] and "probably prevents the cornea and conjunctiva from keratinizing."[3] The desmosomes joining the margins of the fused lids break down during the fifth and sixth month, allowing the eyelids to separate; the lipid secretions of the meibomian glands may be responsible for this disjunction.[3,5]

ORBIT

Orbital fat and connective tissue are derived from neural crest cells. The first evident orbital bone is the maxilla at 6 weeks; the frontal, zygomatic, and palatine bones are apparent at week 7. The lesser wing of the sphenoid bone and the optic canal are present at week 7, the greater wing is evident at week 10, and the wings join at week 16.[72] Most of the orbital bones ossify and fuse between the sixth and seventh months.[3] The angle between the orbits early in development is approximately 180 degrees, decreases to 105 degrees at 3 months, and is 71 degrees at birth and 68 degrees in adulthood (Figure 7-18). The globe reaches its adult size by age 3 years, but the orbit is not of adult size until age 16 years.[3]

EXTRAOCULAR MUSCLES

The **extraocular muscles** are of mesenchymal origin (Figure 7-19). The muscle cells are derived from mesoderm, whereas the connective tissue components originate in neural crest.[1,44] Extraocular muscles once were thought to develop in stages, first posteriorly near the

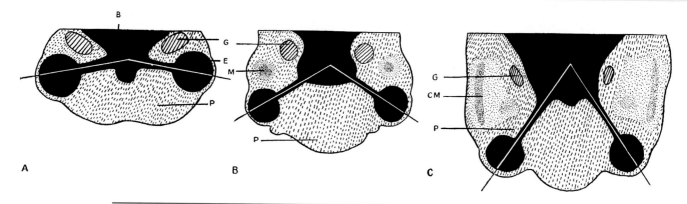

FIGURE 7-18
Sections through developing eyes and optic stalks of human embryos of various stages. **A,** Nine-millimeter embryo (approximately 37 days); 160-degree angle. **B,** Sixteen-millimeter embryo (approximately 48 days); 120-degree angle. **C,** Forty-millimeter embryo (approximately 8 weeks); 72-degree angle. Decrease in angle between optic axes is obvious. *B, Brain; E, eye; P, paraxial mesoderm; M, maxillary mesoderm; G, gasserian ganglion; CM, temporal condensation in maxillary mesoderm.* (From Mann I: *The development of the human eye,* New York, 1964, Grune & Stratton. Copyright 1964, British Medical Association.)

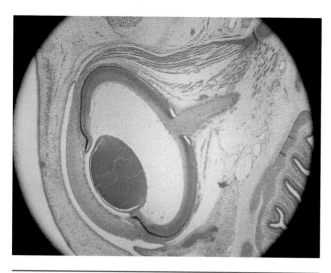

FIGURE 7-19
Light micrograph of 45-mm pig embryo; corneal layers are present, pigment is evident in outer layer of optic cup, eyelids, extraocular muscle, and optic nerve are evident.

orbital apex and then grow forward,[4] but recent investigation suggests that muscle origin, belly, and insertion develop simultaneously.[73] The muscles innervated by cranial nerve III are derived from the first pair of somites at approximately day 26. The lateral rectus muscle, innervated by cranial nerve VI, develops from the mesenchyme of the maxillomandibular area at about day 27. The superior oblique muscle, innervated by cranial nerve IV, is derived from the second pair of somites at day 29.[1] The tendinous sheaths at the scleral insertions are not fully formed until 18 months of age.[1] The

newborn exhibits poorly coordinated eye movements during the early years, indicating that the extraocular muscles are not fully developed and early visual experience can influence the development of normal binocular eye movements.[74]

NASOLACRIMAL SYSTEM

The main lacrimal gland has long been thought to develop from epithelial buds that arise from the temporal portion of the conjunctiva of the superior fornix.[3] Some investigators question this origin and suggest a neural crest origin.[75] The lacrimal gland continues to develop after birth and is not fully developed until age 3 or 4 years.[3]

The nasolacrimal drainage system develops from a cord of surface ectodermal cells that becomes buried below the maxillary mesenchyme. This cord may fragment and form the canaliculi, the nasolacrimal duct, and the lacrimal sac, or the canaliculi might be formed from a later epithelial cord.[3]

BLOOD VESSEL PERMEABILITY AND BARRIERS

The blood-retinal and blood-aqueous barriers are recognizable early in development in the tight junctions formed in the RPE, the non pigmented ciliary epithelium, and the capillaries of the iris and retina. Fenestrations that establish vessel permeability in the capillaries of the ciliary processes and the choriocapillaris also are evident early in the gestational period.

GENETIC IMPLICATIONS

With the current interest in the human genome, the field is growing exponentially and numerous studies are exploring and identifying genes expressed by ocular structures and the mechanisms by which cellular characteristics and processes are governed by those genes. The PAX6 gene is considered the master control gene and is necessary for normal development of ocular structures.[76,77] An increase in PAX6 in mice is associated with multiple lens defects, including abnormal fiber shape and fiber-to-fiber and fiber-to-cell interactions.[53] The PAX6 gene is expressed in the corneal and conjunctival epithelium and may regulate and maintain cell structure; it may also have a role in the proliferation and maintenance of corneal and conjunctival stem cells.[76,77]

Myriad speculations surround genes and the proteins they encode. Some interesting theories concerning ocular structures include: clusterin might be the factor essential for preserving the nonkeratinized state of corneal epithelial cells and may also provide some protection against apoptosis;[78] the gene, ALDH3, may provide some protection against UVR damage to corneal epithelium;[78] there may be a connection between atherosclerosis and drusen formed in AMD through the same or similar extracellular matrix genes;[79] and genes identified in the aqueous outflow tissues are usually associated with lymphatic tissue, perhaps suggesting additional function for the trabecular meshwork.[79]

In addition to providing further information about embryologic development, gene expression profiling can further explain cellular physiology as well as pathophysiology affecting ocular structures. Identifying and understanding the genetic regulation of normal cellular process brings us closer to understanding, treating, and possibly preventing ocular disease and dysfunction.

Marfan's syndrome is a disease affecting connective tissue structures throughout the body. Several genetic mutations have been identified, which lead to faulty production or a reduction in the secretion or assembly of fibrillin molecules.[80] Marfan's related disorders are also associated with abnormalities in extracellular matrix formation. An individual with Marfan's often has tall and thin body stature and can be at increased risk for aortic enlargement. Ocular structures can be affected; high myopia is often present and can increase the risk of retinal detachment; zonular malformation or dysfunction can result in a dislocated lens.

The gene called RAX is thought to be a major factor in the early stages of ocular development and mutations in RAX have been identified as causative in some cases of anophthalmia.[81] Mutations in the PAX2 gene have been implicated in papillorenal syndrome, which is characterized by renal hypoplasia and optic nerve head coloboma.[82]

REFERENCES

1. Barishak YR: *Embryology of the eye and its adnexae*, New York, 2001, Karger.
2. Moore KL: *Before we are born: essentials of embryology and birth defects*, ed 5, Philadelphia, 1998, Saunders.
3. Cook CS, Ozanics V, Jakobiec FA: Prenatal development of the eye and its adnexa. In Tasman W, Jaeger EA, editors: *Duane's foundations of clinical ophthalmology*, vol 1, Philadelphia, 1994, Lippincott.
4. Mann I: *Development of the human eye*, New York, 1964, Grune & Stratton.
5. Barishak YR: Embryology of the eye and its adnexae. In Straub W, editor: *Developments in ophthalmology*, New York, 1992, Karger.
6. Barber AN: *Embryology of the human eye*, St Louis, 1955, Mosby.
7. Morrison DA, FitzPatrick DR, Fleck BW: Iris coloboma with iris heterochromia: a common association, *Arch Ophthalmol* 118(11):1590, 2000.
8. Trachimowicz RA: Review of embryology and its relation to ocular disease in the pediatric population, *Optom Vis Sci* 71(3):154, 1994.
9. Smelser GK: Embryology and morphology of the lens, *Invest Ophthalmol* 4:398, 1965.
10. Matsuo T: The genes involved in the morphogenesis of the eye, *Jpn J Ophthalmol* 37(3):215, 1993:(abstract).
11. Harrington L, Klintworth GK, Seror TE, et al: Developmental analysis of ocular morphogenesis in alpha A-crystallin/diphtheria toxin transgenic mice undergoing ablation of the lens, *Dev Biol* 148(2):508, 1991.
12. Coulombre AJ: Regulation of ocular morphogenesis, *Invest Ophthalmol* 8:25, 1969.
13. McKeehan MS: Induction of portions of the chick lens without contact with the optic cup, *Anat Rec* 132:297, 1958.
14. Grainger RM, Henry JJ, Saha MS, et al: Recent progress on the mechanisms of embryonic lens formation, *Eye* 6(pt 2):117, 1992.
15. Marshall J, Beaconsfield M, Rothery S: The anatomy and development of the human lens and zonules, *Trans Ophthalmol Soc UK* 102:423–440, 1982.
16. Coulombre JL, Coulombre AJ: Lens development: fiber elongation and lens orientation, *Science* 142:1489, 1963.
17. Coulombre JL, Coulombre AJ: Lens development. IV. Size, shape and orientation, *Invest Ophthalmol* 8:251, 1969.
18. O'Rahilly R: The prenatal development of the human eye, *Exp Eye Res* 2:93, 1975.
19. Amaya L, Taylor D, Russell-Eggitt IR, et al: The morphology and natural history of childhood cataracts, *Surv Ophthalmol* 48(2):125, 2003.
20. Nelson LB, Folberg R: Ocular development anomalies. In Tasman W, Jaeger EA, editors: *Duane's foundations of clinical ophthalmology*, vol 1, Philadelphia, 1991, Lippincott.
21. Kanski JJ: *Clinical ophthalmology*, ed 2, Oxford, UK, 1989, Butterworth-Heinemann, p 238.
22. Mutlu F, Leopard IH: The structure of the fetal hyaloid system and tunica vasculosa lentis, *Arch Ophthalmol* 71:102, 1964.
23. Jack RL: Ultrastructural aspects of hyaloid vessel development, *Arch Ophthalmol* 87:427, 1972.
24. Zhu M, Madigan MC, van Driel D, et al: The human hyaloid system: cell death and vascular regression, *Exp Eye Res* 70:767, 2000.
25. Warwick R: *Eugene Wolff's anatomy of the eye and orbit*, ed 7, Philadelphia, 1976, Saunders, p 418.
26. Duke-Elder S, Cook C: Normal and abnormal development. In Duke-Elder S, editor: *System of ophthalmology, Embryology*, vol 3, St Louis, 1963, Mosby.
27. Hollenberg MJ, Spira AW: Early development of the human retina, *Can J Ophthalmol* 7:472, 1972.
28. Mund ML, Rodrigues MM, Fine BS: Light and electron microscopic observations on the pigmented layers of the developing human eye, *Am J Ophthalmol* 73:167, 1972.

29. Smelser GK, Ozanics V, Rayborn M, et al: The fine structure of the retinal transient layer of Chievitz, *Invest Ophthalmol* 12:504, 1973.

30. Uga S, Smelser GK: Electron microscopic study of the development of retinal Müllerian cells, *Invest Ophthalmol* 12:295, 1973.

31. Isenmann S, Kretz A, Cellerino A: Molecular determinants of retinal ganglion cell development, survival, and regeneration, *Prog Retin Eye Res* 22(4):483, 2003:(abstract).

32. Oster SF, Sretavan DW: Connecting the eye to the brain: the molecular basis of ganglion cell axon guidance, *Br J Ophthalmol* 87:639, 2003:(abstract).

33. Narayanan K, Wadhwa S: Photoreceptor morphogenesis in the human retina: a scanning electron microscopic study, *Anat Rec* 252:133, 1998.

34. Willbold E, Layer PG: Müller glia cells and their possible roles during retina differentiation in vivo and in vitro, *Histol Histopathol* 13(2):531, 1998.

35. Smelser GK, Ozanics V, Rayborn M, et al: Retinal synaptogenesis in the primate, *Invest Ophthalmol* 13:340, 1974.

36. Sharma RK, Ehinger EJ: Development and structure of the retina. In Kaufman PL, Alm A, editors: *Adler's physiology of the eye*, St Louis, 2003, Mosby, p 319.

37. Vrabec F: The temporal raphée of the human retina, *Am J Ophthalmol* 62:926, 1966.

38. O'Connor AR, Wilson CM, Fielder AR: *Ophthalmological problems associated with preterm birth Eye* 21:1254–1260, 2007.

39. Yuodelis C, Hendrickson A: A qualitative and quantitative analysis of the human fovea during development, *Vision Res* 26(6):847, 1986.

40. Jeffery G: The retinal pigment epithelium as a developmental regulator of the neural retina, *Eye* 12:499, 1998.

41. Dorrell MI, Aguilar E, Friedlander M: Retinal vascular development is mediated by endothelial filopodia, a preexisting astrocytic template and specific R-cadherin adhesion, *Invest Ophthalmol Vis Sci* 43(11):3500, 2002.

42. Provis JM: Development of the primate retinal vasculature, *Prog Retin Eye Res* 20(6):799, 2001:(abstract).

43. Patz A, Payne JW: Retrolental fibroplasia. In Duane TD, Jaeger EA, editors: *Clinical ophthalmology*, vol 3, Philadelphia, 1982, Harper & Row.

44. Gage JE, Rhoades W, Prucka SK, et al: Fate maps of neural crest and mesoderm in the mammalian eye, *Invest Ophthalmol Vis Sci* 46:4200–4208, 2005.

45. Tisdale AS, Spurr-Michaud SJ, Rodrigues M, et al: Development of the anchoring structures of the epithelium in rabbit and human fetal corneas, *Invest Ophthalmol Vis Sci* 29(5):727, 1988.

46. Zinn KM, Mockel-Pohl S: Fine structure of the developing cornea, *Int Ophthalmol Clin* 15(1):19, 1975.

47. Wulle KG: Electron microscopy of the fetal development of the corneal endothelium and Descemet's membrane of the human eye, *Invest Ophthalmol* 11:897, 1972.

48. Wulle KG, Ruprecht KW, Windrath LC: Electron microscopy of the development of the cell junctions in the embryonic and fetal human corneal endothelium, *Invest Ophthalmol* 13:923, 1974.

49. Lesueur L, Arne JL, Mignon-Conte M, et al: Structural and ultrastructural changes in the developmental process of premature infants' and children's corneas, *Cornea* 13(4):331, 1994.

50. Bahn CF, Falls HF, Varley GA, et al: Classification of corneal endothelial disorders based on neural crest origin, *Ophthalmology* 91:558, 1984.

51. Ozanics V, Rayborn M, Sagun D: Some aspects of corneal and scleral differentiation in the primate, *Exp Eye Res* 22:305, 1976.

52. Wulle KG, Richter J: Electron microscopy of the early embryonic development of the human corneal epithelium, *Albrecht Von Graefes Arch Klin Exp Ophthalmol* 209(1):39, 1978.

53. Duncan MK, Kozmik Z, Cveklova K, et al: Overexpression of PAX6(5a) in lens fiber cells results in cataract and upregulation of (alpha)5(beta)1 integrin expression, *J Cell Sci* 113:3173, 2000.

54. Heinmann K: The development of the choroid in man: choroidal vascular system, *Ophthalmol Res* 3:257, 1971.

55. Wulle KG: The development of the productive and drainage system of the aqueous humor in the human eye, *Adv Ophthalmol* 26:296, 1972.

56. Loewenfeld IE: *The pupil: anatomy, physiology, and clinical applications*, Boston, 1999, Butterworth-Heinemann.

57. Tamura T, Smelser GK: Development of the sphincter and dilator muscles of the iris, *Arch Ophthalmol* 89:332, 1973.

58. Carlson BM: *Human embryology and developmental biology*, St Louis, 1994, Mosby, p 265.

59. Matsuo N, Smelser GK: Electron microscopic studies on the pupillary membrane: the fine structure of the white strands of the disappearing stage of the membrane, *Invest Ophthalmol* 10:108, 1971.

60. Edelhauser HF, Ubels JL: Cornea and sclera. In Kaufman PL, Alm A, editors: *Adler's physiology of the eye*, St Louis, 2003, Mosby, pp 47.

61. Burian HM, Braley AE, Allen L: A new concept of the development of the angle of the anterior chamber of the human eye, *Arch Ophthalmol* 53:439, 1956.

62. Smelser GK, Ozanics V: The development of the trabecular meshwork in primate eyes, *Am J Ophthalmol* 71:366, 1971.

63. Rodrigues MM, Katz SI, Foidart JM: Collagen factor VIII antigen, and immunoglobulins in the human aqueous drainage channels, *Ophthalmology* 87:337, 1980.

64. Tripathi BJ, Tripathi RC: Neural crest origin of human trabecular meshwork and its implications for the pathogenesis of glaucoma, *Am J Ophthalmol* 107:583, 1989.

65. Tripathi BJ, Tripathi RC: Embryology of the anterior segment of the human eye. In Ritch R, Shields MB, Krupin T, editors: *The glaucomas*, St Louis, 1989, Mosby.

66. Kupfer C, Ross K: The development of outflow facility in human eyes, *Invest Ophthalmol* 10:513, 1971.

67. Hansson HA, Jerndal T: Scanning electron microscopic studies on the development of the iridocorneal angle in human eyes, *Invest Ophthalmol* 10:252, 1971.

68. Coulombre AJ, Coulombre JL: Mechanisms of ocular development, *Int Ophthalmol Clin* 15(1):7, 1975.

69. Sadun AA, Glaser JS: Anatomy of the visual sensory system. In Tasman W, Jaeger EA, editors: *Duane's foundations of clinical ophthalmology*, vol 1, Philadelphia, 1994, Lippincott.

70. Kikkawa DO, Lucarelli MJ, Shovlin JP, et al: Ophthalmic facial anatomy and physiology. In Kaufman PL, Alm A, editors: *Adler's physiology of the eye*, St Louis, 2003, Mosby, pp 16.

71. Anderson H, Ehlers N, Matthiessen ME, et al: Histochemistry and development of the human eyelids. II. A cytochemical and electron microscopical study, *Acta Ophthalmol (Copenh)* 45:288, 1967.

72. Sires BS, Gausas R, Cook BE, et al: Orbit. In Kaufman PL, Alm A, editors: *Adler's physiology of the eye*, St Louis, 2003, Mosby.

73. Sevel D: Reappraisal of the origin of human extraocular muscles, *Ophthalmology* 88:1330, 1981.

74. Porter JD, Andrade FH, Baker RS: The extraocular muscles. In Kaufman PL, Alm A, editors: *Adler's physiology of the eye*, St Louis, 2003, Mosby, pp 787.

75. Tripathi BJ, Tripathi RC: Evidence of neuroectodermal origin of the human lacrimal gland, *Invest Ophthalmol Vis Sci* 31:393, 1990.

76. Koroma BM, Yang JM, Sundin OH: The PAX6 homeobox gene is expressed throughout the corneal and conjunctival epithelia, *Invest Ophthalmol Vis Sci* 38(1):108, 1997.

77. Secker GA, Daniels JT: Corneal epithelial stem cells: deficiency and regulation, *Stem Cell Res* 4:159–168, 2008.

78. Kinoshita S, Adachi W, Sotozono C, et al: Characteristics of the human ocular surface epithelium, *Prog Retin Eye Res* 20(5):639, 2001.

79. Wistow G: The NEI Bank project for ocular genomics: data-mining gene expression in human and rodent eye tissues, *Prog Retin Eye Res* 25:43–77, 2006.

80. Bonetti MI: Microfibrils: a cornerstone of extracellular matrix and a key to understand Marfan syndrome, *Ital J Anat Embryol* 114:201–224, 2009.

81. Lequeux L, Rio M, Vigouroux A, et al: Confirmation of RAX gene involvement in human anophthalmia, *Clin Genet* 74:392–395, 2008.

82. Martinovic-Bouriel J, Benachi A: PAX2 mutations in fetal renal hypodysplasia, *Am J Med Genet* 152A:830–835, 2010.

8 *Bones of the Skull and Orbit*

The skull can be divided into two parts: the cranium and the face. The cranium consists of two parietal bones, the occipital bone, two temporal bones, the sphenoid bone, and the ethmoid bone. The face is made up of two maxillary bones, two nasal bones, the vomer, two inferior conchae, two lacrimal bones, two palatine bones, two zygomatic bones, and the mandible. The single frontal bone is a part of both the cranium and the face.

Generally, the bones of the skull unite at sutures that form immovable joints. The exception is the movable temporomandibular joint, which attaches the mandible to the temporal bones. Air-filled cavities called sinuses are contained within several of the bones.

After a brief description of the bones of the skull, this chapter presents a more detailed presentation of the orbital bones. The reader is advised to have a skull available for reference while reading this chapter, particularly for distinguishing the relationships and articulations between bones and identifying foramina and fissures.

BONES OF THE CRANIUM

The paired **parietal bones** form the roof and sides of the cranium (Figure 8-1). The parietal bones articulate with each other at the midline in the sagittal suture, with the occipital bone posteriorly in the lambdoid suture, and with the frontal bone anteriorly at the coronal suture. The parietal bone articulates inferiorly with the temporal bone and the greater wing of the sphenoid bone.

The **occipital bone** forms the posterior aspect of the skull and posterior floor of the cranial cavity. A prominence, the external occipital protuberance, or *inion*, is found on the external surface at the posterior midline (Figure 8-2). The large foramen magnum is found in the inferior aspect of the occipital bone. The inner surface of the bone forms the posterior cranial fossa, in which there are depressions where the lobes of the cerebellum lie. Figure 8-3 shows the inner aspect of the cranial floor. The occipital bone articulates with the temporal bones, parietal bones, and sphenoid bone.

Clinical Comment: Inion

THE INION, located just outer to the posterior pole of the occipital cortex, is a useful landmark in the placement of the electrodes used to record a visual-evoked response (VER). This electrodiagnostic test records responses from the visual cortex. Clinical applications include the determination of visual acuity in a patient unable to respond to the typical eye chart and the assessment of impulse conduction in the patient with suspected multiple sclerosis.

Each of the **temporal bones** is composed of two portions: a large, flat plate, the *squamous portion;* and a thickened, wedge-shaped area, the *petrous portion.* The squamous portion forms the side of the cranium and articulates with the parietal bone and the sphenoid bone. An anterior projection, the *zygomatic process,* articulates with the zygomatic bone (see Figure 8-1). The petrous portion extends within the cranium and houses the middle and inner ear structures. The *mastoid process* and *styloid process* project from the inferior aspect, and between these two processes is the *stylomastoid foramen,* through which the facial nerve exits the skull. The petrous portion articulates with the occipital bone in the floor of the skull. The *carotid canal* runs superiorly and anteriorly through the petrous portion and provides an entrance for the internal carotid artery into the cranial cavity (Figure 8-3).

The single **frontal bone** forms the anterior portion of the cranium, anterior floor of the cranial cavity, and superior part of the face (Figure 8-4). At the top of the skull, the frontal bone articulates with the parietal bones; inferiorly it articulates with the sphenoid bone, ethmoid bone, and lacrimal bones. Inferoanteriorly, it articulates with the nasal bones, maxillary bones, and zygomatic bones. The inner surface of the cranial cavity portion of the frontal bone forms the anterior cranial fossa (see Figure 8-3), in which the frontal lobes of the cerebral hemispheres lie. The frontal sinuses are located within the anterior portion of the frontal bone.

The **sphenoid bone** is a single bone, the body of which lies in the midline and articulates with the occipital bone and the temporal bones to form the

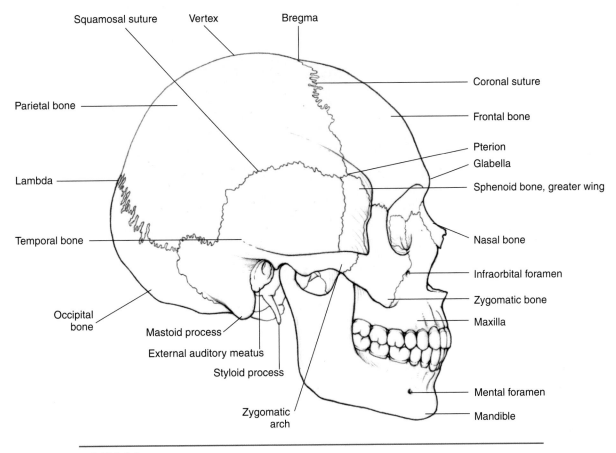

FIGURE 8-1
Lateral view of skull. (From Mathers LH, Chase RA, Dolph J et al: *Clinical anatomy principles*, St Louis, 1996, Mosby.)

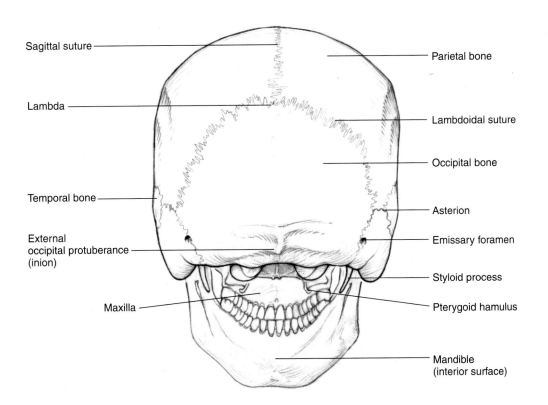

FIGURE 8-2
Posterior view of skull. (From Mathers LH, Chase RA, Dolph J, et al: *Clinical anatomy principles*, St Louis, 1996, Mosby.)

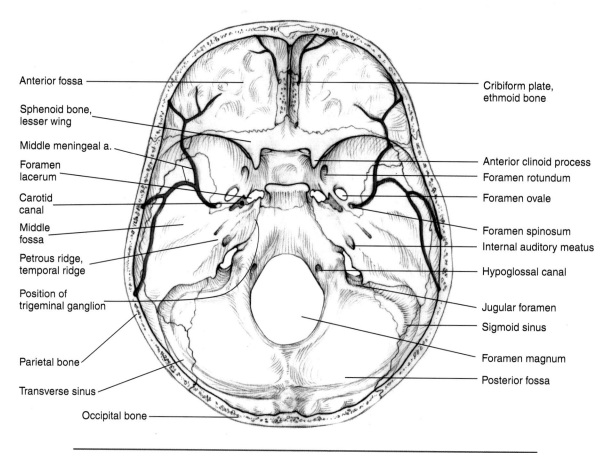

Anterior fossa

Sphenoid bone, lesser wing

Middle meningeal a.

Foramen lacerum

Carotid canal

Middle fossa

Petrous ridge, temporal ridge

Position of trigeminal ganglion

Parietal bone

Transverse sinus

Occipital bone

Cribiform plate, ethmoid bone

Anterior clinoid process

Foramen rotundum

Foramen ovale

Foramen spinosum

Internal auditory meatus

Hypoglossal canal

Jugular foramen

Sigmoid sinus

Foramen magnum

Posterior fossa

FIGURE 8-3
Floor of skull. (From Mathers LH, Chase RA, Dolph J, et al: *Clinical anatomy principles*, St Louis, 1996, Mosby.)

FIGURE 8-4
Anterior view of skull. (From Mathers LH, Chase RA, Dolph J, et al: *Clinical anatomy principles*, St Louis, 1996, Mosby.)

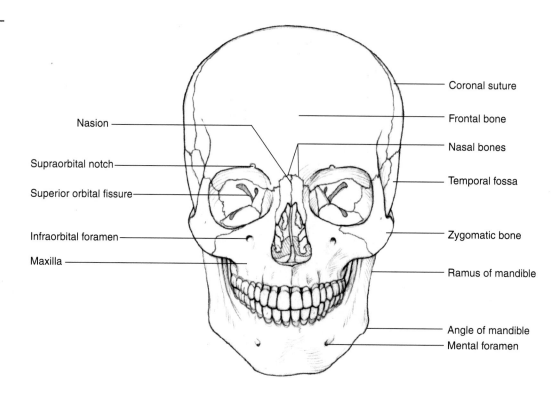

Nasion

Supraorbital notch

Superior orbital fissure

Infraorbital foramen

Maxilla

Coronal suture

Frontal bone

Nasal bones

Temporal fossa

Zygomatic bone

Ramus of mandible

Angle of mandible

Mental foramen

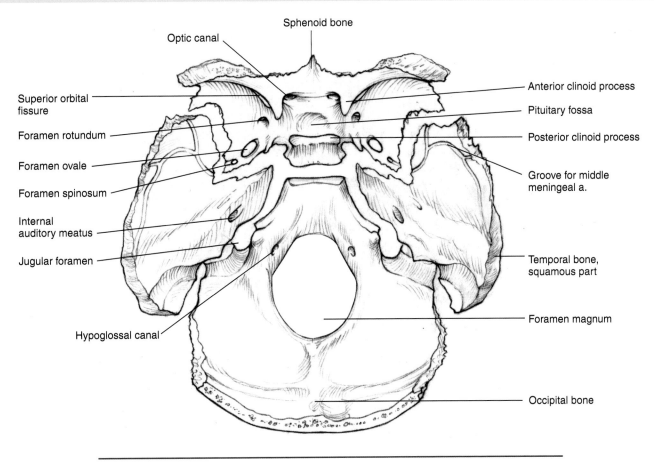

FIGURE 8-5
Disarticulated view of base of skull. (From Mathers LH, Chase RA, Dolph J, et al: *Clinical anatomy principles*, St Louis, 1996, Mosby.)

base of the cranium (see Figure 8-3). The sphenoid bone joins the zygomatic bones to form the lateral walls of the orbits. Anteriorly and inferiorly the sphenoid bone articulates with the maxillary and palatine bones, superiorly with the parietal bones, and anteriorly and superiorly with the ethmoid and frontal bones. The depression on the superior cranial surface of the body of the sphenoid bone, the *hypophyseal fossa* (or the *sella turcica*), houses the pituitary gland; a portion of the body is hollow, forming the sphenoid sinus cavity.

Two pairs of wings project from the body of the sphenoid bone. The **lesser wings** project from the anterior aspect of the body and are more superior and smaller than the greater wings (see Figure 8-3). The lesser wings are attached to the body by small roots or struts. The gap between the lesser wing and the sphenoid body forms the *optic foramen (canal)* through which the optic nerve exits the orbit. The lesser wings articulate with the frontal and ethmoid bones.

The **greater wings** project from the lateral aspects of the body and articulate with the frontal bone, the

parietal bones, squamous portions of the temporal bones, and the zygomatic bones. The *pterygoid process* projects from the base of the greater wing and articulates with the vertical stem of the palatine bone; each contributes to a shallow depression, the *pterygopalatine fossa*. Three important foramina are located in the greater wing (Figure 8-5): the *foramen rotundum*, through which the maxillary nerve passes; the *foramen ovale*, through which the mandibular nerve passes; and the *foramen spinosum*, through which the middle meningeal artery passes.

The single **ethmoid bone** resembles a rectangular box that contains a midline perpendicular plate. This plate bisects the top of the box, the horizontal *cribriform plate*, which is perforated for the passage of the olfactory nerves. The sides of the box parallel to the perpendicular plate are the orbital plates and are separated from the perpendicular plate by the ethmoid air cells. The ethmoid bone articulates with the sphenoid and frontal bones superiorly and with the vomer inferiorly; the orbital plates also articulate with the maxillary and lacrimal bones.

BONES OF THE FACE

The single **frontal bone** forms the forehead and articulates with the nasal bones, maxillae, and zygomatic bones in formation of the face (see Figure 8-4). The sutures joining adjacent bones of the face generally are named according to the names of the two bones that are connected (e.g., the suture between the frontal bone and the zygomatic bone is the *frontozygomatic* suture).

The two **maxillae,** or **maxillary bones,** form the upper jaw, the hard palate, the lateral walls of the nasal cavity, and the floor of both orbits (see Figure 8-4). Each maxillary bone articulates with the frontal, nasal, lacrimal, ethmoid, sphenoid, palatine, and zygomatic bones. That portion of the maxillary bone forming the cheek contains the maxillary sinus.

The two **nasal bones** form the bridge of the nose and articulate with each other, with the frontal bone, and with the frontal processes of the maxillary bones (see Figure 8-4). The **vomer** is a single bone that forms the posterior part of the nasal septum. It articulates with the palatine and maxillary bones inferiorly and with the ethmoid bone superiorly. The **inferior conchae** are separate bones located along the lateral walls of the nasal cavity.

The **lacrimal bone** (one in each orbit) is the smallest bone of the face and articulates with the maxillary bone, ethmoid bone, and frontal bone.

There are two **palatine bones.** Each is an L-shaped bone that extends from the hard palate at the back of the mouth to the orbit. The horizontal plate is found in the oral cavity; the vertical stem runs along the posterior aspect of the nasal cavity and articulates with the pterygoid process of the sphenoid bone. A small, flattened area at the top of the vertical stem is located in the orbital floor at the posterior edge of the orbital plate of the maxilla.

The paired **zygomatic bones** form the lateral part of the cheekbones and articulate with the zygomatic process of the temporal bones to form the *zygomatic arches* (see Figure 8-1). The zygomatic bones also articulate with the maxillary bones and with the greater wings of the sphenoid bone.

The **mandible** forms the movable lower jaw. It is a horseshoe-shaped bone consisting of a curved horizontal body and two perpendicular processes, the rami.

THE ORBIT

The orbits are bony cavities on either side of the midsagittal plane of the skull below the cranium. They contain the globes, the extraocular muscles, and orbital nerves, blood vessels, and connective tissue.

The orbit is shaped like a four-sided pyramid, the base of which is at the anterior orbital margin and the apex at the posterior margin within the skull. The orbital walls are referred to as the roof, floor, and medial and lateral walls. The medial walls run approximately parallel to each other, whereas the two lateral walls, if extended posteriorly, would form approximately a 90-degree angle with each other[1,2] (Figure 8-6). The orbit has also been described as pear shaped, having its widest portion 1.5 cm inside the orbital margin.[1] The orbital floor extends to approximately two-thirds the depth of the orbit; the other three sides extend to the apex.

Each orbit is composed of seven bones—the frontal, maxillary, zygomatic, sphenoid, ethmoid, palatine, and lacrimal bones (Figure 8-7). The frontal, sphenoid, and ethmoid are each a single bone and take part in the formation of both orbits.

ORBITAL WALLS

Roof

The roof is triangular and is composed primarily of the **orbital plate of the frontal bone** in front (Figure 8-8). The **lesser wing of the sphenoid** contributes a small posterior portion. The orbital plate of the frontal bone is thin in the area that separates the orbit from the anterior cranial fossa. In an elderly adult, bone in this area may resorb, leaving only the periosteal connective tissue in contact with the dural covering of the frontal lobe of the brain. The small area of the lesser wing of the sphenoid that is involved in this wall runs slightly downward, and an oval foramen, the **optic canal,** lies between it and the body of the sphenoid (see Figure 8-7). This optic foramen is located roughly at the apex of the orbit.

The frontal bone forms the ridge of the superior orbital margin. Behind the lateral aspect of this margin is an indentation in the frontal bone: the **fossa for the lacrimal gland.** A U-shaped piece of cartilage, the **trochlea,** is attached to the orbital plate of the frontal bone approximately 2 mm behind the medial aspect of the superior orbital margin. The tendon of the superior oblique muscle passes through this pulleylike structure.

Floor

The floor is also triangular and is composed of the **orbital plate of the maxillary bone** and the **orbital plate of the zygomatic bone** in front and the small **orbital process of the palatine bone** behind (Figure 8-9). The maxillary bone makes up the largest part of the floor, and most of the remainder is provided by the zygomatic bone. The orbital process of the palatine bone is a small, flattened area at the top of the vertical arm and is located at the most posterior edge of the orbital plate of the maxilla. Often in the adult skull, the

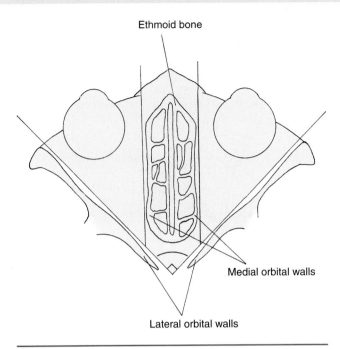

Ethmoid bone

Medial orbital walls

Lateral orbital walls

FIGURE 8-6
Angular relationship of orbital walls. Medial walls are approximately parallel to each other; if lateral walls were extended, an approximate right angle would be formed.

suture between the orbital process of the palatine bone and the maxilla is indistinguishable.

The floor does not reach all the way to the apex and is separated from the lateral wall posteriorly by the **inferior orbital fissure.** The **infraorbital groove** runs across the floor from the inferior orbital fissure and anteriorly is bridged by a thin plate of bone, thus becoming a canal running within the maxillary bone. This canal opens on the facial surface of the maxilla below the inferior orbital margin as the **infraorbital foramen** (see Figure 8-7). The inferior orbital margin is composed of the maxilla and the maxillary process of the zygomatic bone.

Clinical Comment: Blow-Out Fracture of the Orbit

The orbital rim is strong and can withstand considerable impact. However, a blow to the orbital rim can cause compression of the orbital contents, and such a sudden increase in intraorbital pressure might cause a fracture in one of the orbital walls. In the classic blow-out fracture, the orbital rim remains intact. The floor of the orbit is particularly susceptible to such a fracture, which usually occurs in the thin region along the infraorbital canal[2-4] (Figure 8-10). Clinical signs and symptoms accompanying this damage include orbital swelling, ecchymosis, anesthesia of the area innervated by the infraorbital nerve, and diplopia caused by restriction of ocular motility (particularly

noted in upward gaze).[4] Limitations in ocular motility are caused by damage to the inferior extraocular muscles, either from bruising or hematoma or from entrapment of the muscle or adjoining connective tissue within the fracture.[3,5,6]

Medial Wall

The medial wall is rectangular. From front to back, it is formed by the **frontal process of the maxilla,** the **lacrimal bone,** the **orbital plate of the ethmoid,** and a part of the **body of the sphenoid** (Figure 8-11). A ridge on the frontal process of the maxilla that forms the anterior part of the medial orbital margin also forms the **anterior lacrimal crest,** which demarcates one border of the **fossa for the lacrimal sac.** The lacrimal bone, a small bone approximately the size of a thumbnail, together with the frontal process of the maxillary bone, forms the wall of this fossa. The lower portion of the fossa is a groove that is continuous inferiorly with the **nasolacrimal canal,** which continues into the nasal cavity. A ridge in the lacrimal bone forms the **posterior lacrimal crest** and is continuous superiorly with the prominence of the frontal bone, forming the posterior part of the medial margin of the orbit.

The ethmoid bone forms most of the medial wall. The orbital plate of the ethmoid sometimes is said to be "paper thin" (lamina papyracea); thus the medial wall is the thinnest of the orbital walls. The small part of the sphenoid bone present in this wall is part of the body and is located at the posterior end adjacent to the wall of the optic canal. The floor is joined to the medial wall at the sutures connecting the bones of the two walls, and the anterior and posterior ethmoidal canals are located within the frontoethmoidal suture at the junction of the roof and medial wall.

Lateral Wall

The lateral wall is roughly triangular and is composed of the **zygomatic bone** in front and of the greater **wing of the sphenoid bone** behind (Figure 8-12). The zygomatic bone separates the orbit from the temporal fossa. One or more foramina may be present in the zygomatic bone as a conduit for nerves and vessels between the orbit and facial areas. The lateral or marginal orbital tubercle (Whitnall's tubercle) is a small, bony prominence located on the orbital surface of the zygomatic bone and is the attachment site for the aponeurosis of the superior palpebral levator muscle, the lateral palpebral ligament, and the lateral check ligament.[7]

The greater wing of the sphenoid separates the orbit from the middle cranial fossa. The roof is separated from the lateral wall in back by the **superior orbital fissure** and in front by the frontozygomatic and

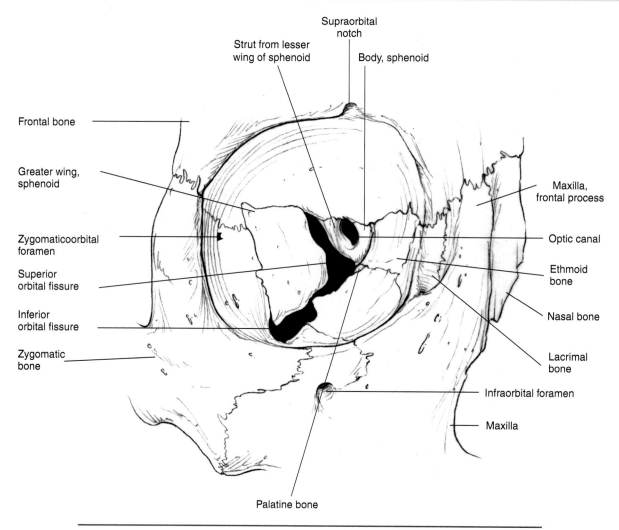

FIGURE 8-7
Anterior view of bones of orbit. (From Mathers LH, Chase RA, Dolph J, et al: *Clinical anatomy principles*, St Louis, 1996, Mosby.)

frontosphenoidal sutures. The **inferior orbital fissure** separates the posterior part of the floor from the lateral wall (see Figure 8-7).

ORBITAL MARGINS

Although dimensions of the orbit vary widely, the average horizontal diameter of the orbital margin is 4 cm, the average vertical diameter is 3.5 cm, and the average depth is 4.5 cm.[1,2,8] The frontal bone forms the superior orbital margin. The highest point of this arch is located one-third the way along the margin from the superior medial corner of the orbit. The *supraorbital notch* (see Figure 8-7) is located just medial to the center of the superior orbital margin and is the conduit for the supraorbital vessels and nerves. This notch can be palpated easily. In 25% of orbits, the supraorbital notch is enclosed to form a foramen.[2,9]

At the superior medial corner is a less well-defined groove, the *supratrochlear notch,* through which pass the nerve and vessels of the same name. The supratrochlear notch remains a notch or groove in the majority of orbits, becoming a foramen in just 3%.[9]

The lateral orbital margin is the orbital region most exposed to possible injury and therefore is the strongest area of the orbital margin. It is formed by the zygomatic process of the frontal bone superiorly and by the frontal process of the zygomatic bone inferiorly.

The inferior orbital margin usually is formed equally by the maxillary bone and the zygomatic bone. The zygomaticomaxillary suture can often be easily palpated through the skin along the inferior orbital edge. The *infraorbital foramen* (the opening from the infraorbital canal) is found in the anterior surface of the maxillary bone below the inferior orbital margin.

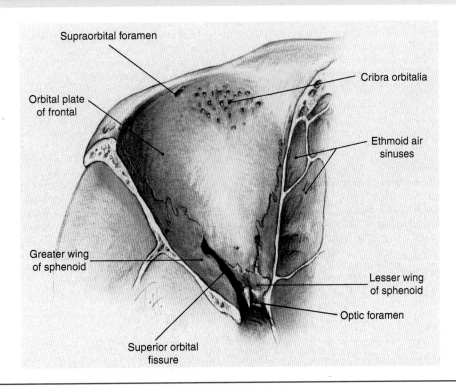

FIGURE 8-8
Bones of orbital roof. (From Doxanas MT, Anderson RL: *Clinical orbital anatomy*, Baltimore, 1984, Williams & Wilkins.)

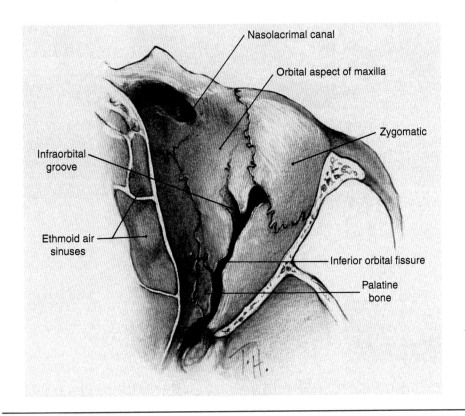

FIGURE 8-9
Bones of orbital floor. (From Doxanas MT, Anderson RL: *Clinical orbital anatomy*, Baltimore, 1984, Williams & Wilkins.)

Blowout fracture

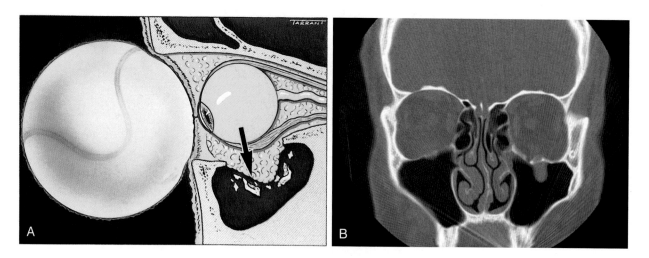

FIGURE 8-10

A, Mechanism of blow-out fracture. Arrow indicates that the force damages the weakest orbital wall, the floor. **B,** Coronal computed tomography (CT) scan showing blow-out fracture of left orbital floor. (**A** from Kanski JJ: *Clinical ophthalmology: a systematic approach*, ed 5, Oxford, UK, 2003, Butterworth-Heinemann; **B** courtesy Dr. Weon Jun, Portland VA Medical Center, Portland, Ore.)

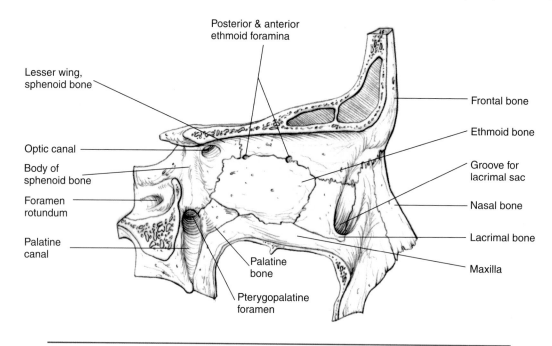

FIGURE 8-11

Bones of medial orbital wall. (From Mathers LH, Chase RA, Dolph J, et al: *Clinical anatomy principles*, St Louis, 1996, Mosby.)

The frontal process of the maxillary bone articulates with the frontal bone and forms part of the medial rim of the orbital margin. This process articulates posteriorly with the lacrimal bone and anteriorly with the nasal bone. The medial margin is not continuous.

Starting from the inferior nasal aspect, which is the anterior lacrimal crest, the orbital margin forms a spiral (Figure 8-13). The posterior lacrimal crest completes the superior curve of the medial orbital margin.

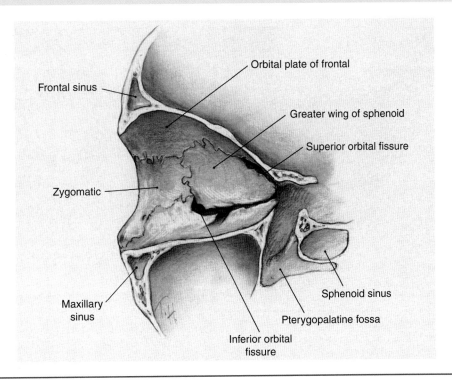

FIGURE 8-12
Bones of lateral orbital wall. (From Doxanas MT, Anderson RL: *Clinical orbital anatomy*, Baltimore, 1984, Williams & Wilkins.)

ORBITAL FORAMINA AND FISSURES

A number of foramina and fissures exist between the orbit and the middle cranial fossa, sinuses, and face to allow the entrance and exit of vessels and nerves that supply the globe and orbital structures. The **optic foramen** or the **optic canal** (see Figure 8-7) is formed by a bridge of bone called the "optic strut," which extends from the lesser wing to the sphenoid body.[10] The canal lies just lateral to the body of the sphenoid. The canal often causes an indentation into the bone of the sphenoid sinus.[11] It provides communication between the orbital cavity and the middle cranial fossa and is separated from the medial posterior edge of the superior orbital fissure by the optic strut. The optic nerve exits and the ophthalmic artery enters the orbit through this canal (Figure 8-14).

The **superior orbital fissure** is the gap between the lesser wing and the greater wing of the sphenoid bone and is located between the roof and the lateral wall (see Figure 8-7). As with the optic canal, this fissure is a communication between the orbital cavity and the middle cranial fossa. The fissure usually is widest medially, becoming narrower toward the lateral portion. Approximately midway on the lower aspect is a small sharp spur (the lateral rectus spine) that serves as the attachment for the lateral rectus muscle. A circular band of connective tissue, the **common tendinous ring** (or **annulus of Zinn**), is located anterior to the fissure and the optic canal. This ring is the origin for the four rectus muscles. Figure 8-15 shows the relationships among the superior orbital fissure, the tendinous ring, and the various nerves passing through them. The lacrimal nerve, frontal nerve, trochlear nerve, and superior ophthalmic vein pass through the superior orbital fissure above the circular tendon. The superior and inferior divisions of the oculomotor nerve, the nasociliary nerve, and the abducens nerve pass through the fissure and the ring tendon. The optic nerve and the ophthalmic artery pass through the optic canal and the tendinous ring.

The **inferior orbital fissure** lies between the floor of the orbit and the lateral wall (see Figure 8-7). It allows passage of vessels and nerves between the orbit and the pterygopalatine and temporal fossae. This fissure often is narrowest in its center. The foramen rotundum opens into the pterygopalatine fossa and transmits the maxillary division of the trigeminal nerve to the inferior orbital fissure. Branches of the maxillary nerve, including the infraorbital nerve, join vessels passing through the inferior orbital fissure. Most of these structures continue into the infraorbital groove in the maxillary bone. The inferior ophthalmic vein exits the orbit through the inferior orbital fissure below the ring tendon.

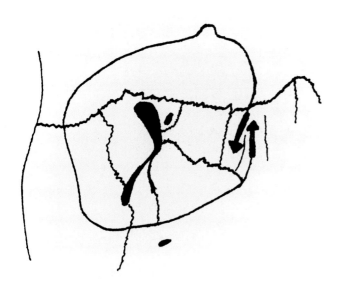

FIGURE 8-13
Orbital margin. Arrows indicate spiral shape formed at nasal margin, note that the start and end of the spiral are along the anterior and posterior crest of the fossa for the lacrimal sac.

Clinical Comment: Optic Nerve Damage

The dura mater lining the optic canal is adherent to both the dura of the optic nerve and the periosteum of the canal. This close confinement of the nerve within the bony passage predisposes the nerve to compression and damage by even very small lesions or tumors of the bony canal.[12]

PARANASAL SINUSES

The paranasal sinuses are mucosa-lined, air-filled cavities located in four of the orbital bones. These hollow spaces decrease the weight of the skull and help add resonance to the voice. The paranasal sinuses communicate with the nasal cavity through small apertures.

The orbit is surrounded on three sides by sinuses (Figure 8-16): the **frontal sinus** above, the **ethmoid** and **sphenoid sinus** cavities medial to, and the **maxillary sinus** below the orbit. Of these, the maxillary sinus is largest. The roof of the maxillary sinus is the orbital plate of the maxilla; this plate, only 0.5 to 1 mm thick, separates the sinus from the orbital contents.[1] The sphenoid sinus is within the body of the sphenoid and, in some individuals, continues into the lesser wing and may surround the optic canal.[1] The ethmoid sinus sometimes continues into the lacrimal bone or into the frontal process of the maxilla.[13] In a high percentage of orbits, the thin bone of both the sphenoid and the ethmoid sinuses makes contact with the dural sheath of the optic nerve.[14,15] Table 8-1 shows the location of each of the sinus cavities.

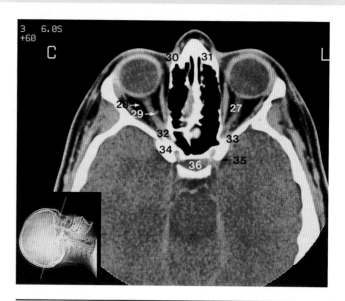

FIGURE 8-14
Horizontal section through the orbits. CT scan through long axis of orbit in horizontal plane. *27,* Optic nerve; *28,* long posterior ciliary artery; *29,* ophthalmic artery; *30,* angular vein; *31,* frontal process of maxilla; *32,* optic canal; *33,* superior orbital fissure; *34,* lesser wing of sphenoid; *35,* anterior clinoid process; *36,* pituitary gland. (From Mathers LH, Chase RA, Dolph J, et al: *Clinical anatomy principles*, St Louis, 1996, Mosby.)

Clinical Comment: Orbital Cellulitis

*The thin walls of the sinus cavities are poor barriers to the passage of infection from the air cavities into the orbit. If pathogens from a sinusitis penetrate the thin, bony barrier, a serious infection involving the orbital contents might ensue. A major infection that involves the orbital connective-tissue contents is called **orbital cellulitis**, and one of its major causes is sinusitis.[2,3,16,17] Signs and symptoms include sudden onset of pain, edema, proptosis, and a decrease in ocular motility. Orbital cellulitis is a serious medical situation because of the relatively easy access to the brain through orbital foramina and fissures and must be treated aggressively; hospitalization may be required.[3,16] Orbital cellulitis also is a possible sequela of a blow-out fracture, which can (but rarely does) provide a pathologic avenue between the sinus cavities and the orbit that results in orbital infection.[18]*

ORBITAL CONNECTIVE TISSUE

The connective tissue of the orbit is arranged in a complex network that serves to line, cover, and separate orbital structures; to anchor soft tissue structures to bone; and to compartmentalize areas. Although this network is continuous, the segments are described here individually according to their position and function.

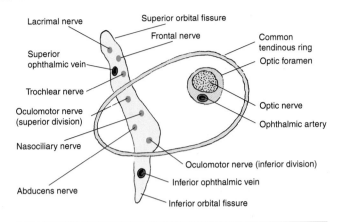

FIGURE 8-15
Nerves and vessels that enter orbit through superior orbital fissure *within*, *above*, and *below* the common tendinous ring.

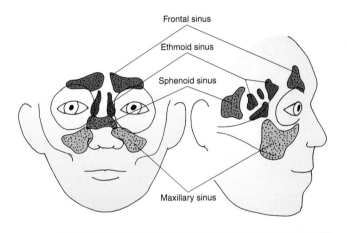

FIGURE 8-16
Location of sinus cavities within orbital walls.

Periorbita

The **periorbita,** also called the **orbital periosteum** or **orbital fascia,** covers the bones of the orbit (Figure 8-17). This dense connective tissue membrane serves as an attachment site for muscles, tendons, and ligaments and is a support structure for the blood supply to the orbital bones. The periorbita is attached only loosely to the underlying bone except at the orbital margins, the sutures, and the edges of fissures and foramina. At the orbital margins it is continuous with the periosteal covering of the bones of the face; at the edges of the superior orbital fissure, the optic canal, and the ethmoid canals, the periorbita is continuous with the periosteal layer of the dura mater. At the anterior portion of the optic canal, the periorbita splits such that a portion becomes continuous with the dura of the optic nerve and another portion reflects forward to take part in the formation of the common tendinous ring. At the inferior orbital fissure the periorbita is continuous

Table 8-1   Paranasal Sinuses

Sinus	Location
Frontal	In frontal bone, on each side of midline, superior to orbits
Ethmoid	Several air cells on both sides of perpendicular plate of ethmoid bone, medial to orbits
Sphenoid	In body of sphenoid bone, posterior and medial to orbits
Maxillary	In each maxillary bone, inferior to orbits

with the periosteum of the skull. At the lacrimal crests a sheet of periorbita covers the lacrimal sac, and the periorbita is continuous with the tissue lining the nasolacrimal canal. Another portion of the periorbita covers the lacrimal gland.

Orbital Septum

At the orbital margins the periorbita is continuous with a connective tissue sheet known as the **orbital septum,** also termed the **palpebral fascia** or **septum orbitale.** This dense connective tissue sheet is circular and runs from the entire rim of the orbit to the tarsal plates, which are embedded in the eyelids. This strong barrier helps prevent facial infections from entering the orbit; it also maintains orbital fat in its place. Figures 8-17 and 8-18 show the relationships between orbital structures and these connective tissue structures. At the lateral margin the orbital septum lies *in front of* the lateral palpebral ligament and the check ligament for the lateral rectus muscle.[7] At the superior orbital margin the orbital septum passes *in front of* the trochlea and bridges the supraorbital and supratrochlear notches. At the medial margin the orbital septum, which attaches *behind* the posterior lacrimal crest, lies *in front of* the check ligament for the medial rectus muscle; it lies *behind* the medial palpebral ligament, Horner's muscle, and the lacrimal sac (see Figure 8-18), isolating the lacrimal sac (which communicates with the nasal cavity) from the orbit proper.

Clinical Comment: Preseptal Cellulitis

PRESEPTAL CELLULITIS is an inflammatory condition that affects the tissue of the eyelid. If an infection of an eyelid gland becomes more serious and involves the tissue around the gland, preseptal cellulitis occurs. The disease can be limited by the location of the orbital septum, which provides a barrier to prevent spread into the orbit, which could result in the development of orbital cellulitis.

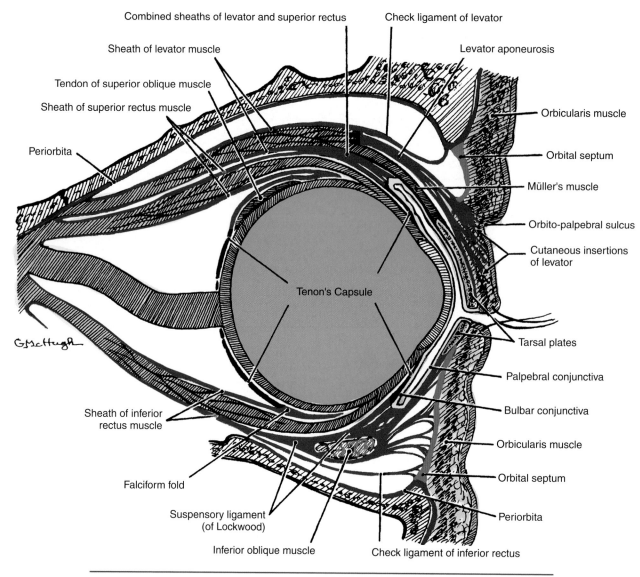

Combined sheaths of levator and superior rectus

Check ligament of levator

Sheath of levator muscle

Levator aponeurosis

Tendon of superior oblique muscle

Sheath of superior rectus muscle

Periorbita

Orbicularis muscle

Orbital septum

Müller's muscle

Orbito-palpebral sulcus

Cutaneous insertions of levator

Tenon's Capsule

Tarsal plates

Palpebral conjunctiva

Bulbar conjunctiva

Sheath of inferior rectus muscle

Orbicularis muscle

Orbital septum

Falciform fold

Periorbita

Suspensory ligament (of Lockwood)

Inferior oblique muscle

Check ligament of inferior rectus

FIGURE 8-17
Fascial system of orbit shown in vertical section through vertical meridian of eyeball, with the latter in primary position, eyelids closed. (From Kronfeld PC: *The human eye*, Rochester, NY, 1943, Bausch & Lomb Press.)

Tenon's Capsule

Tenon's capsule (bulbar fascia) is a sheet of dense connective tissue that encases the globe.[19] It lies between the conjunctiva and the episclera and merges with them anteriorly in the limbal area. Tenon's capsule is pierced by the optic nerve, the vortex veins, the ciliary vessels and nerves, and the extraocular muscles. At the muscle insertions, Tenon's capsule forms sleevelike sheaths that cover the tendons.[2,20] Posteriorly, Tenon's capsule merges with the dural sheath of the optic nerve. This dense connective tissue capsule acts as a barrier to prevent the spread of orbital infections into the globe.

Suspensory Ligament (of Lockwood)

The suspensory ligament (of Lockwood) (see Figure 8-17) is a hammocklike sheet of dense connective tissue that runs from its attachment on the lacrimal bone at the medial orbital wall to the zygomatic bone at the lateral wall. Tissue from several structures—Tenon's capsule, the sheaths of the two inferior extraocular muscles, and the inferior eyelid aponeurosis—contributes to the formation of this ligament. The suspensory ligament helps to support the globe, particularly in the absence of the bones of the orbital floor.

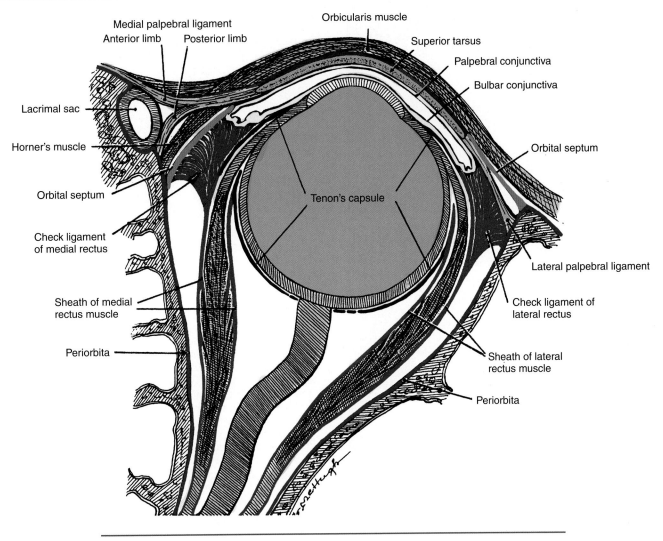

FIGURE 8-18
Fascial system of orbit shown in horizontal section. Plane of section lies slightly above horizontal meridian of eyeball, which is assumed to be in primary position, eyelids closed. (From Kronfeld PC: *The human eye*, Rochester, NY, 1943, Bausch & Lomb Press.)

Orbital Muscle of Müller

The **orbital muscle of Müller** is a small, smooth muscle embedded in the periorbita and covering part of the inferior orbital fissure.[6,21] Its function in humans is unknown.

Orbital Septal System

A complex web of interconnecting connective tissue septa organize the orbital space surrounding the globe into radial compartments. Collagenous strands connect the periorbita to Tenon's capsule and intermuscular membranes. This connective tissue system of "slings" anchors and supports the extraocular muscles and blood vessels, attaching them to adjacent orbital walls.[22] The slings associated with each of the muscles maintain correct positioning of the muscles during eye movements. Varying degrees of connectivity occur throughout the orbit (see Figures 10-11 and 10-12).

Orbital Fat

The spaces not occupied by ocular structures, connective tissue, nerves, or vessels become filled with adipose tissue. Usually, four adipose tissue compartments are located within the muscle cone surrounding the optic nerve and separating it from the extraocular muscles.[6,23] A ring of adipose tissue separates the muscles from the walls of the orbit, and adipose is the predominant tissue near the orbital apex.[6] Because of the close association of the orbital contents, a space-occupying lesion will cause outward displacement of the globe.

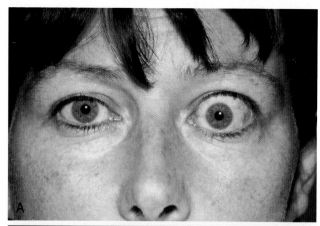

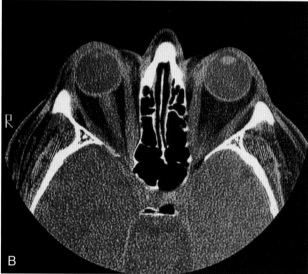

FIGURE 8-19
A, Asymmetric signs in ophthalmic Graves' disease, proptosis of the left eye. **B,** CT scan showing proptosis of the right eye. (**A** from Kanski JJ: *Clinical ophthalmology: a systematic approach,* ed 5, Oxford, UK, 2003, Butterworth-Heinemann; **B** courtesy. Weon Jun, O.D., Portland VA Medical Center, Portland, Ore.)

Clinical Comment: Exophthalmos

*Protrusion of the globe is termed **exophthalmos,** or **proptosis** (Figure 8-19). It can be caused by a number of pathologic conditions, including inflammation, edema, tumors, and injuries.[16] The most common type is thyroid ophthalmopathy (dysthyroid orbitopathy, Graves' disease), which can cause hypertrophy of the extraocular muscles; in some patients the muscles become enlarged to eight times their normal size.[3] Thyroid ophthalmopathy also causes proliferation of orbital fat and connective tissue, and lymphoid infiltration.[3] Because the orbital tissue is encased in immovable bony walls, this increase in volume of the orbital contents produces protrusion of the globe and simulates eyelid retraction. At the first sign of proptosis, investigation is necessary to determine the causative factor.*

AGING CHANGES IN THE ORBIT

In elderly adults the orbital septum often weakens, particularly in the medial inferior area, and herniation of fat and loose connective tissue can occur. The walls of the paranasal sinuses thin, and with age these walls may actually contain perforations that pass into the orbit.

REFERENCES

1. Warwick R: *Eugene Wolff's anatomy of the eye and orbit,* ed 7, Philadelphia, 1976, Saunders, pp 1, 8, 15, 19.
2. Doxanas MT, Anderson RL: *Clinical orbital anatomy,* Baltimore, 1984, Williams & Wilkins, pp 20, 25, 117.
3. Kanski JJ: *Clinical ophthalmology,* ed 3, London, 1994, Butterworth-Heinemann, pp 33, 52.
4. Forrest LA, Schuller DE, Strauss RH: Management of orbital blow-out fractures, *Am J Sports Med* 17(2):217-220, 1989.
5. Taher AA: Diplopia caused by orbital floor blowout fracture, *Oral Surg Oral Med Oral Pathol* 75(4):433-435, 1993.
6. Koornneef L: Orbital connective tissue. In Jakobiec FA, editor: *Ocular anatomy, embryology, and teratology,* Philadelphia, 1982, Harper & Row, p 835.
7. Rosenstein T, Talebzadeh N, Pogrel MA: Anatomy of the lateral canthal tendon, *Oral Surg Oral Med Oral Pathol Oral Radiol Endod* 89(1):24-28, 2000.
8. Reeh MJ, Wobig JL, Wirtschafter JD: *Ophthalmic anatomy,* San Francisco, 1981, American Academy of Ophthalmology, p 11.
9. Webster RC, Gaunt JM, Hamdan US, et al: Supraorbital and supratrochlear notches and foramina: anatomical variations and surgical relevance, *Laryngoscope* 96(3):311-315, 1986.
10. Sires BS, Gausas R, Cook BE Jr, et al: Orbit. In Kaufman PL, Alm A, editors: *Adler's physiology of the eye,* St Louis, 2003, Mosby, p 11.
11. Goldberg RA, Hannai K, Toga AW: Microanatomy of the orbital apex. Computed tomography and microcryoplaning of soft and hard tissue, *Ophthalmology* 99(9):1447-1452, 1992.
12. Lang J, Kageyama I: The ophthalmic artery and its branches, measurements, and clinical importance, *Surg Radiol Anat* 12(2):83-90, 1990.
13. Blaylock WK, Moore CA, Linberg JV: Anterior ethmoid anatomy facilitates dacryocystorhinostomy, *Arch Ophthalmol* 108(12):1774-1777, 1990.
14. Bansberg SF, Harner SG, Forbes G: Relationship of the optic nerve to the paranasal sinuses as shown by computed tomography, *Otolaryngol Head Neck Surg* 96(4):331-335, 1987.
15. Cheung DK, Attia EL, Kirkpatrick DA, et al: An anatomic and CT scan study of the lateral wall of the sphenoid sinus as related to the transnasal transethmoid endoscopic approach, *J Otolaryngol* 22(2):63-68, 1993.
16. Berkow R, editor: *The Merck manual,* ed 14, Rahway, NJ, 1982, Merck, p 1984.
17. Mills RP, Kartush JM: Orbital wall thickness and the spread of infection from the paranasal sinuses, *Clin Otolaryngol* 10(4):209-216, 1985.
18. Silver HS, Fucci MJ, Flanagan JC, et al: Severe orbital infection as a complication of orbital fracture, *Arch Otolaryngol Head Neck Surg* 118(8):845-848, 1992.
19. Tenon JR, Naus J, Blanken R: Anatomical observations on some parts of the eye and eyelids, *Strabismus* 11(1):63-68, 2003.
20. Eggers HM: Functional anatomy of the extraocular muscles. In Tasman W, Jaeger EA, editors: *Duane's foundations of clinical ophthalmology,* vol 1, Philadelphia, 1994, Lippincott.
21. Rodríguez-Vázquez JF, Mérida-Velasco JR, Jiménez-Collado J: Orbital muscle of Müller: observations on human fetuses measuring 35-150 mm, *Acta Anat (Basel)* 139:300-303, 1990.
22. Dutton JJ: Clinical and surgical orbital anatomy, *Ophthalmol Clin North Mm* 9(4):527, 1996.
23. Wolfram-Gabel R, Kahn JL: Adipose body of the orbit, *Clin Anat* 15(3):186-192, 2002.

The ocular adnexa includes the structures situated in proximity to the globe. This chapter discusses the eyebrows, structures of the eyelids, the conjunctiva, and the lacrimal system, which consists of a secretory system, for tear production, and an excretory system, for tear drainage.

EYEBROWS

The eyebrows consist of thick skin covered by characteristic short, prominent hairs extending across the superior orbital margin, usually arching slightly but sometimes merely running horizontally. Generally, in men the brows run along the orbital margin, whereas in women the brows run above the margin.[1] The first body hairs produced during embryologic development are those of the eyebrow.[2]

The muscles located in the forehead—the frontalis, procerus, corrugator superciliaris, and orbicularis oculi—produce eyebrow movements, an important element in facial expression (Figure 9-1). The **frontalis** muscle originates high on the scalp and inserts into connective tissue near the superior orbital rim. The fibers are oriented vertically and raise the eyebrow, causing a look of surprise or attention. The **corrugator** originates on the frontal bone and inserts into skin superior to the medial eyebrow. It is characterized as the muscle of trouble or concentration, and its fibers are oriented obliquely; it moves the brow medially, toward the nose, creating vertical furrows between the brows. The **procerus,** the muscle of menace or aggression, originates on the nasal bone and inserts into the medial side of the frontalis. It pulls the medial portion of the eyebrow inferiorly and produces horizontal furrows over the bridge of the nose.[2,3] The orbicularis oculi (described later) lowers the entire brow. The fibers of these muscles blend with one another and are difficult to separate.[2] All are innervated by the facial nerve—cranial nerve VII.

EYELIDS

The eyelids, or palpebrae, are folds of skin and tissue that, when closed, cover the globe. The eyelids have four major functions: (1) cover the globe for protection,

(2) move the tears toward drainage at the medial canthus on closure, (3) spread the tear film over the anterior surface of the eye on opening, and (4) contain structures that produce the tear film. On closure the upper eyelid moves down to cover the cornea, whereas the lower eyelid rises only slightly. When the eyes are closed gently, the eyelids should cover the entire globe.

Clinical Comment: Lagophthalmos

LAGOPHTHALMOS refers to incomplete closure of the eyelids (Figure 9-2). Its cause may be physiologic, mechanical (e.g., scarring), or paralytic. Lagophthalmos is most evident during sleep, when drying of the inferior cornea may result. Scratchy, irritated eyes are evident on awakening, and punctate keratitis can occur.[4-6] Clinical assessment of the inferior cornea will show varying degrees of epithelial disruption, manifested as staining with fluorescein dye.

PALPEBRAL FISSURE

The **palpebral fissure** is the area between the open eyelids. Although numerous variations exist in the positional relationship of the lid margins to the limbus, generally the upper lid just covers the superior limbus when one's eyes are open and looking straight ahead. The lower lid position is more variable, usually lying within 1 mm of the inferior limbus.[7-9]

The upper and lower eyelids meet at the corners of the palpebral fissure in the lateral and medial canthi. The **lateral canthus** is located approximately 5 to 7 mm medial to the bony orbital margin and lies directly on the globe.[9] The **medial canthus** is at the medial orbital margin but is separated from the globe by a reservoir for the pooling of tears, the **lacrimal lake.** The floor of the lacrimal lake is the **plica semilunaris** (Figure 9-3). This narrow, crescent-shaped fold of conjunctiva, located in the medial canthus, allows for lateral movement of the eye without stretching the bulbar conjunctiva. The **caruncle** is a small, pink mass of modified skin located just medial to the plica. It is covered with epithelium that contains goblet cells and fine hairs and their associated sweat and sebaceous glands.

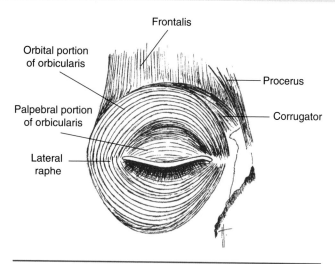

FIGURE 9-1
Forehead muscles that control the eyebrows. These are called the muscles of expression.

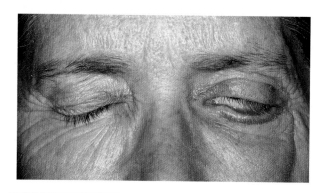

FIGURE 9-2
Lagophthalmos: inability to oppose the eyelids on attempted lid closure. In this patient, left seventh cranial nerve palsy caused a lower lid paralytic ectropion and lagophthalmos. (From Krachmer JH, Palay DA: *Cornea color atlas,* St Louis, 1995, Mosby.)

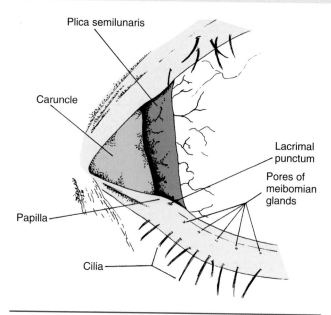

FIGURE 9-3
Structures located in left medial canthus.

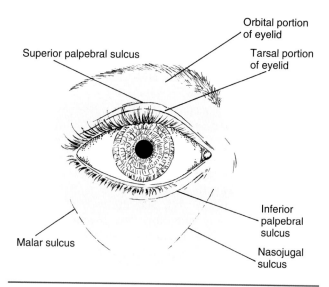

FIGURE 9-4
Surface anatomy of the right eyelid.

EYELID TOPOGRAPHY

The upper eyelid extends to the eyebrow and is divided into the tarsal and the orbital (or preseptal) parts. The **tarsal portion** lies closest to the lid margin, rests on the globe, and contains the tarsal plate. The skin is thin, and the underlying loose connective tissue is devoid of adipose tissue. The **orbital portion** extends from the tarsus to the eyebrow, and a furrow—the **superior palpebral sulcus**—separates the tarsal portion from the orbital portion (Figure 9-4). This sulcus separates the pretarsal skin, which is tightly adherent to the underlying tissue, from the preseptal skin, which is only loosely adherent to its underlying tissue, which contains a cushion of fat. In the eyelids of those of Eastern Asian descent, the orbital septum fuses with the levator aponeurosis below the upper tarsal border, allowing the fat to descend further into the lid[10] and eliminating the superior palpebral sulcus.[2,11-13]

In the lower eyelid the **inferior palpebral sulcus,** which separates the lower lid into tarsal and orbital parts, is often not very distinct. The tarsal portion rests against the globe, and the orbital portion extends from the lower border of the tarsus onto the cheek, extending just past the inferior orbital margin to the nasojugal and malar sulci (see Figure 9-4). These furrows occur at the attachment of the skin to the underlying connective tissue and become more prominent with age.

EYELID MARGIN

The eyelid margin rests against the globe and contains the eyelashes and the pores of the meibomian glands. The cilia (eyelashes) are arranged at the lid margin in a double or triple row, with approximately 150 in the upper eyelid and 75 in the lower lid.[14] The lashes curl upward on the upper and downward on the lower lid. Replacement lashes grow to full size in approximately 10 weeks, and each lash is replaced approximately every 5 months.[9] The eyelashes are richly supplied with nerves, causing them to be sensitive to even the slightest unexpected touch, which will elicit a protective response—a blink.

Clinical Comment: Abnormalities Affecting the Cilia

Various epithelial diseases can cause madarosis (loss of eyelashes) or trichiasis (misdirected growth of eyelashes), in which the eyelashes grow toward rather than away from the palpebral fissure. Contact with the cornea can cause irritation and painful abrasions and can lead to ulceration.[4] The problem lashes can be removed by epilation.

The pores of the meibomian glands are located posterior to the cilia (see Figure 9-3), and the transition from skin to conjunctiva, the mucocutaneous junction, occurs just posterior to these openings.[15] A groove called the gray line runs along the eyelid margin between the cilia insertions and the pores of the meibomian glands. This groove is the location of a surgical plane that divides the lid into anterior and posterior portions.[2]

The eyelid margin can be divided into two parts: the medial one sixth is the *lacrimal portion*, and the lateral five sixths is the *ciliary portion*. The division occurs at the *lacrimal papilla*, a small elevation containing the *lacrimal punctum*, the opening that carries the tears into the nasolacrimal drainage system (see Figure 9-3). Usually, no cilia or meibomian pores are found medial to the punctum, in the lacrimal portion of the lid margin.

Clinical Comment: Epicanthus

EPICANTHUS is a vertical fold of skin at the nasal canthus, arising in the medial area of the upper eyelid and terminating in the nasal canthal area. It is common in the newborn and may cause the appearance of esotropia (Figure 9-5). A parent of an infant with epicanthus might worry that the child's eyes are crossed; however, a cover test will identify a true esotropia. As the bridge of the nose develops, epicanthus gradually disappears. A form of epicanthus arising from the tarsal fold and extending into the medial canthal area is common in those of Eastern Asian descent.[2]

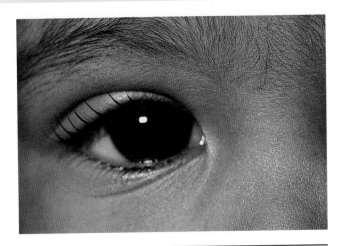

FIGURE 9-5
Epicanthal fold may give rise to pseudoesotropia. (From Kanski JJ, Nischal KK: *Ophthalmology: clinical signs and differential diagnosis*, St Louis, 1999, Mosby.)

EYELID STRUCTURES

Orbicularis Oculi Muscle

The striated fibers of the **orbicularis oculi** muscle are located below the subcutaneous connective tissue layer and encircle the palpebral fissure from the eyelid margin to overlap onto the orbital margin. The muscle can be divided into two regions: palpebral and orbital.

Palpebral Portion

The **palpebral portion** of the orbicularis oculi muscle occupies the area of the eyelid that rests on the globe and is closest to the eyelid margin. It sometimes is divided further into pretarsal and preseptal parts. The palpebral portion is composed of semicircles of muscle fibers that run from the medial orbital margin and the medial palpebral ligament[16] to the *lateral palpebral raphe*, where the superior and inferior fibers interdigitate with one another (see Figure 9-1). The lateral palpebral raphe overlies the lateral palpebral ligament.

Some fibers arise from deeper attachments on the posterior lacrimal crest. This section of the palpebral part of the orbicularis, the **muscle of Horner** or **lacrimal part (pars lacrimalis)**, encircles the lacrimal canaliculi.[9,11,16,17] Contraction of the orbicularis assists in moving tears through the canaliculi into the nasolacrimal drainage system.[18] Another section of the palpebral orbicularis, the **muscle of Riolan** or **ciliary part (pars ciliaris)**, lies near the lid margin on both sides of the meibomian gland openings; it maintains the lid margins close to the globe.[19]

Clinical Comment: Ectropion and Entropion

*Eversion of the eyelid margin is called **ectropion** (Figure 9-6), the common cause of which is loss of muscle tone, a normal occurrence in the aging process. As the lid margin falls away from its position against the globe, the lacrimal punctum is no longer in position to drain the tears from the lacrimal lake. **Epiphora**, an overflow of tears onto the cheek, may occur, causing maceration of the delicate skin in this area.*

*Inversion of the lid margin is called **entropion** and may result from spasm of the orbicularis oculi muscle causing the lid margin to turn inward (Figure 9-7). This inward turning puts the eyelashes in contact with the globe and, unless relieved, can cause corneal abrasion. Scarring of the lid after trauma or disease may also cause entropion. Both ectropion and entropion are more common in the lower lid and can be corrected surgically, if necessary. The anatomic relationship of the muscular and connective tissue components is an important consideration when repair is done.[20-22]*

Orbital Portion

The **orbital portion** of the orbicularis oculi muscle is attached superiorly to the orbital margin, medial to the supraorbital notch. The fibers encircle the area outer to the palpebral portion and attach inferiorly to the orbital margin, medial to the infraorbital foramen.[2] These concentric circular fibers extend throughout the rest of the lid and over the orbital rim.

Orbicularis Action

The orbicularis oculi muscle is innervated by cranial nerve VII (the facial nerve). Contraction of the palpebral portion closes the eyelid gently, and the palpebral orbicularis is the muscle of action in an involuntary blink and a voluntary wink; relaxation of the levator

muscle follows.[23] Spontaneous involuntary blinking renews the precorneal tear film. A reflex blink is protective and may be elicited by a number of stimuli—a loud noise; corneal, conjunctival, or cilial touch; or the sudden approach of an object. When the orbital portion of the orbicularis contracts, the eye is closed tightly, and the areas surrounding the lids—the forehead, temple, and cheek—are involved in the contraction. Such eyelid closure is often a protective mechanism against ocular pain or after injury, and is called reflex blepharospasm. If the lids are closed tightly in a strong contraction, forces compressing the orbital contents can significantly increase the intraocular pressure.[24]

The antagonist to the palpebral portion of the orbicularis is the levator muscle. The antagonist to the orbital portion is the frontalis muscle.

Superior Palpebral Levator Muscle

The **superior palpebral levator muscle,** the retractor of the upper eyelid, is located within the orbit above the globe and extends into the upper lid. It originates on the lesser wing of the sphenoid bone above and in front of the optic foramen, and its sheath blends with the sheath of the superior rectus muscle. As the levator approaches the eyelid from its posterior origin at the orbital apex, a ligament, the **superior transverse ligament (Whitnall's ligament)** may act as a fulcrum, changing the anteroposterior direction of the levator to superoinferior[10,12,25-28] (Figure 9-8). The superior transverse ligament is a fibrous band that spans the anterior superior orbit from the trochlea to the lacrimal gland fascia. It provides support for the upper lid and orbital structures as well as acting as a fulcrum. The ligament is located at the point where the levator muscle fibers end and the aponeurosis begins.[29]

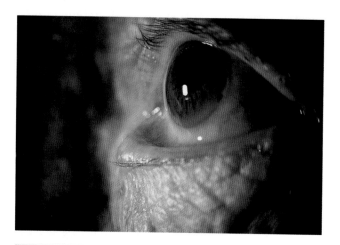

FIGURE 9-6
Severe involutional (senile) ectropion. (From Kanski JJ: *Clinical ophthalmology: a systematic approach,* ed 5, Oxford, UK, 2003, Butterworth-Heinemann.)

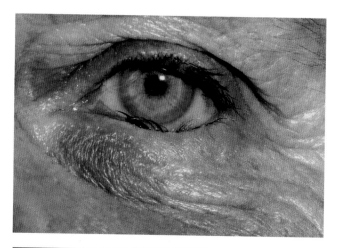

FIGURE 9-7
Involutional (senile) entropion. (From Kanski JJ: *Clinical ophthalmology: a systematic approach,* ed 5, Oxford, UK, 2003, Butterworth-Heinemann.)

Levator Aponeurosis

As it enters the eyelid, the levator becomes a fan-shaped tendinous expansion, the **levator aponeurosis.** Unlike a typical tendon, the aponeurosis spreads out into an extensive sheet posterior to the orbital septum. The fibers of the aponeurosis penetrate the orbital septum and extend into the upper lid, fanning out across its entire width. These tendinous fibers pass through the submuscular connective tissue; the posterior fibers insert into the lower anterior surface of the tarsal plate, and the anterior fibers run between the muscle bundles of the orbicularis to insert primarily into the skin of the eyelid, although some insert into the intermuscular septa of the orbicularis[9,11,25-28] (see Figure 9-8). This attachment of the fibers from the levator aponeurosis anchors the skin to the underlying tissues in the pretarsal area of the eyelid and creates the palpebral sulcus. In those of Eastern Asian descent, the orbital septum attaches to the tarsal plate more inferiorly, and the aponeurotic fibers do not attach as extensively to the cutaneous tissue.[2,11]

The two side extensions of the aponeurosis are referred to as horns. The *lateral horn* helps to support the lacrimal gland by holding it against the orbital roof, dividing the gland into orbital and palpebral lobes (Figure 9-9). The lateral horn then attaches to the lateral palpebral ligament and lateral orbital tubercle. The *medial horn* is attached to the medial palpebral ligament and medial orbital rim.

Levator Action

Contraction of the levator muscle causes elevation of the eyelid. The connection between the sheath of the levator and sheath of the superior rectus coordinates eyelid position with eye position so that as the eye is elevated, the lid is raised.[27,28] The levator is innervated by the superior division of the oculomotor nerve, cranial nerve III.

The eyelids are closed by relaxation of the levator and contraction of the orbicularis oculi muscles. The tonic activity of the levator and the relaxation of the orbicularis holds the eyelid open. In a blink, tonic activity of the levator is suspended, and with a burst of activity the orbicularis rapidly lowers the lid, followed by a cessation of orbicularis activity and resumption of levator tonicity.[30]

Retractor of Lower Eyelid

The retractor of the lower lid is the **capsulopalpebral fascia (lower eyelid aponeurosis).**[2,10] The capsulopalpebral fascia, an anterior extension from the sheath of the inferior rectus muscle and the suspensory ligament, inserts into the inferior edge of the tarsal plate.[11,27,28] This insertion coordinates lid position with globe movement. The lower eyelid is depressed on globe depression, and the lower eyelid elevates slightly on upward movement of the globe.[8] The capsulopalpebral fascia also fuses with the orbital septum and sends some fibers to insert into the inferior fornix.[2,21,28]

Tarsal Muscle (of Müller)

The **superior tarsal muscle (muscle of Müller)** is composed of smooth muscle and originates on the posteroinferior aspect of the levator muscle. These smooth muscle fibers begin to appear within the striated muscle at the point at which the muscle becomes aponeurotic.[2,9,27,28] The superior tarsal muscle inserts on the superior edge of the tarsal plate (see Figures 9-8 and 9-9). Contraction of Müller's muscle can provide 2 mm of additional lid elevation.[10]

A similar smooth muscle, the inferior tarsal muscle, is found in the lower eyelid. It arises from the inferior

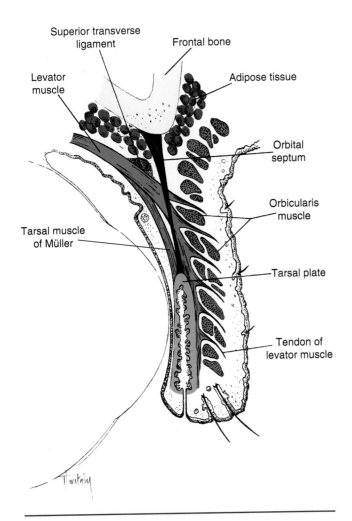

FIGURE 9-8
Sagittal section of upper eyelid.

Superior transverse ligament
Frontal bone
Levator muscle
Adipose tissue
Orbital septum
Orbicularis muscle
Tarsal muscle of Müller
Tarsal plate
Tendon of levator muscle

FIGURE 9-9
Orbital area viewed from in front, with skin, subcutaneous tissue, and orbital septum removed. Levator tendon sectioned before its insertion on tarsal plate; origin and insertion of Müller's muscle evident.

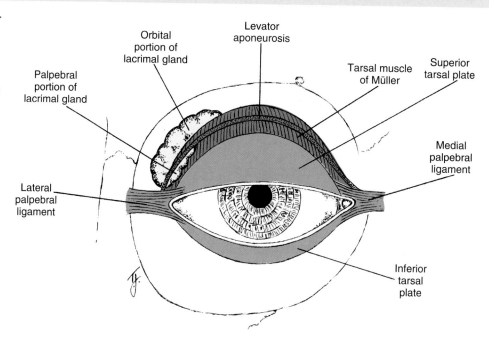

rectus muscle sheath and inserts into the lower conjunctiva and lower border of the tarsal plate.[2,9,24] Investigators disagree about whether the inferior tarsal muscle actually inserts into the tarsal plate[2,9,27] or inserts into the tissue below the tarsal plate.[31] Both tarsal muscles are innervated by sympathetic fibers that widen the palpebral fissure when activated (as in situations associated with fear or surprise).[9,28]

Clinical Comment: Ptosis

> *PTOSIS is a condition in which the upper eyelid droops or sags. It can be caused by weakness or paralysis of the levator or Müller's muscle. If Müller's muscle alone is affected, a less noticeable form of ptosis occurs than when the levator is involved.[32] An individual with ptosis might attempt to raise the lid by using the frontalis muscle, which results in elevation of the eyebrow and wrinkling of the forehead (Figure 9-10).*

Tarsal Plate

Each eyelid contains a **tarsal plate (tarsus)** that gives the lid rigidity and structure and shapes it to the curvature of the globe. The tarsal plate in the upper lid is approximately 11 mm high, and the inferior tarsal plate is approximately 5 mm high.[9] The anterior surface is adjacent to the submuscular connective tissue. The posterior surface is adherent to the palpebral conjunctiva. The orbital border of the tarsus is attached to the orbital septum, whereas the marginal border lies at the lid

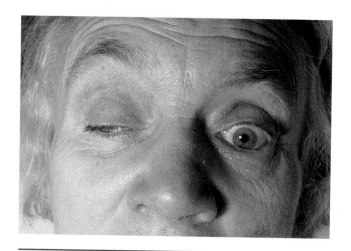

FIGURE 9-10
Unilateral ptosis. Note elevation of brow. (From Kanski JJ, Nischal KK: *Ophthalmology: clinical signs and differential diagnosis*, St Louis, 1999, Mosby.)

margin. The sides of the tarsal plates are attached to the bony orbital margin by the palpebral or tarsal ligaments (see Figure 9-9).

Clinical Comment: Eyelid Eversion

> *When attempting to evert the upper lid, one should place the cotton-tipped applicator or fingertip above the superior edge of the tarsal plate. The novice experiences difficulty in everting the eyelid if the applicator is placed in the middle of the tarsal plate.*

Palpebral Ligaments

The palpebral or tarsal ligaments are bands of dense connective tissue connecting the tarsal plates to the orbital rim and holding the tarsal plates in position against the globe during eye and lid movements. The **medial palpebral ligament** runs from the medial edge of each tarsal plate to the medial orbital rim, where it divides into two limbs. One limb attaches to the posterior lacrimal crest and the other to the anterior lacrimal crest. Both limbs lie anterior to the orbital septum[33] (see Figure 8-18).

The **lateral palpebral ligament** is located posterior to the orbital septum and attaches the lateral edges of the tarsal plates to the lateral orbital margin at the lateral orbital tubercle[34] (see Figure 8-18). Fibrous connections between the lateral palpebral ligament and the check ligament for the lateral rectus muscle allow a slight lateral displacement of the lateral canthus with extreme abduction.[35]

The upper borders of both the medial and the lateral ligaments are joined to the expansion of the levator tendon, and their lower borders are joined to an expansion of the ligament of Lockwood.[9] The connective tissue structures at the canthi have been described as a retinaculum that is made up of the palpebral ligaments, the horns of the levator aponeurosis, the suspensory ligament, the check ligaments, and the superior transverse ligament.[2]

Glands of the Lids

The **meibomian glands (tarsal glands)** are sebaceous glands embedded in the tarsal plate. These long, multi-lobed glands resemble a large bunch of grapes and are arranged vertically such that their openings are located in a row along the lid margin posterior to the cilia (Figure 9-11). Approximately 30 to 40 meibomian glands are found in the upper lid and 20 to 30 in the lower lid.[14] On eyelid eversion the vertical rows of the meibomian glands can sometimes be seen as yellow streaks through the palpebral conjunctiva. These glands secrete the outer lipid layer of the tear film.

Clinical Comment: Contact Lens Wear

Some studies have identified a loss in both the number and the length of meibomian glands in the contact lens wearer (Figure 9-12). Loss does not appear to be dependent on the type of lens but rather on the duration of wear and is speculated to be due to chronic irritation.[36]

The sebaceous **glands of Zeis** secrete sebum into the hair follicle of the cilia, coating the eyelash shaft to keep it from becoming brittle.[9]

The **glands of Moll** have been called modified sweat glands but are more accurately described as specialized apocrine glands.[37] They are located near the lid margin and their ducts empty into the hair follicle, into the Zeis gland duct, or directly onto the lid margin. Similar glands found in the axillae are scent organs, but that is likely not the function of the Moll glands.[9,14]

The **accessory lacrimal glands of Krause** are located in the stroma of the conjunctival fornix, and the **accessory lacrimal glands of Wolfring** are located along the orbital border of the tarsal plate[2,9] (see Figure 9-11). These glands are oval and display numerous acini. In the upper fornix, 20 to 40 glands of Krause are found, although only six to eight such glands appear in the lower fornix.[2] The glands of Wolfring are less numerous. The secretion of the accessory lacrimal glands appears similar to that of the main lacrimal gland and contributes to the aqueous layer of the tear film.

HISTOLOGIC FEATURES

Skin

The skin of the eyelid contains many fine hairs, sebaceous glands, and sweat glands. It is the thinnest skin in the body, easily forms folds and wrinkles, and is almost transparent in the very young.[2] The epidermal layer consists of a basal germinal layer, a granular layer, and a superficial layer that is cornified. The underlying dermis is abundant in elastic fibers. A very sparse areolar connective tissue layer, the subcutaneous tissue, lies below the dermis. This thin layer is devoid of adipose tissue in the tarsal portion. A pad of fat often is located in this region in the orbital portion that separates the orbicularis from the skin.[9]

Clinical Comment: Fluid Accumulation

The loose connective tissue layer of the eyelid can be separated easily from the underlying tissue and is the site of accumulation of blood or edema in injuries or accumulation of exudates in inflammatory conditions. The thinness of the skin and the fine underlying adjacent tissue allow this area to be greatly distensible, as evidenced in patients with periorbital cellulitis or ecchymosis (a black eye). This skin recovers rapidly after distention because of the elasticity of the dermis. With advancing age, however, the skin loses its elasticity, and stretching will cause exaggerated skin folds.

Muscles

The **orbicularis oculi** lies deep to the subcutaneous layer. These striated muscle bundles run throughout the eyelid. In a sagittal section of the lid prepared

FIGURE 9-11
Sagittal section of eyelid, illustrating palpebral muscles and glands.

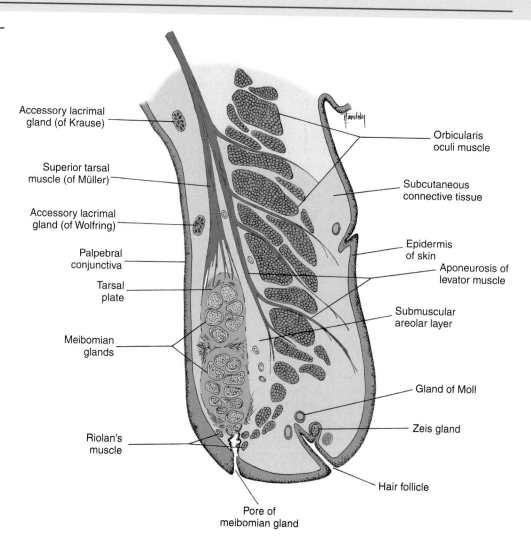

Accessory lacrimal gland (of Krause)

Superior tarsal muscle (of Müller)

Accessory lacrimal gland (of Wolfring)

Palpebral conjunctiva

Tarsal plate

Meibomian glands

Riolan's muscle

Pore of meibomian gland

Orbicularis oculi muscle

Subcutaneous connective tissue

Epidermis of skin

Aponeurosis of levator muscle

Submuscular areolar layer

Gland of Moll

Zeis gland

Hair follicle

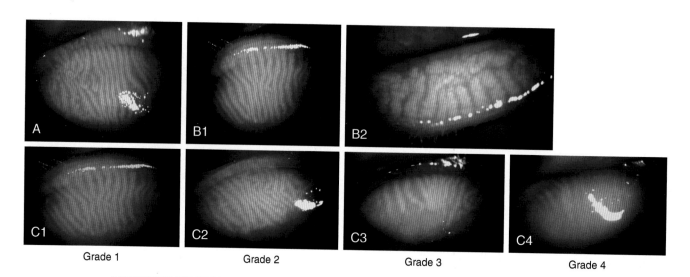

A

B1

B2

C1

Grade 1

C2

Grade 2

C3

Grade 3

C4

Grade 4

FIGURE 9-12

Infrared digital photography of meibomian glands. A, Normal meibomian gland anatomy; **B,** normal meibomian glands, upper and lower lids; **C,** grading scales for meibomian gland loss. (Courtesy Patrick Caroline, C.O.T., Pacific University College of Optometry, Forest Grove, Ore.)

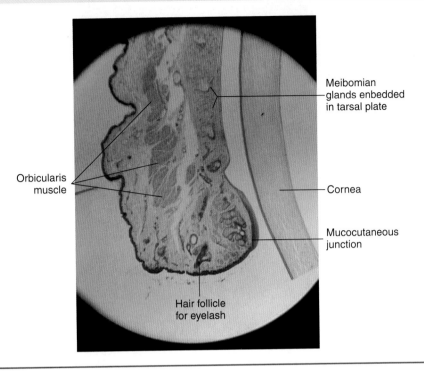

Meibomian glands enbedded in tarsal plate

Orbicularis muscle

Cornea

Mucocutaneous junction

Hair follicle for eyelash

FIGURE 9-13
Light micrograph of upper lid and cornea section.

for microscopic examination, the orbicularis bundles are cut in cross section (Figure 9-13). Along the lid margin, small muscle bundles located on both sides of the meibomian gland represent a specific part of the orbicularis, the ciliary part **(Riolan's muscle),** which holds the lid margin against the globe (see Figure 9-11).

Posterior to the orbicularis lies another layer of loose connective tissue, the submuscular areolar layer, which separates the muscle from the tarsal plate. Between this layer and the tarsal plate is a potential space, the pretarsal space, that contains the vessels of the palpebral arcades. The preseptal space is located between the orbicularis and the orbital septum; directly above is the preseptal cushion of fat.[9]

Tendinous fibers of the **levator aponeurosis** run through the submuscular tissue layer between the orbicularis and the superior tarsal muscle to insert into the tarsal plate and the skin of the lid (see Figure 9-11). It is this insertion of fibers that anchors the skin so firmly in the tarsal portion of the lid. There is no such attachment of the aponeurosis in the preseptal area. The smooth muscle fibers of the **superior tarsal muscle** are located above the superior tarsal plate and insert into its upper edge. Both the aponeurosis and the superior tarsal muscle are cut longitudinally in a microscope slide of a sagittal section of the lid.

Tarsal Plates

The **tarsal plates** are composed of dense connective tissue. The collagen fibrils of this tissue are of uniform size and run both vertically and horizontally to surround the meibomian glands.

Palpebral Conjunctiva

The **palpebral conjunctiva** is composed of two layers, a stratified epithelial layer and a connective tissue stromal layer, the submucosa. The **epithelial layer** of the conjunctiva is continuous with the skin epithelium at the mucocutaneous junction of the lid margin (see Figure 9-12). As the conjunctiva lines the lid, squamous cells are replaced by cuboidal and columnar cells, forming a stratified columnar mucoepithelial layer, the granular and keratinized layers having been discontinued.[14,38] At the **mucocutaneous junction,** the epithelial layer is approximately five cells thick and may be a location for stem cells that repopulate the palpebral conjunctival epithelium.[39] Over much of the upper lid the conjunctival epithelium is two or three cells thick, whereas over much of the lower lid, the epithelium is three or four cells thick.[9] This stratified columnar epithelium continues throughout the fornices into the bulbar conjunctiva, where it changes to a stratified squamous layer near the limbus, becoming continuous with the corneal epithelium.

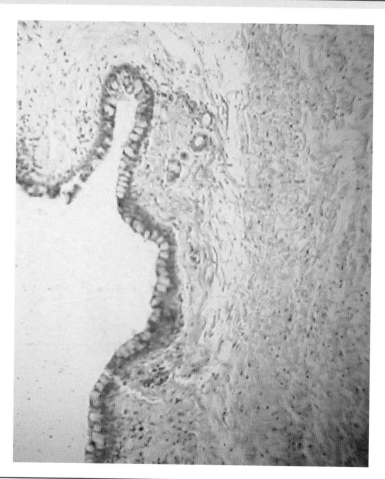

FIGURE 9-14
Light micrograph of conjunctival palpebral epithelium showing goblet cells.

The surface of the superficial conjunctival cells and their microvilli and microplicae are covered with a *glycocalyx* similar to that of the corneal surface.[40,41] Melanin granules often are found in the cytoplasm of conjunctival epithelial cells, especially near the limbus; these are particularly prevalent in individuals with heavily pigmented skin. Goblet cells, which produce the mucous component of the tear film, also are located in the epithelium. Subsurface vesicles, found below the outer membrane of the superficial conjunctival cell, may be an additional source of mucous material. As these vesicles fuse with the epithelial cell membrane, chains extend outward to form a chemical bond with the mucous layer secreted by the goblet cells. These chains increase the adherence of the tear film to the globe. These vesicle membranes may also contribute to the microvilli present on the surface epithelial cells.[42]

The **goblet cells,** which produce, store, and secrete the innermost mucous layer of the tear film, are scattered throughout the stratified columnar conjunctival epithelium (Figure 9-14). These cells are most numerous in the inferior nasal aspect of the tarsal conjunctiva.[43] Their number decreases with advancing age and increases in inflammatory conditions. A goblet cell produces mucin droplets that accumulate, causing the cell to swell and become goblet shaped. The surface of the cell finally ruptures, releasing mucus. Parasympathetic and sympathetic nerves have been associated with goblet cells and may play a role in their secretion.[44] Invaginations of conjunctival epithelium, often located near the fornix, are called **crypts of Henle.** Goblet cells release their mucus into the cavity formed by these invaginations, and the mucus may become trapped if the opening to the crypt is narrow. This accumulation of mucoid material may account for the application of the misnomer "glands" of Henle to describe these structures.

Clinical Comment: Vitamin A Deficiency

VITAMIN A DEFICIENCY has been associated with a loss of goblet cells. In dry-eye disorders showing a decrease in the number of goblet cells, treatment with vitamin A therapy can induce the reappearance of goblet cells.[45] In acute disease cellular proteins may be activated causing keratinization of the surface epithelia.[46]

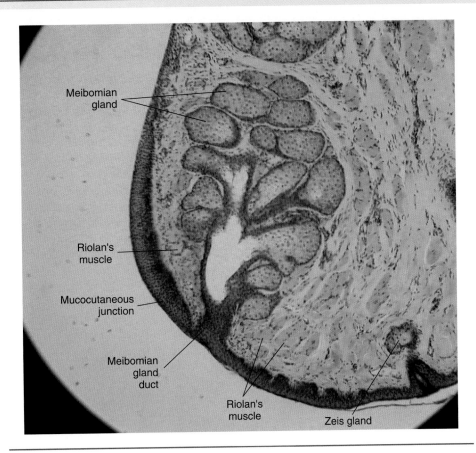

FIGURE 9-15
Light micrograph of meibomian glands embedded in tarsal plate. Duct and pore are shown.

The **submucosa (stroma, substantia propria)** of the palpebral conjunctiva is very thin in the tarsal portion of the eyelid but becomes increasingly thick in the orbital portion. It is composed of loose, vascularized connective tissue that can be subdivided into an outer lymphoid layer and a deep fibrous layer. In addition to the normal connective tissue components (collagen fibrils, fibroblasts, ground substance, and a few fine elastic fibers), the lymphoid layer contains macrophages, mast cells, polymorphonuclear leukocytes, eosinophils, accumulations of lymphocytes, and occasional Langerhans cells.[47] Immunoglobulin A (IgA) is found in the lymphoid layer, making the conjunctiva an immunologically active tissue.[48-50] More lymphoid tissue is found in palpebral conjunctiva than in bulbar conjunctiva.[51]

The deep fibrous layer connects the conjunctiva to underlying structures and contains a random network of collagen fibrils and numerous fibroblasts, blood vessels, nerves, and accessory lacrimal glands. This fibrous layer merges and is continuous with the dense connective tissue of the tarsal plate. The conjunctiva is so richly supplied with blood vessels that a pale palpebral conjunctiva may be a clinical sign of anemia.

Clinical Comment: Conjunctival Cysts and Concretions

CLEAR CONJUNCTIVAL CYSTS, either intraepithelial or subepithelial, are filled with mucoid material and are found most often in the palpebral conjunctiva.[52] Conjunctival concretions are small, yellow-white nodules about the size of a pinhead and most often are located in the tarsal conjunctiva. They are composed of fine granular material and membranous debris, products of cellular degeneration. These nodules are hardened but contain no calcium deposits.[53] Concretions are found more often in elderly patients and can be removed if they produce foreign body irritation.[50]

Glands

The **meibomian glands** are large sebaceous glands occupying the length of the tarsal plate. Each consists of 10 to 15 lobes or acini attached to a large central duct.[54,55] The duct is arranged vertically such that the opening is located at the edge of the tarsal plate corresponding to the eyelid margin (Figure 9-15).

Meibomian glands are *holocrine glands;* their secretion is produced by the decomposition of the entire cell. Each acinus is surrounded by a layer of myoepithelial cells and is filled with actively dividing cells. The daughter cells become large and polyhedral, they begin to synthesize lipids and fill with lipid droplets.[56] As each cell degenerates, the nucleus begins to diminish in size, and the cell membrane disintegrates.

Cells in varying stages of decomposition pack each saccule. Decomposed cells move down the duct toward the opening. The pressure exerted by a blink releases the secretion into the tear film,[57] at which point the secretion (lipid droplets and cell debris) forms the outermost lipid layer of the tear film.[15,54,55,58] The predominant innervation of meibomian glands is parasympathetic and may act to alter the lipid production or cause cell rupture.[59,60]

The secretion of the meibomian glands has been called meibum to distinguish it from sebum secreted by the sebaceous glands of the skin and hair follicles. Meibum is much more viscous than sebum; sebum is more polar and if mixed with the tear film will contaminate and disrupt it.[61]

Histologically, the sebaceous Zeis glands are similar to the meibomian glands. The **Zeis glands,** however, are composed of just one or two acini and are associated with the eyelash follicle (Figure 9-16). Generally, two Zeis glands are present per follicle. They release sebum into the follicle, thereby preventing the cilia from becoming dry and brittle.[54]

Glands of Moll, *modified apocrine glands,* are also located near the eyelash follicle. They consist of a spiral that begins as a large cavity, the neck of which becomes narrow as it forms a duct. The large lumen often appears empty and is surrounded by a layer of cuboidal to columnar secretory cells (Figure 9-17).[54] Myoepithelial cells surround these cells. As the Moll gland is an apocrine gland, its secretion is composed not of the whole cell but of parts of cellular cytoplasm. The duct might empty into the duct of a Zeis gland, or it might open directly onto the lid margin between cilia.[37] Recent histochemical studies have identified antimicrobial peptides and proteins in Moll gland secretions that suggest a role in immune defense protecting the lash shaft and ocular surface.[37,62]

Accessory lacrimal glands are groups of secretory cells with a truncated-pyramid shape arranged in an oval pattern around a central lumen[38] (Figure 9-18). The acini are surrounded, sometimes incompletely, by a row of

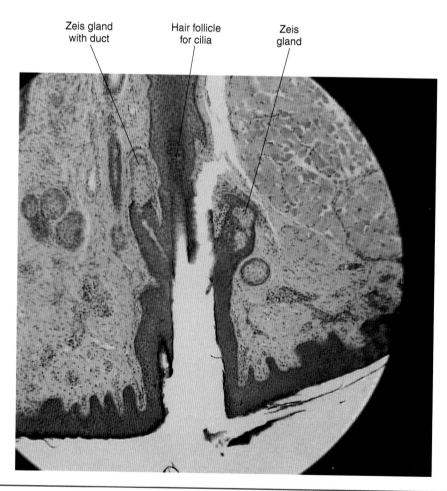

Zeis gland with duct   Hair follicle for cilia   Zeis gland

FIGURE 9-16

Light micrograph of lid margin. Zeis gland is located next to hair follicle; duct is evident.

myoepithelial cells.[2] Animal studies suggest that the ducts of Wolfring glands have a tortuous course and open onto the palpebral conjunctiva.[63] These are *merocrine glands*— that is, the cell remains intact and secretes a product— and they have the same histologic makeup as the main lacrimal gland.[63] The secretion contains antibacterial agents, lysozyme, lactoferrin, and immunoglubulins.[58] The accessory lacrimal glands are densely innervated, as is the main lacrimal gland.[64]

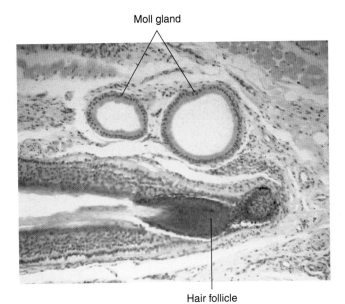

Moll gland

Hair follicle

FIGURE 9-17
Light micrograph of hair follicle for cilia. Two Moll glands are seen.

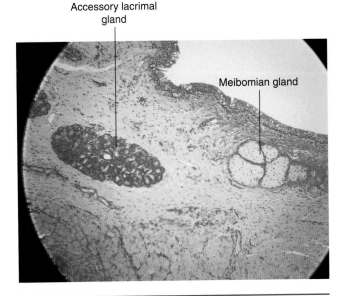

Accessory lacrimal gland

Meibomian gland

FIGURE 9-18
Light micrograph of lower lid. Accessory lacrimal gland is seen distal to tarsal plate, which has meibomian gland within it.

Clinical Comment: Common Eyelid Conditions

A ***hordeolum*** *is an acute inflammation of an eyelid gland, usually caused by staphylococci.[4] An infected Zeis or Moll gland is called an external hordeolum, or common stye, and usually comes to a head on the skin of the eyelid (Figure 9-19). A localized infection of a meibomian gland usually drains from the inside surface of the lid and thus is called an internal hordeolum. Mild cases usually resolve with hot compress treatment, but more severe cases might require antibiotic treatment.*

A ***chalazion*** *is a localized, noninfectious, and sometimes painless swelling of a meibomian gland, often caused by an obstructed duct (Figure 9-20). The gland may extrude its secretion into surrounding tissue, setting up a granulomatous inflammation. Medical or surgical therapy sometimes is necessary.[65]*

Blepharitis *is an inflammatory disease of the lid; meibomian gland dysfunction is often the cause. Blockage of the gland pores can result in inflammation, sometimes complicated by bacterial infection.[66] Clinical presentation might include crusting at the lash base and erythematosus of the lid margin. It can become a chronic condition that requires periodic treatments with hot packs, lid scrubs, and antibiotic ointment. Long-term inflammation can lead to hyperkeratinization and fibrosis of the glands and hyperemia and telangiectasia of the lid margin.[67]*

INNERVATION OF EYELIDS

The ophthalmic and maxillary divisions of the trigeminal nerve provide sensory innervation of the eyelids. The upper lid is supplied by the supraorbital, supratrochlear, infratrochlear, and lacrimal nerves, branches of the ophthalmic division. The supply to the lower

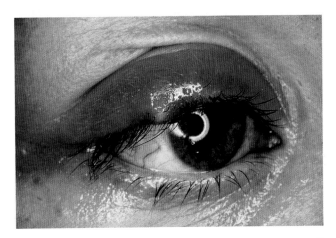

FIGURE 9-19
External hordeolum. (From Kanski JJ: *Clinical ophthalmology: a systematic approach*, ed 5, Oxford, UK, 2003, Butterworth-Heinemann.)

lid is by the infratrochlear branch of the ophthalmic nerve and the infraorbital nerve, a branch of the maxillary division (Figure 9-21). Motor control of the orbicularis muscle is through the temporal and zygomatic branches of the facial nerve, and that of the levator muscle is through the superior division of the oculomotor nerve. The tarsal smooth muscles are innervated by sympathetic fibers from the superior cervical ganglion.

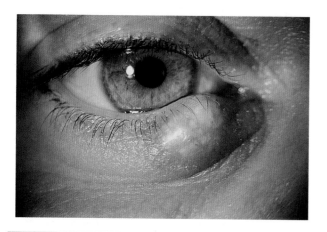

FIGURE 9-20
Painless chalazion. (From Kanski JJ, Nischal KK: *Ophthalmology: clinical signs and differential diagnosis*, St Louis, 1999, Mosby.)

BLOOD SUPPLY OF EYELIDS

The blood vessels are located in a series of arcades or arches in each eyelid. The marginal palpebral arcade lies near the lid margin, and the peripheral palpebral arcade lies near the orbital edge of the tarsal plate (Figure 9-22). The vessels forming these arcades are branches from the medial and lateral palpebral arteries. The medial and lateral palpebral arteries are branches of the ophthalmic and lacrimal arteries, respectively. Normal variations occur in the blood supply, and the most common variation is a lack of the peripheral arcade in the lower lid.

CONJUNCTIVA

The **conjunctiva** is a thin, translucent mucous membrane that runs from the limbus over the anterior sclera, forms a cul-de-sac at the superior and inferior fornices, and turns anteriorly to line the eyelids. It ensures smooth movement of the eyelids over the globe. The conjunctiva can be divided into three sections that are continuous with one another: (1) the tissue lining the eyelids is the **palpebral conjunctiva,** or tarsal conjunctiva; (2) the **bulbar conjunctiva** covers the sclera; and (3) the **conjunctival fornix** is the cul-de-sac connecting palpebral and bulbar sections (Figure 9-23). Conjunctival stem cells are scattered in the basal layer throughout the conjunctiva, but are more numerous in the fornix region.[68,69]

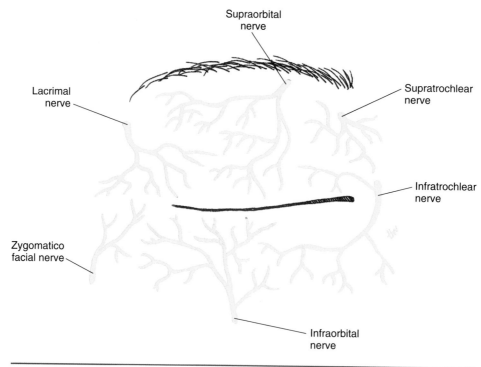

FIGURE 9-21
Palpebral innervation.

At the **mucocutaneous junction** of the lid margin (see Figure 9-15), the nonkeratinized squamous palpebral conjunctival epithelium is continuous with the keratinized squamous epithelium of the epidermis of the eyelid. The conjunctiva forming the fornices is attached loosely to the fascial extensions of the levator, tarsal, and extraocular muscles, providing coordination of conjunctival movement with movement of the globe and lids. The fornices are present superiorly, inferiorly, and laterally, easing movement of the globe without creating undue stretching of the conjunctiva. The lateral fornix is the deepest and extends posterior to the equator of the globe.

The bulbar conjunctiva is translucent, allowing the sclera to show through, and is colorless except when its blood vessels are engorged. Bulbar conjunctiva is loosely adherent to the underlying tissue up to within 3 mm of the cornea, where it becomes tightly adherent and merges with the underlying Tenon's capsule and sclera.

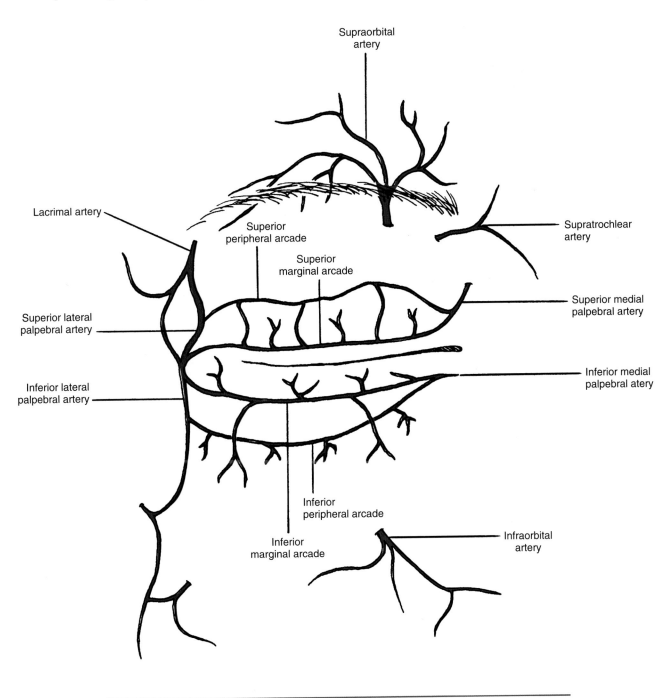

FIGURE 9-22
Palpebral blood supply.

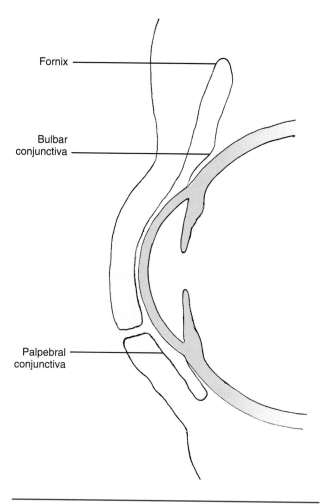

FIGURE 9-23
Three partitions of conjunctiva.

Labels on figure: Fornix, Bulbar conjunctiva, Palpebral conjunctiva

PLICA SEMILUNARIS

The **plica semilunaris** is a crescent-shaped fold of conjunctiva located at the medial canthus (see Figure 9-3). (It might be a remnant of the nictitating membrane seen in lower vertebrates.) The epithelium is 8 to 10 cells thick and contains numerous goblet cells, and the stroma is highly vascularized, containing smooth muscle fibers and adipose tissue.[70] Because there is no deep fornix at the medial side as there is at the lateral side, the evident function of the plica is to allow full lateral movement of the eye without tissue stretching.

CARUNCLE

The function of the **caruncle,** a mound of tissue that overlies the medial edge of the plica semilunaris (see Figure 9-3), is poorly understood. The caruncle is similar to conjunctiva in that it contains nonkeratinized epithelium and accessory lacrimal glands, but it also has

skin elements: hair follicles and sebaceous and sweat glands.[70,71] The sebaceous glands are a likely source for the occasional accumulation of matter in the medial canthus of the healthy eye.

CONJUNCTIVAL BLOOD VESSELS

The palpebral conjunctiva receives its blood supply from the palpebral arcades. Branches from the arcades anastomose on both sides of the tarsal plate; vessels from the posterior network supply the palpebral conjunctiva in both upper and lower lids.

The fornices are supplied by branches from the peripheral arcades, which then branch again and enter the bulbar conjunctiva, forming a plexus of vessels, the posterior conjunctival arteries. These anastomose with the plexus of anterior conjunctival arteries formed by branches from the anterior ciliary arteries. Conjunctival veins parallel the arteries but are more numerous. They drain into the palpebral and ophthalmic veins.

CONJUNCTIVAL LYMPHATICS

The conjunctival lymphatic vessels are arranged in superficial and deep networks within the submucosa. These vessels drain into the lymphatics of the eyelids; those from the lateral aspect empty into the parotid lymph node, and those from the medial aspect empty into the submandibular lymph node (see Figure 11-14).

CONJUNCTIVAL INNERVATION

Sensory innervation of the bulbar conjunctiva is through the long ciliary nerves. Sensory innervation of the superior palpebral conjunctiva is provided by the frontal and lacrimal branches of the ophthalmic nerve. Innervation of the inferior palpebral conjunctiva is provided by the lacrimal nerve and the infraorbital branch of the maxillary nerve. All sensory information is carried in the trigeminal nerve.

Clinical Comment: Biomicroscopic Examination

The normal bulbar conjunctiva is clear and displays a fine network of blood vessels. The blood flow in an individual vessel may be seen under high magnification. The conjunctival surface is not as smooth as the cornea, and thus a small amount of fluorescein pooling might be evident in the normal eye. The palpebral conjunctiva is examined by everting the eyelids and should appear bright pink in color. The blood vessel network is evident, and arteries can be seen that run at right angles to the lid margins. The meibomian gland ducts, if seen, will appear as fine yellow lines.

Clinical Comment: Conjunctivitis

CONJUNCTIVITIS is any inflammation of the conjunctiva and can be caused by a variety of factors. Among the common causative agents are bacterial or viral invasion and allergic reaction. In inflammatory conditions, fluids often accumulate in the loose stromal tissue; this conjunctival edema is called **chemosis.** *Dilation and engorgement of the conjunctival blood vessels also occur with inflammation and irritation; this vascular change is known as* **conjunctival injection.** *Both chemosis and injection are present to varying degrees in diseases and irritations of the conjunctiva. In viral conjunctivitis the preauricular lymph node often is prominent on the involved side.*

Clinical Comment: Giant Papillary Conjunctivitis

GIANT PAPILLARY CONJUNCTIVITIS (GPC) is a common complication often seen in the contact lens wearer. The patient has hyperemic palpebral conjunctiva with large papilla, so large they are described as "cobblestone." The cause is thought to be an allergic reaction either to substances in the lens material, in the cleaning solutions, or to buildup of material on the lens surface. Treatment might include changing lens material, changing solution, or perhaps discontinuation of wear temporarily.

Clinical Comment: Pingueculae and Pterygia

A PINGUECULA consists of an opaque, slightly elevated mass of modified conjunctival tissue in the interpalpebral area, usually at the 3-o'clock or 9-o'clock position. Pingueculae may vary considerably in size and appearance but usually are round or oval and yellowish (Figure 9-24). Two histologic changes occur in the submucosal layers, whereas the epithelial layers remain unchanged. The first submucosal change is hyalinization, which occurs in a zone just below the epithelium. This zone contains degenerating collagen and a granular material that probably results from the breakdown of connective tissue components.[72,73] The second submucosal change in development of pinguecula is the formation of abnormal elastic fibers. Precursors of elastic fibers and abnormally immature forms of newly synthesized elastic fibers are found beneath the zone of hyalinization. These fibers degenerate, and elastic myofibrils are greatly reduced, which prevents normal assembly of elastic fibers.[72,73] Fibroblasts in these regions show extensive alteration.

A pterygium is a fibrovascular overgrowth of bulbar conjunctiva onto cornea and is usually progressive. As with pinguecula, pterygium occurs in the 3-o'clock or 9-o'clock position of the interpalpebral area (Figure 9-25). The triangular pterygium may be gray in appearance, and its apex (often called the head) invades the cornea. This leading edge is composed of a zone of limbal epithelial tissue arising from altered basal stem cells. A zone of cells follows the head, migrates along the corneal basement membrane, and dissolves Bowman's layer.[72,74] The head is the only site of firm attachment to the corneal surface. Fibrovascular tissue with the same abnormal characteristics seen in pingueculae underlie the epithelium of a pterygium.[74-76] An extensive network of blood vessels is evident.[72]

Pingueculae and pterygia show many of the same connective tissue changes but are different diseases. If mutational changes occur in the limbal epithelium at the corneal edge of a pinguecula, it may become a pterygium.[76] Exposure to irritants such as wind and dust might initiate hyperplasia and be a precursor of both these degenerative changes. Molecular damage produced by chronic solar radiation, particularly high-energy ultraviolet rays, is the primary causal factor in pterygium, with irritants being predisposing factors.[74,77-79] Biochemical studies have shown that oxidative stress can result in biochemical cellular changes that cause cellular proliferation, vascularization, and the adhesion to the corneal surface that occurs in pterygium.[80-82]

Pingueculae rarely are treated unless inflamed. Pterygia are surgically removed (1) when the apex approaches the visual axis, (2) if significant corneal astigmatism is induced, or (3) for cosmetic concerns. Complete removal is difficult because the altered cells appear as normal cornea, and the abnormal cell can only be discerned histologically.[75] Thus pterygia often recur. Patients with either condition should be advised of the relationship of these conditions to irritants and sun exposure, and ultraviolet-filtering protective lenses should be prescribed, as well as artificial tears and ocular lubricants as needed.

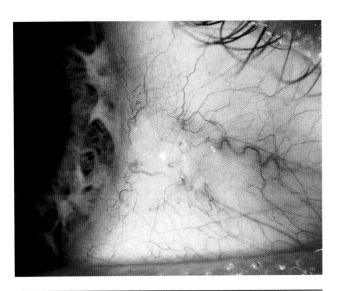

FIGURE 9-24
Pinguecula. (From Krachmer JH, Palay DA: *Cornea color atlas,* St Louis, 1995, Mosby.)

TENON'S CAPSULE

Below the conjunctival stroma is a thin, fibrous sheet called **Tenon's capsule (fascia bulbi).** Tenon's capsule serves as a fascial cavity within which the globe can move. It protects and supports the globe and attaches it to the orbital connective tissue.

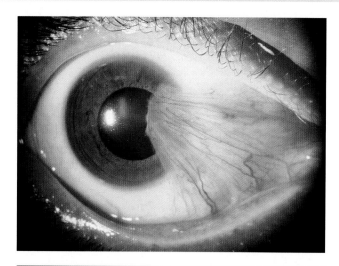

FIGURE 9-25
Pterygium. (From Krachmer JH, Palay DA: *Cornea color atlas*, St Louis, 1995, Mosby.)

The collagen fibrils that form Tenon's capsule are arranged in a three-dimensional network of longitudinal, horizontal, and oblique groups.[83] In young people, Tenon's capsule contains collagen fibrils of uniform shape and diameters of 70 to 110 nm; in older individuals there is greater variation in fibril shape, and diameters vary from 30 to 160 nm.[83,84] Few fibroblasts and some elastic fibers are present, but in a very small ratio compared with the number of collagen fibrils.[84]

TEAR FILM

The tear film, which covers the anterior surface of the globe, has several functions: (1) keeps the surface moist and serves as a lubricant between the globe and eyelids; (2) traps debris and helps remove sloughed epithelial cells and debris; (3) is the primary source of atmospheric oxygen for the cornea; (4) provides a smooth refractive surface necessary for optimum optical function[85]; (5) contains antibacterial substances (lysozyme, beta-lysin, lactoferrin, immunoglobulins) to help protect against infection[86]; (6) helps to maintain corneal hydration by changes in tonicity that occur with evaporation[87]; and (7) contains various growth factors and peptides that can regulate ocular surface wound repair.[58]

The tear film is composed of three layers (Figure 9-26). The outermost is a **lipid layer** containing waxy esters, cholesterol, and free fatty acids, primarily produced by the meibomian glands. The lipid layer retards evaporation and provides lubrication for smooth eyelid movement. The middle or **aqueous layer** contains inorganic salts, glucose, urea, enzymes, proteins, glycoproteins, and most of the antibacterial substances.[2] It is secreted by the main and accessory lacrimal glands. The innermost or **mucous layer** acts as an interface that

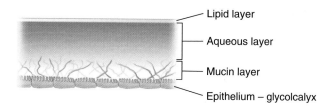

FIGURE 9-26
Schematic representation of tear film.

facilitates adhesion of the aqueous layer of the tears to the ocular surface.[88,89] It is composed of the glycocalyx secretion from the surface epithelia and mucin produced and secreted by the conjunctival goblet cells. Mucins can also bind and entrap bacteria and viruses blocking binding sites on microbes and preventing them from penetrating the ocular surface.[58]

According to some sources, the tear film is 7 to 10 μm thick, with the aqueous layer accounting for 90% of the thickness.[9,90] However, measurements using laser interferometry suggest that the full thickness of the mucous layer was not recognized using conventional measuring methods. Some have estimated tear layer thickness in the range of 34 to 45 μm, with the mucous layer the thickest.[91-93] The mucous and aqueous portions are not static and may not remain as separate and distinct layers but may form a sort of gradient hampering accurate measurements.[58]

LACRIMAL SECRETORY SYSTEM

The secretory system includes the main lacrimal gland, the accessory lacrimal glands, meibomian glands, and the conjunctival goblet cells. The main **lacrimal gland** is located in a fossa on the temporal side of the orbital plate of the frontal bone, just posterior to the superior orbital margin.

The lacrimal gland is divided into two portions, *palpebral* and *orbital*, by the aponeurosis of the levator muscle (see Figure 9-9). The superior orbital portion is larger and almond shaped. The superior surface lies against the periorbita of the lacrimal fossa, the inferior surface rests against the aponeurosis, the medial edge lies against the levator, and the lateral edge lies on the lateral rectus muscle. The palpebral lobe is one third to one half the size of the orbital lobe and is subdivided into two or three sections.[38] If the upper lid is everted, the lacrimal gland can be seen above the edge of the upper tarsal plate. Ducts from both portions of the gland exit through the palpebral lobe.

The lacrimal gland consists of lobules made up of numerous acini. Each acinus is an irregular arrangement of secretory cells around a central lumen surrounded by an incomplete layer of myoepithelial cells.[94] (Histologically, the main lacrimal gland is identical to the accessory lacrimal glands.) A network of ducts connects the acini and drains into one of the main excretory ducts. There are approximately 12 of these ducts, which empty into the conjunctival sac in the superior fornix.[49] The secretion is composed of water, electrolytes, and antibacterial agents including lysozyme, lactoferrin, and immunoglobulins. The accessory glands are located in the subconjunctival tissue from the fornix area to near the tarsal plate. Basic secretion maintains the normal volume of the aqueous portion of the tears, and reflex secretion increases the volume in response to a stimulus. Both main and accessory glands play a role in basic and reflex secretion.

The lacrimal gland is supplied by the lacrimal artery, a branch of the ophthalmic artery. Sensory innervation is through the lacrimal nerve, a branch of the ophthalmic division of the trigeminal nerve. The gland receives vasomotor sympathetic innervation and secretomotor parasympathetic innervation.[95] Reflex tearing occurs with stimulation of branches of the ophthalmic nerve or in response to external stimuli, such as intense light; the afferent pathway is through the trigeminal nerve, and the parasympathetic pathway is through the facial nerve.

Disagreement still exists regarding the relative contributions of the main and accessory lacrimal glands. In the traditional view, accessory glands provide basic secretion, and the main lacrimal gland is primarily active during reflex or psychogenic stimulation.[95] A more recent view holds that all lacrimal glands produce the aqueous layer and that production is stimulus driven, with the rate of production ranging from low levels in sleep to high levels under conditions of stimulation.[58,96]

Clinical Comment: Tear Film Assessment

Various clinical tests are used to assess the extent of tear abnormalities, although no single test is thought to be diagnostically effective.[97] The Schirmer test is a clinical measure of the adequacy of the aqueous portion of the tears. A special piece of filter paper is inserted over the inferior eyelid margin. Normally the strip should be moistened by at least 5 mm after 5 minutes.[86,98] This test can be done with or without topical anesthesia; the test without topical anesthetic measures both reflex and basic secretion, and the test with anesthetic measures only basic secretion. The phenol red thread test, which uses a thread treated with a pH indicator, may be used in place of the Schirmer strips.

In another clinical assessment method, fluorescein dye is instilled into the lower cul-de-sac and it spreads throughout the tear film. After a blink the thin lipid upper layer begins to break down, and dry spots appear. The time between the completion of the blink and the first appearance of a dry spot is termed the tear film breakup time (TBUT) and gives an indirect measure of the evaporative rate. Normally the TBUT is greater than 10 seconds and longer than the time between blinks.[2,98-100] A short TBUT can occur if

irregularities or disturbances in the corneal surface prevent complete tear film adherence or if abnormalities exist in the lipid layer causing increased evaporation.[101]

Clinical Comment: Dry Eye

Alteration in any of the layers of the tear film or in normal lid anatomy and closure can result in depletion of the tear film and cause dry eye, one of the most common disorders seen in clinical eye care practice. Dry eye syndrome has a complex etiology and may be caused by a deficiency or alteration of any of the layers of the tear film or by an abnormal interaction between the layers.[102] Aqueous deficiencies are common, and normal aging can cause a decrease of aqueous tear production. Patients with rheumatoid arthritis often develop Sjögren syndrome, an autoimmune disease that affects the lacrimal gland, causing a deficiency in the aqueous layer. This can cause an uncomfortable gritty, sandy feeling.[103,104] Inflammation of the meibomian glands, meibomianitis, can modify the composition of the secretion producing a more viscous meibum that does not flow as easily through the pores.[105,106] Loss of lipid secretion can lead to alterations in the lipid layer, allowing increased evaporation of the tear film and leading to dry eye symptoms of irritation and corneal epithelial compromise.[36,67] Conditions with deficient secretion of mucus are associated with reduced goblet cell populations, such as chemical burns, Stevens-Johnson syndrome, and ocular pemphigoid.[99,107] Complaints associated with dry eye include scratchy and foreign body sensations.

The diagnosis of dry eye is not usually based on a single definitive finding. The instillation of dye (fluorescein, lissamine green, or rose Bengal) can indicate tissue damage that occurs because of a defective tear film but does not indicate the reason.[97] The tear film can be augmented by the application of ocular lubricants, consisting of artificial tears during the day and ointments at night. More serious dry eye problems can be treated with procedures that decrease tear drainage; punctual plugs are a temporary solution, and electrocautery can produce permanent closure of the punctum. Recent clinical studies suggest that a subclinical inflammatory condition contributing to dry eye may be successfully treated with topical antiinflammatory agents such as cyclosporin A.[108-111]

TEAR FILM DISTRIBUTION

The lacrimal gland fluid is secreted into the lateral part of the upper fornix and descends across the anterior surface of the globe. Contraction of the orbicularis forces meibum out of the pores and lid motion can spread the thin lipid layer across the surface. Each blink reforms the tear film, spreading it over the ocular surface.

At the posterior edge of both upper and lower eyelid margins, there is a meniscus of tear fluid. The meniscus at the lower lid is more easily seen. The upper tear meniscus is continuous with the lower meniscus at the lateral canthus, whereas at the medial canthus the tear menisci lead directly to the puncta and drain into them.[112] The

lacrimal lake, a tear reservoir, is located in the medial canthus. The plica semilunaris makes up the floor of the lake, and the caruncle is located at its medial side.

NASOLACRIMAL DRAINAGE SYSTEM

Some tear fluid is lost by evaporation and some by reabsorption through conjunctival tissue, but approximately 75% passes through the nasolacrimal drainage system.[86] The nasolacrimal drainage system consists of the puncta, canaliculi, lacrimal sac, and nasolacrimal duct, which empties into the nasal cavity (Figure 9-27).

Puncta and Canaliculi

A small aperture, the **lacrimal punctum,** is located in a slight tissue elevation, the **lacrimal papilla,** at the junction of the lacrimal and ciliary portions of the eyelid margin. Both upper and lower lids have a punctum. The puncta are turned toward the globe and normally can be seen only if the eyelid edge is everted slightly. Each punctum opens into a tube, the **lacrimal canaliculus.**

The canaliculi are tubes in the upper and lower lids that join the puncta to the lacrimal sac. The walls of the canaliculi contain elastic tissue and are surrounded by fibers from the lacrimal portion of the orbicularis muscle (Horner's muscle). The first portion of the canaliculus is vertical and extends approximately 2 mm; a slight dilation, the ampulla, is at the base of the vertical portion of the canaliculus.[9,14,113] The canaliculus then turns horizontally to run along the lid margin for approximately 8 mm (see Figure 9-27). The canaliculi join to form a

single common canaliculus that pierces the periorbita covering the lacrimal sac and enters the lateral aspect of the sac.[114] The angle at which the canaliculus enters the sac produces a physiologic valve that prevents reflux.[2,113-116]

Lacrimal Sac and Nasolacrimal Duct

The **lacrimal sac** lies within a fossa in the anterior portion of the medial orbital wall. This fossa is formed by the frontal process of the maxillary bone and the lacrimal bone. The sac is surrounded by fascia, continuous with the periorbita, which runs from the anterior to the posterior lacrimal crests. The two limbs of the medial palpebral ligament straddle the sac to attach to the posterior and anterior crests.[117] The orbital septum and the check ligament of the medial rectus muscle lie behind the lacrimal sac (see Figure 8-18).

The lacrimal sac empties into the **nasolacrimal duct** just as it enters the nasolacrimal canal in the maxillary bone. The duct is approximately 15 mm long and terminates in the inferior meatus of the nose. At this point the **valve of Hasner** is found. This fold of mucosal tissue prevents retrograde movement of fluid up the duct from the nasal cavity.[9,17,113]

TEAR DRAINAGE

During closure the eyelids meet first at the temporal canthus; closure then moves toward the medial canthus, where the tears pool in the lacrimal lake. The tear menisci are pushed toward the lacrimal puncta into which they drain. Theories explaining tear drainage report that the state of the lacrimal sac is either distended or compressed by contraction of the orbicularis muscle. According to some, contraction of the lacrimal part of the orbicularis compresses the canaliculi, forcing the tears into the lacrimal sac.[118] Coincidentally, contraction of the muscle pulls on the fascial sheath attached to the lacrimal sac,[16,118] which causes lateral displacement of the lateral wall, expanding the sac and creating negative pressure within it—in effect, pulling tears in from the canaliculus. On relaxation of the orbicularis, the lacrimal sac collapses, and the tears are driven into the nasolacrimal duct. In addition, the canaliculi open and act as siphons to pull tears in through the puncta.[118] The tears drain into the nasolacrimal duct mainly by gravity, where most are absorbed by the mucosal lining before the remaining tears enter the inferior meatus.[2]

A number of studies, however, have measured an increase in pressure within the lacrimal sac during lid closure.[119] Using high-speed photography, the medial edges of the eyelids have been observed to meet, halfway into a blink, occluding the puncta.[112] According to this theory, the canaliculi and lacrimal sac are compressed,

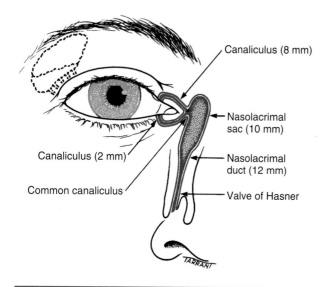

FIGURE 9-27
Anatomy of lacrimal drainage system. (From Kanski JJ: *Clinical ophthalmology,* ed 3, Oxford, UK, 1995, Butterworth-Heinemann.)

forcing all fluids into the nasolacrimal duct. As the eyelids open, compression of the canaliculi decreases, but the puncta remain occluded, creating a negative pressure in the canaliculi. When the puncta finally are opened, the negative pressure pulls the tears in immediately after the blink.[2,120]

The primary difference in these two theories is the state of the lacrimal sac. In the first scenario the sac is dilated, whereas in the second case the sac is compressed with orbicularis contraction. Capillary attraction plays a role in moving tears into the puncta and down into the canaliculi between blinks.[86]

AGING CHANGES IN ORBITAL ADNEXA AND LACRIMAL SYSTEM

The eyebrow position heightens in both genders with increasing age.[120]

The aging process is apparent in the eyelids as tissue atrophies, the skin loses elasticity, and wrinkles appear. With age the distance between the center of the pupil and the lower eyelid margin increases due to sagging of the lower lid; this change is greater in males than females.[120] More pronounced changes in lid margin position, including ectropion and entropion (previously described), increase in incidence with age-related changes in the orbicularis muscle tone.

Tearing may be caused by eversion of the lower punctum due to eyelid position or by stenosis of the passages in the lacrimal drainage system; both occur more frequently in elderly persons. Some studies find that the basal rate of tear secretion diminishes after age 40, contributing to dry eye, the incidence of which increases with age.[121,122] Others have determined that tear reflex secretion decreases.[123] The goblet cell population may decrease over age 80 and a decrease in lysozyme and lactoferrin are noted.[123] Causative factors include loss of glandular tissue and a change in composition of the meibomian secretion forming a more viscous material that does not flow as easily.[36,66] The incidence of vascular engorgement at the lid margin and plugged meibomian gland pores also increase with age.[66]

REFERENCES

1. McCord CD, Doxanas MT: Browplasty and browpexy: an adjunct to blepharoplasty, *Plast Reconstr Surg* 86(2):248, 1990.
2. Doxanas MT, Anderson RL: *Clinical orbital anatomy*, Baltimore, 1984, Williams & Wilkins, p 89.
3. Tarbet KJ, Lemke BN: Clinical anatomy of the upper face, *Int Ophthalmol Clin* 37(3):11, 1997.
4. Bartlett JD, Jaanus SD: *Clinical ocular pharmacology*, ed 3, Boston, 1995, Butterworth-Heinemann, p 583.
5. Katz J, Kaufman HE: Corneal exposure during sleep (nocturnal lagophthalmos), *Arch Ophthalmol* 95:449, 1977.
6. Sturrock GD: Nocturnal lagophthalmos and recurrent erosion, *Br J Ophthalmol* 60:97, 1976.
7. Jelks GW, Jelks EB: The influence of orbital and eyelid anatomy on the palpebral aperture, *Clin Plast Surg* 18(1):183, 1991.
8. Fox SA: The palpebral fissure, *Am J Ophthalmol* 62:73, 1966.
9. Warwick R: *Eugene Wolff's anatomy of the eye and orbit*, ed 7, Philadelphia, 1976, Saunders, p 181.
10. Stewart JM, Carter SR: Anatomy and examination of the eyelids, *Int Ophthalmol Clin* 42(2):1, 2002.
11. Dailey RA, Wobig JL: Eyelid anatomy, *J Dermatol Surg Oncol* 18:1023, 1993.
12. Goldberg RA, Wu JC, Jesmanwicz A, et al: Eyelid anatomy revisited. Dynamic high-resolution magnetic resonance images at Whitnall's ligament and upper eyelid structures with the use of a surface coil, *Arch Ophthalmol* 110(11):1598, 1992.
13. Jeong S, Lemke BN, Dortzbach RK, et al: The Asian upper eyelid: an anatomical study with comparison to the Caucasian eyelid, *Arch Ophthalmol* 117:907, 1999.
14. Jakobiec FA, Iwamoto T: The ocular adnexa: lids, conjunctiva, and orbit. In Fine BS, Yanoff M, editors: *Ocular histology*, ed 2, New York, 1979, Harper & Row, p 290.
15. Jester JV, Nicolaides N, Smith RE: Meibomian gland studies: histologic and ultrastructural investigations, *Invest Ophthalmol Vis Sci* 20(4):537, 1981.
16. Ahl NC, Hill JC: Horner's muscle and the lacrimal system, *Arch Ophthalmol* 100:488, 1982.
17. Fernandez-Valencia R, Pellico LG: Functional anatomy of the human saccus lacrimalis, *Acta Anat (Basel)* 139:54, 1990.
18. Shinohara H, Kominami R, Yasutaka S, et al: The anatomy of the lacrimal portion of the orbicularis oculi muscle (tensor tarsi or Horner's muscle), *Okajimas Folia Anat Jpn* 77(6):225, 2001:(abstract).
19. Lipham WJ, Tawfik HA, Dutton JJ: A histologic analysis and three-dimensional reconstruction of the muscle of Riolan, *Ophthal Plastic Reconst Surg* 18(2):93, 2002.
20. Morax S, Herdan ML: The aging eyelid, *Schweiz Rundsch Med Prax* 9(48):1506, 1990:(abstract).
21. Dryden RM, Leibsohn J, Wobig J: Senile entropion. Pathogenesis and treatment, *Arch Ophthalmol* 96:1978, 1883.
22. Fox SA: Primary congenital entropion, *Arch Ophthalmol* 56:839, 1956.
23. Kikkawa DO, Lucarelli MJ, Shovlin JP, et al: Ophthalmic facial anatomy and physiology. In Kaufman PL, Alm A, editors: *Adler's physiology of the eye*, ed 10, St Louis, 2003, Mosby.
24. Hart WM Jr: The eyelids. In Hart WM Jr, editor: *Adler's physiology of the eye*, ed 9, St Louis, 1992, Mosby.
25. Wobig JL: Surgical technique for ptosis repair, *Aust N Z J Ophthalmol* 17(2):125, 1989.
26. Anderson RL, Beard C: The levator aponeurosis. Attachments and their clinical significance, *Arch Ophthalmol* 95:1437, 1977.
27. Kuwabara T, Cogan DG, Johnson CC: Structure of the muscles of the upper eyelid, *Arch Ophthalmol* 93:1189, 1975.
28. Wobig JL: The eyelids. In Reeh MJ, Wobig JL, Wirtschafter JD, editors: *Ophthalmic anatomy*, San Francisco, 1981, American Academy of Ophthalmology, p 38.
29. Lim HW, Paik DJ, Lee YJ: A cadaveric anatomical study of the levator aponeurosis and Whitnall's ligament, *Korean J Ophthalmol* 23:183–187, 2009.
30. Evinger C, Manning KA, Sibony PA: Eyelid movements: mechanisms and normal data, *Invest Ophthalmol Vis Sci* 32:387, 1991.
31. Hawes MJ, Dortzbach RK: The microscopic anatomy of the lower eyelid retractors, *Arch Ophthalmol* 100:1313, 1982.
32. Small RG, Sabates NR, Burrows D: The measurement and definition of ptosis, *Ophthalmol Plast Reconstr Surg* 5(3):171, 1989.
33. Anderson RL: Medial canthal tendon branches out, *Arch Ophthalmol* 95:2051, 1977.

34. Rosenstein T, Talebzadeh N, Pogrel MA: Anatomy of the lateral canthal tendon, *Oral Surg Oral Med Oral Pathol Oral Radiol Endod* 89(1):24, 2000.

35. Gioia VM, Linberg JV, McCormick SA: The anatomy of the lateral canthal tendon, *Arch Ophthalmol* 105:529, 1987.

36. Arita R, Itoh K, Inoue K, et al: Contact lens wear is associated with decrease of meibomian glands, *Ophthalmology* 116:379–384, 2009.

37. Stoeckelhuber M, Stoeckelhuber BM, Welsch U: Human glands of Moll: histochemical and ultrastructural characterization of the glands of Moll in the human eyelid, *J Invest Dermatol* 121(1):28, 2003.

38. Iwamoto T, Jakobiec FA: Lacrimal glands. In Tasman W, Jaeger EA, editors: *Duane's foundations of clinical ophthalmology*, vol 1, Philadelphia, 1994, Lippincott.

39. Wirtschafter JD, Ketcham JM, Weinstock RJ, et al: Mucocutaneous junction as the major source of replacement palpebral conjunctival epithelial cells, *Invest Ophthalmol Vis Sci* 40(13):3138, 1999.

40. Gipson IK, Yankauckas M, Spurr-Michaud SJ, et al: Characteristics of a glycoprotein in the ocular surface glycocalyx, *Invest Ophthalmol Vis Sci* 33:218, 1992.

41. Nichols B, Dawson CR, Togni B: Surface features of the conjunctiva and cornea, *Invest Ophthalmol Vis Sci* 24:570, 1983.

42. Dilly PN: On the nature and the role of the subsurface vesicles in the outer epithelial cells of the conjunctiva, *Br J Ophthalmol* 69:477, 1985.

43. Kessing SV: Investigations of the conjunctival mucin. (Quantitative studies of the goblet cells of conjunctiva). (Preliminary report). *Acta Ophthalmol (Copenh)* 44:439, 1966.

44. Diebold Y, Rios JD, Hodges RR, et al: Presence of nerves and their receptors in mouse and human conjunctival goblet cells, *Invest Ophthalmol Vis Sci* 42(10):2270, 2001.

45. Sullivan WR, McCulley JP, Dohlman CH: Return of goblet cells after vitamin A therapy in xerosis of the conjunctiva, *Am J Ophthalmol* 75:720, 1973.

46. Kruse FE, Tseng SC: Retinoic acid regulates clonal growth and differentiation of cultured limbal and peripheral corneal epithelium, *Invest Ophthalmol Vis Sci* 35:2405–2420, 1994.

47. Steuhl KP, Sitz U, Knorr M, et al: [Age-dependent distribution of Langerhans cells within human conjunctival epithelium], [German] *Ophthalmologe* 92(1):21–25, 1995.

48. Hogan MJ, Alvarado JA: *Histology of the human eye*, Philadelphia, 1971, Saunders, p 112.

49. Allensmith MR, Greiner JV, Baird RS: Number of inflammatory cells in the normal conjunctiva, *Am J Ophthalmol* 86:250, 1978.

50. Jakobiec FA, Iwamoto T: Ocular adnexa: introduction to lids, conjunctiva, and orbit. In Tasman W, Jaeger EA, editors: *Duane's foundations of clinical ophthalmology*, vol 1, Philadelphia, 1994, Lippincott.

51. Knop N, Knop E: Conjunctiva-associated lymphoid tissue in the human eye, *Invest Ophthalmol Vis Sci* 41:1270–1279, 2000.

52. Srinivasan BD, Jakobiec FA, Iwamoto T, et al: Epibulbar mucogenic subconjunctival cysts, *Arch Ophthalmol* 96:857, 1978.

53. Chin GN, Chi EY, Bunt A: Ultrastructure and histochemical studies of conjunctival concretions, *Arch Ophthalmol* 98:720, 1980.

54. Weingeist TA: The glands of the ocular adnexa. In Zinn KM, editor: *Ocular structure for the clinician*, Boston, 1973, Little, Brown, p 243.

55. Sirigu P, Shen RL, Pinto-da-Silva P: Human meibomian glands: the ultrastructure of acinar cells as viewed by thin section and freeze-fracture transmission electron microscopes, *Invest Ophthalmol Vis Sci* 33(7):2284, 1992.

56. Efron N, Al-Dossarit M, Pritchard N: in vivo confocal microscopy of the palpebral conjunctiva and tarsal plate, *Optom Vis Sci* 86: 1303–1308, 2009.

57. Butovich IA, Millar TJ, Ham BM: Understanding and analyzing meibomian lipids—A review, *Curr Eye Res* 33:405–420, 2008.

58. Dartt DA, Hodges RR, Zoukhri D: *Tears and their secretion*. In *The biology of the eye Fischbarg J*, vol 10, Amsterdam, 2006, Elsevier, 18–82.

59. Butovich IA: The meibomian puzzle: combining pieces together, *Prog Retin Eye Res* 28:483–498, 2009.

60. LeDoux MS, Zhou Q, Murphy RB, et al: Parasympathetic innervation of the meibomian glands in rats, *Invest Ophthalmol Vis Sci* 42(11):2434, 2001.

61. Krachmer JH, Mannis MJ, Holland EJ: Seborrhea and meibomian gland dysfunction. In Krachmer JH, Mannis MJ, Holland EJ, editors: *Cornea, vol 1*, St Louis, 2005, Mosby.

62. Stoeckelhuber M, Messmer EM, Schubert C, et al: Immunolocalization of defensins and cathelicidin in human glands of Moll, *Ann Anat* 190:230–237, 2008.

63. Bergmanson JP, Doughty MJ, Blocker Y: The acinar and ductal organization of the tarsal accessory lacrimal gland of Wolfring in rabbit eyelid, *Exp Eye Res* 68(4):411, 1999.

64. Seifert P, Stuppi S, Spitznas M: Distribution pattern of nervous tissue and peptidergic nerve fibers in accessory lacrimal glands, *Curr Eye Res* 16:298, 1997.

65. Kanski JJ: *Clinical ophthalmology*, ed 3, London, 1994, Butterworth-Heinemann.

66. Den S, Shimizu K, Ikeda T, et al: Association between meibomian gland changes and aging, sex, or tear function, *Cornea* 25:651–655, 2006.

67. McCann LC, Tomlinson A, Pearce EI, et al: Tear and meibomian gland function in blepharitis and normals, *Eye Contact Lens* 35:203–208, 2009.

68. Pe'er J, Zajicek G, Greifner H, et al: Streaming conjunctiva, *Anat Rec* 245(1):36, 1996.

69. Revoltella RP, Papini S, Poselinni A, et al: Epithelial stem cells of the eye surface, *Cell Prolif* 40:445–461, 2007.

70. Fine BS, Yanoff M: *Ocular histology*, ed 2, Hagerstown, Md, 1979, Harper & Row, p 310.

71. Shields CL, Shields JA: Tumors of the caruncle, *Int Ophthalmol Clin* 33(3):31, 1993.

72. Austin P, Jakobiec FA, Iwamoto T: Elastodysplasia and elastodystrophy as the pathologic bases of ocular pterygia and pinguecula, *Ophthalmology* 90:96, 1983.

73. Li ZY, Wallace RN, Streeten BW, et al: Elastic fiber components and protease inhibitors in pinguecula, *Invest Ophthalmol Vis Sci* 32(5):1573, 1991.

74. Dushku N, John MK, Schultz GS, et al: Pterygia pathogenesis: corneal invasion by matrix metalloproteinase expressing altered limbal epithehal basal cells, *Arch Ophthalmol* 119:695, 2001.

75. Dushku N, Reid TW: P53 expression in altered limbal basal cells of pingueculae, pterygia, and limbal tumors, *Curr Eye Res* 16:1179, 1997.

76. Dushku N, Reid TW: Immunohistochemical evidence that human pterygia originate from an invasion of vimentin-expressing altered limbal epithelial basal cells, *Curr Eye Res* 13:473, 1994.

77. Taylor HR, West SK, Rosenthal FS, et al: Corneal changes associated with chronic UV radiation, *Arch Ophthalmol* 107:1481, 1989.

78. Mackenzie FD, Hirst LW, Battistutta D, et al: Risk analysis in the development of pterygia, *Ophthalmology* 99(7):1056, 1992.

79. Young RW: The family of sunlight-related eye diseases, *Optom Vis Sci* 71(2):125, 1994.

80. John-Aryankalayil M, Dushku N, Jaworski CJ, et al: Microarray and protein analysis of human pterygium, *Mol Vis* 12:55–64, 2006.

81. Kase S, Osaki M, Sato I, et al: Immunolocalisation of E-cadherin and beta-catenin in human pterygium, *Br J Ophthalmol* 91:1209–1212, 2007.

82. Kau HC, Tsai CC, Lee CF, et al: Increased oxidative DNA damage, 8-hydroxydeoxy- guanosine, in human pterygium, *Eye* 20:826–831, 2006.

83. Shauly Y, Miller B, Lichtig C: Tenon's capsule: ultrastructure of collagen fibrils in normals and infantile esotropia, *Invest Ophthalmol Vis Sci* 33:651, 1992.

84. Meyer E, Ludatscher RN, Miller B, et al: Connective tissue of the orbital cavity in retinal detachment: an ultrastructural study, *Ophthal Res* 24:365, 1992.

85. Reiger G: The importance of the precorneal tear film for the quality of optical imaging, *Br J Ophthalmol* 76:157, 1992.

86. Lemp MA, Wolfley DE: The lacrimal apparatus. In Hart WM Jr, editor: *Adler's physiology of the eye*, ed 9, St Louis, 1992, Mosby.

87. Mishima S, Maurice DM: The effect of normal evaporation on the eye, *Exp Eye Res* 1:46, 1961.

88. Lemp MA, Holly FJ, Iwata S: The precorneal tear film, *Arch Ophthalmol* 83:89, 1970.

89. Watanabe H, Fabricant M, Tisdale AS, et al: Human corneal and conjunctival epithelia produce a mucin-like glycoprotein for the apical surface, *Invest Ophthalmol Vis Sci* 36(2):337, 1995.

90. Ehlers N: The thickness of the precorneal tear film. Factors in spreading and maintaining a continuous tear film over the corneal surface, *Acta Ophthalmol (Copenh)* 8(suppl 81):92, 1965.

91. Prydal JI, Artal P, Woon H, et al: Study of human precorneal tear film thickness and structure using laser interferometry, *Invest Ophthalmol Vis Sci* 33(6):1992, 2006.

92. Prydal JI, Campbell FW: Study of precorneal tear film thickness and structure by interferometry and confocal microscopy, *Invest Ophthalmol Vis Sci* 33(6):2006, 1992.

93. Peral A, Pintor J.: Ocular mucin visualization by confocal laser scanning microscopy, *Cornea* 27:395–401, 2008.

94. Egeberg J, Jenson OA: The ultrastructure of the acini of the human lacrimal gland, *Acta Ophthalmol (Copenh)* 47:400, 1969.

95. Jones LT: Anatomy of the tear system, *Int Ophthalmol Clin* 13(1):3, 1973.

96. Jordan A, Baum JL: Basic tear flow. Does it exist? *Ophthalmology* 95:1, 1980.

97. Khanal S, Tomlinson A, McFayden A, et al: *Dry eye diagnosis Invest Ophthalmol Vis Sci* 49:1407–1414, 2008.

98. Cho P, Yap M: Schirmer test. A review, *Optom Vis Sci* 70(2):152, 1993.

99. Lemp MA, Dohlman CH, Kuwabara T, et al: Dry eye secondary to mucous deficiency, *Trans Am Acad Ophthalmol Otolaryngol* 75:1223, 1971.

100. Lemp MA, Hamill JR Jr: Factors affecting tear film breakup in normal eyes, *Arch Ophthalmol* 89:103, 1973.

101. Mai G, Yang S: Relationship between corneal dellen and tear film breakup time, *Yen Ko Hsueh Pao (Eye Sci)* 7(1):43, 1991:(abstract).

102. Khurana AK, Chaudhary R, Ahluwalia BK, et al: Tear film profile in dry eye, *Acta Ophthalmol (Copenh)* 69(1):79, 1991.

103. Friedlaender MH: Ocular manifestations of Sjögren's syndrome: keratoconjunctivitis sicca, *Rheum Dis Clin North Am* 18(3):591, 1992.

104. Roberts DK: Keratoconjunctivitis sicca, *J Am Optom Assoc* 62(3):187, 1991.

105. Borchman D, Yappert MC, Foulks G.N.: Changes in human meibum lipid with meibomian gland dysfunction using principal component analysis, *Exp Eye Res* 91:246–256, 2010.

106. Ibrahim OMA, Matsumoto Y, Dogru M, et al: The efficacy, sensitivity, and specificity of in vivo laser confocal microscopy in the diagnosis of meibomian gland dysfunction, *Ophthalmology* 117:665–672, 2010.

107. Ralph RA: Conjunctival goblet cell density in normal subjects and in dry eye syndromes, *Invest Ophthalmol* 14(4):299, 1975.

108. Cross WD, Lay LF Jr, Walt JG, et al: Clinical and economic implications of topical cylosporin A for the treatment of dry eye, *Manag Care Interface* 15(9):44, 2002.

109. Calonge M: The treatment of dry eye, *Surv Ophthalmol* (Suppl 2):S227, 2001.

110. Stevenson D, Tauber J, Reis BL: Efficacy and safety of cyclosporin: A ophthalmic emulsion in the treatment of moderate-to-severe dry eye disease: a dose-ranging, randomized trial, The Cyclosporin A Phase 2 Study Group, *Ophthalmology* 107(5):967, 2000.

111. Sall K, Stevenson OD, Mundorf TK, et al: Two multicenter, randomized studies of the efficacy and safety of cyclosporin ophthalmic emulsion in moderate-to-severe dry eye disease. The Cyclosporin A Phase 3 Study Group, *Ophthalmology* 107(4):631, 2000.

112. Doane MG: Blinking and the mechanics of the lacrimal drainage system, *Ophthalmology* 88(8):844, 1981.

113. Wobig JL: The lacrimal apparatus. In Reeh MJ, Wobig JL, Wirtschafter JD, editors: *Ophthalmic anatomy*, San Francisco, 1981, American Academy of Ophthalmology, p 55.

114. Yazici B, Yazici Z: Frequency of the common canaliculus: a radiological study, *Arch Ophthalmol* 118:1381, 2000.

115. Doane MG: Interactions of eyelids and tears in corneal wetting and the dynamics of the normal human eye blink, *Am J Ophthalmol* 89:507, 1980.

116. Tucker NA, Tucker SM, Linberg JV: The anatomy of the common canaliculus, *Arch Ophthalmol* 114:1231, 1996.

117. Milder B, Demorest BH: Dacryocystography. The normal lacrimal apparatus, *Arch Ophthalmol* 51:181, 1954.

118. Jones LT, Marquis MM: Lacrimal function, *Am J Ophthalmol* 73:658, 1972.

119. Lucarelli MJ, Dartt DA, Cook BE, et al: The lacrimal system. In Kaufman PL, Alm A, editors: *Adler's physiology of the eye*, ed 10, St Louis, 2003, Mosby.

120. van den Bosch WA, Leenders I, Mulder P: Topographic anatomy of the eyelids, and the effects of sex and age, *Br J Ophthalmol* 83:347, 1999.

121. Lin PY, Tsai SY, Cheng CY, et al: Prevalence of dry eye among an elderly Chinese population in Taiwan: the Shihpai Eye study, *Ophthalmology* 110(6):1096, 2003.

122. Schaumberg DA, Sullivan DA, Buring JE, et al: Prevalence of dry eye syndrome among US women, *Am J Ophthalmol* 136(2):318, 2003.

123. Van Haeringen NJ: Aging and the lacrimal system, *Br J Ophthalmol* 81:824–826, 1997.

The muscles of the globe can be divided into two groups: the involuntary intrinsic muscles and the voluntary extrinsic muscles. The intrinsic muscles—the ciliary muscle, the iris sphincter, and the iris dilator—are located within the eye; these muscles control the movement of internal ocular structures. The extrinsic muscles—the six extraocular muscles—attach to the sclera and control movement of the globe.

This chapter begins with a brief review of the microscopic and macroscopic anatomy of striated muscle, then discusses eye movements and describes the characteristics and actions of each extraocular muscle. (The smooth intrinsic muscles are discussed in Chapter 3.)

MICROSCOPIC ANATOMY OF STRIATED MUSCLE

Striated muscle is surrounded by a connective tissue sheath known as the *epimysium;* continuous with this sheath is a connective tissue network, the *perimysium,* which infiltrates the muscle and divides it into bundles. The individual muscle fiber within the bundle is surrounded by a delicate connective tissue enclosure, the *endomysium* (Figure 10-1). The individual muscle fiber is comparable to a cell; however, each fiber is multinucleated, with the nuclei arranged at the periphery of the fiber. The plasma cell membrane surrounding each muscle fiber, the *sarcolemma,* forms a series of invaginations into the cell, the *transverse tubules (T tubules),* which allow ions to spread quickly through the cell in response to an action potential. The cell cytoplasm, *sarcoplasm,* contains normal cellular structures and special muscle fibers, the myofibrils.

Myofibrils comprise two types, thick and thin. The thick myofibrils are composed of hundreds of *myosin* subunits. Each subunit is a long, slender filament with two globular heads attached by arms at one end. These filaments lie next to each other and form the "backbone" of the myofibril, with the heads projecting outward in a spiral (Figure 10-2, *A*). The thin myofibrils are formed by the protein *actin* arranged in a double-helical filament, with a molecular complex of troponin and tropomyosin lying within the grooves of the double helix (Figure 10-2, *B*).

The alternating light and dark bands characteristic of striated muscle are produced by the manner in which these two types of myofibrils are arranged. The light band is the I (isotropic) band, and the dark band is the A (anisotropic) band. These names describe the birefringence to polarized light exhibited by the two areas.[1]

The I band contains two sets of actin filaments connected to each other at the Z line, a dark stripe bisecting the I band. Only actin myofibrils are found in the I band. The A band contains both myosin and actin; the central lighter zone of the A band—the H zone—contains only myosin. Overlapping actin and myosin filaments form the outer darker edges of the A band (Figure 10-3). The M line bisects the H zone and contains proteins that interconnect the myosin fibrils.

A *sarcomere* extends from Z line to Z line and is the contractile unit of striated muscle. With muscle contraction, a change in configuration occurs; the H zone width decreases as the actin filaments slide past the myosin filaments. The sarcomere is shortened; as this occurs along the muscle, muscle length is decreased. The length of the actin and myosin filaments remain constant as does the A band, the I band and the H zone shorten.

SLIDING RATCHET MODEL OF MUSCLE CONTRACTION

The process of muscle contraction and sarcomere shortening is explained by the sliding ratchet model[2-4] (Figure 10-4). The initiation of a muscle contraction occurs when a nerve impulse causes the release of acetylcholine into the neuromuscular junction. The sarcolemma depolarizes and an action potential passes along the surface and is carried into the muscle fiber through the system of T-tubules. Ionic channels are opened and calcium ions are released from the sarcoplasmic reticulum into sarcoplasm. Ca^{2+} binds to the troponin-tropomyosin complex, resulting in a configurational change, allowing an active site on the actin protein to be available for binding with a myosin head. Coincidentally, adenosine triphosphate (ATP) attached to the myosin head is broken down and released, allowing a cross-bridge to bind with the active actin site. Once this bond is formed, the head tilts toward the shaft of the myosin filament, pulling the actin filament along with it.

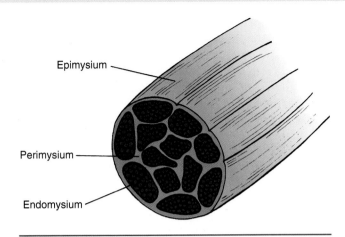

FIGURE 10-1
Connective tissue network of striated muscle.

The junction between the actin and myosin is broken by the attachment of a new ATP molecule to the myosin head. The head then rights itself, and the cross-bridge is ready to bind with the next actin site along the chain. This ratchet type of movement occurs along the length of the fiber, moving the filaments past one another with the overall effect of shortening the sarcomere and the entire muscle.

Clinical Comment: Myasthenia Gravis

MYASTHENIA GRAVIS is a chronic autoimmune neuromuscular disease caused by a defect in transmission of the nerve impulse to muscle fibers. Antibodies are formed that either block or destroy the acetylcholine receptors at the neuromuscular junction. Muscle weakness and fatigue worsens throughout the day and is particularly evident with repetitive movements. Often the first clinical symptom is ptosis; sometimes during a vision examination, the upper lid begins to droop and by the end of the examination is quite evident. Ocular myasthenia gravis is limited to eye and lid muscles, resulting in diplopia and ptosis.

STRUCTURE OF THE EXTRAOCULAR MUSCLES

The extraocular muscles have a denser blood supply, and their connective tissue sheaths are more delicate and richer in elastic fibers than is skeletal muscle.[5] Fewer muscle fibers are included in a motor unit in extraocular muscle than are found in skeletal muscle elsewhere. Striated muscle of the leg can contain several hundred muscle fibers per motor unit[6]; in the extraocular muscles, each axon innervates 3 to 10 fibers.[7] This dense innervation provides for precise fine motor control of the extraocular muscles resulting in high velocity ocular movements,

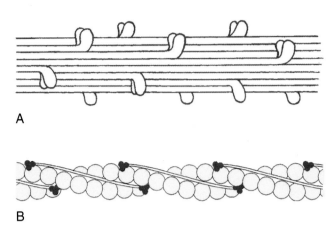

FIGURE 10-2
Myosin and actin myofibrils. **A,** Myosin fibril is composed of two-headed filaments, with heads arranged in a spiral. **B,** Actin myofibril is composed of double-helix filament to which troponin-tropomyosin complex is attached.

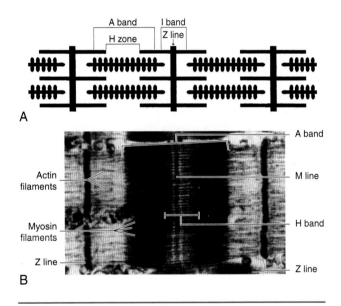

FIGURE 10-3
A, Arrangement of thick and thin filaments in sarcomere.
B, Photomicrograph of striated muscle, with parts of sarcomere indicated. (**B** from Krause WJ, Cutts JH: *Concise text of histology,* Baltimore, 1981, Williams & Wilkins.)

necessary in saccades, (up to 1000 degrees per second) and very accurate pursuits (velocities of 100 degrees per second) and fixations.[8] Singly innervated fibers have the classic end plate *(en plaque)* seen in skeletal muscle; multiply innervated fibers have a neuromuscular junction resembling a bunch of grapes *(en grappe).*[9,10]

The extraocular muscles have a range of fiber sizes, with the fibers closer to the surface generally having smaller diameters (5 to 15 μm) and those deeper within

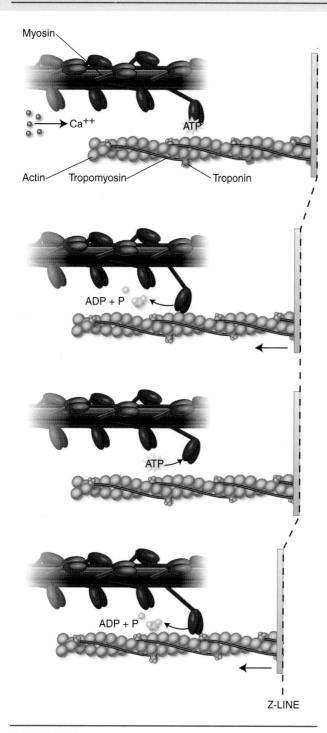

Myosin

Ca++

ATP

Actin Tropomyosin Troponin

ADP + P

ATP

ADP + P

Z-LINE

FIGURE 10-4
Sliding ratchet model of muscle contraction.

the muscle generally having larger diameters (10 to 40 μm).[11-14] They can be divided into groups based on characteristics such as location, size, morphology, neuromuscular junction type, or various biochemical properties.[5,12,13,15,16] The fibers range from typical twitch fibers at one end of the spectrum to typical slow fibers at the other end, with gradations in between.

It would seem that the fast-twitch fibers should produce quick saccadic movements and the slow fibers should produce slower pursuit movements and provide muscle tone. However, all fibers apparently are active at all times and share some level of involvement in all ocular movements.[12,14,16,17] Extraocular muscles are among the fastest and most fatigue-resistant of striated muscle.[18]

Muscle spindles and Golgi tendon organs of typical striated muscle have been identified in human extraocular muscle, although it is unclear whether these structures provide any useful proprioceptive information relative to the extraocular muscles.[19,20] Afferent information regarding extraocular muscle proprioception is thought to be mediated by a receptor that is unique to extraocular muscle, the *myotendinous cylinder (palisade ending)*.[16,21]

EYE MOVEMENTS

FICK'S AXES

Before a discussion of the individual muscles and the resultant eye movements caused by their contraction, it is necessary to define certain terms. All eye movement can be described as rotations around one or more axes. According to Fick, these axes divide the globe into quadrants and intersect at the center of rotation, a fixed nonmoving point[22] and the approximate geometric center of the eye. For convenience, it is assumed that the eye rotates around this fixed point, located 13.5 mm behind the cornea; this point varies in ametropia, is slightly more posterior in myopia, and is slightly more anterior in hyperopia.[5] The **x-axis** is the **horizontal** or **transverse axis** and runs from nasal to temporal. The **y-axis** is the **sagittal axis** running from the anterior pole to the posterior pole. The **z-axis** is the **vertical axis** and runs from superior to inferior (Figure 10-5). When the front of the eye moves up, the back moves down. When the front of the eye moves right, the back of the eye moves left. The anterior pole of the globe is the reference point used in the description of any eye movement. Eye movements are described and based on the movement of the muscle insertion towards its origin.

DUCTIONS

Movements involving just one eye are called **ductions** (Figure 10-6). Rotations around the vertical axis move the anterior pole of the globe medially—**adduction**—or laterally—**abduction.** Rotations around the horizontal axis move the anterior pole of the globe up—**elevation (supraduction)**—or down—**depression (infraduction)**.

Torsions or cyclorotations are rotations around the sagittal axis and are described in relation to a point at the 12-o'clock position on the superior limbus. **Intorsion (incyclorotation)** is the rotation of that point nasally,

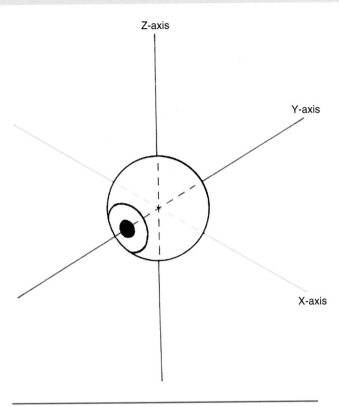

FIGURE 10-5
Fick axes: *x*-axis is horizontal; *y*-axis is sagittal; and *z*-axis is vertical.

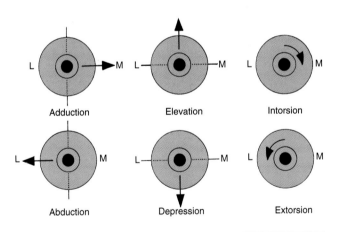

FIGURE 10-6
Movements of the eye in duction. Anterior pole is point of reference. *L,* Lateral; *M,* medial.

and **extorsion (excyclorotation)** is the rotation of that point temporally. Torsional movements may occur in an attempt to keep the horizontal retinal raphe parallel to the horizon.[23] With a head tilt of 30 degrees, the ipsilateral eye is intorted approximately 7 degrees, and the contralateral eye is extorted approximately 8 degrees.[24]

Torsional movements have been questioned by some investigators who believe that true torsion occurs only in pathologic conditions.[25] Others have documented torsion in normal eye movements and with head tilt.[26-29]

VERGENCES AND VERSIONS

Movements involving both eyes are either vergences or versions, depending on the relative directions of movement. In **vergence** movements, the eyes move in opposite left-right directions; these are disjunctive movements. In **convergence** each eye is adducted, and in **divergence** each eye is abducted. **Version** movements are conjugate movements and occur when the eyes move in the same direction. **Dextroversion** is right gaze, and **levoversion** is left gaze. In **supraversion** both eyes are elevated, and in **infraversion** both eyes are depressed. Table 10-1 lists terms for monocular and binocular eye movements and some combination movements.

POSITIONS OF GAZE

The primary position of gaze is defined as the position of the eye with the head erect, the eye located at the intersection of the sagittal plane of the head and the horizontal plane passing through the centers of rotation of both eyes, and the eye focused for infinity.[17] Secondary positions of gaze are rotations around either the vertical axis or the horizontal axis; tertiary positions are rotations around both the vertical and the horizontal axes.

MACROSCOPIC ANATOMY OF THE EXTRAOCULAR MUSCLES

The six extraocular muscles are medial rectus, lateral rectus, superior rectus, inferior rectus, superior oblique, and inferior oblique (Figure 10-7). From longest to shortest, the rectus muscles are the superior, the medial, the lateral, and the inferior.[30]

ORIGIN OF THE RECTUS MUSCLES

The four rectus muscles have their origin on the **common tendinous ring (annulus of Zinn).** This oval band of connective tissue is continuous with the periorbita and is located at the apex of the orbit anterior to the optic foramen and the medial part of the superior orbital fissure. The upper and lower areas are thickened bands and sometimes are referred to as the upper and lower tendons or limbs. The medial and lateral rectus muscles take their origin from both parts of the tendinous ring. The superior rectus is attached to the upper limb, and the inferior rectus is joined to the lower (Figure 10-8). The medial rectus and the superior rectus also attach to the dural sheath of the optic nerve.[30]

Table 10-1   Ocular Movement Terminology

MONOCULAR		BINOCULAR	
Eye Movement*	**Term**	**Eye Movement**	**Term**
Medial	Adduction	Right	Dextroversion
Lateral	Abduction	Left	Levoversion
Up	Elevation, supraduction, or sursumduction	Up	Supraversion or sursumversion
Down	Depression, infraduction, or deorsumduction	Down	Infraversion or deorsumversion
Rotation of 12-o'clock position medially	Intorsion, incyclorotation, or incycloduction	Up and right	Dextroelevation
Rotation of 12-o'clock position laterally	Extorsion, excyclorotation, or excycloduction	Up and left	Levoelevation
Anterior out of orbit	Protrusion or exophthalmos	Down and right	Dextrodepression
Posterior into orbit	Retraction or enophthalmos	Down and left	Levodepression
		Both eyes adduct	Convergence
		Both eyes abduct	Divergence
		Both eyes extort	Excyclovergence
		Both eyes intort	Incyclovergence
		Rotation of 12-o'clock position to right	Dextrocycloversion
		Rotation of 12-o'clock position to left	Levocycloversion

*For all movements the anterior pole of the globe is the reference point unless otherwise noted.

Clinical Comment: Retrobulbar Optic Neuritis

> *RETROBULBAR OPTIC NEURITIS is an inflammation affecting the sheaths of the optic nerve. Generally, there are no observable fundus changes in this condition, but pain with extreme eye movement can be one of the early presenting signs.[1,30] The optic nerve sheath is supplied with a dense sensory nerve network and because of the close association of muscle sheath and optic nerve sheath, eye movement can cause stretching of the optic nerve sheath, resulting in a sensation of pain.[31]*

The area enclosed by the tendinous ring is called the **oculomotor foramen,** and several blood vessels and nerves pass through the foramen, having entered the orbit either through the optic canal or the superior orbital fissure (see Figure 10-8). The optic nerve and ophthalmic artery enter the oculomotor foramen from the optic canal; the superior and inferior divisions of the oculomotor nerve, the abducens nerve, and the nasociliary nerve enter the oculomotor foramen from the superior orbital fissure (see Figure 10-8). These structures lie within the muscle cone, the area enclosed by the four rectus muscles and the connective tissue joining them. Thus the motor nerve to each rectus muscle can enter the surface of the muscle that lies within the muscle cone.

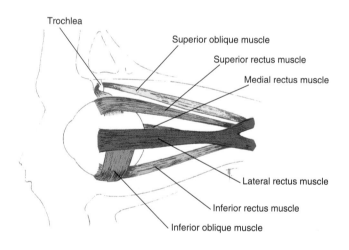

Trochlea
Superior oblique muscle
Superior rectus muscle
Medial rectus muscle
Lateral rectus muscle
Inferior rectus muscle
Inferior oblique muscle

FIGURE 10-7
Globe in orbit as viewed from lateral side.

In 1887, Motais described a common muscle sheath between the rectus muscles enclosing the space within the muscle cone.[5] More recently, dissections by Koornneef[32] revealed no definitive, continuous muscle sheath between the rectus muscles in the retrobulbar region.

The lacrimal and frontal nerves and the superior ophthalmic vein lie above the common ring tendon, and the inferior ophthalmic vein lies below. They are outside the muscle cone (see Figure 8-15).

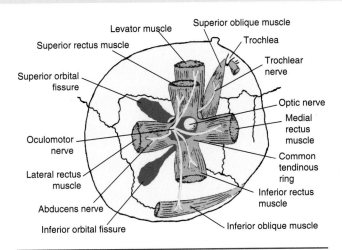

FIGURE 10-8
Orbital apex with globe removed. The origin of the rectus muscles at the anulus of Zinn. Motor innervation of the extraocular muscles and the relationship between superior orbital fissure and common tendinous ring is shown.

INSERTIONS OF THE RECTUS MUSCLES: SPIRAL OF TILLAUX

The four rectus muscles insert into the globe anterior to the equator. A line connecting the rectus muscle insertions forms a spiral, as described by Tillaux. This spiral starts at the medial rectus, the insertion that is closest to the limbus, and proceeds to the inferior rectus, the lateral rectus, and finally the superior rectus, the insertion farthest from the limbus[5] (Figure 10-9). In a recent study, variations were found from person to person in specific measurements, but the **spiral of Tillaux** was always observed.[33] The tendons of insertion pierce Tenon's capsule and merge with scleral fibers. A sleeve of the capsule covers the tendon for a short distance, and the muscle can slide freely within this sleeve.[5,13] Connective tissue extends from the insertions joining them to each other.

MEDIAL RECTUS MUSCLE

The **medial rectus muscle** is the largest of the extraocular muscles, with its size probably resulting from the frequency of its use in convergence.[30] Its *origin* is from both the upper and the lower parts of the common ring tendon and from the sheath of the optic nerve. The medial rectus muscle parallels the medial orbital wall until it passes through a connective tissue pulley just posterior to the equator of the globe; at this point it follows the curve of the globe to its *insertion*.[34] The *insertion* of the medial rectus is about 5.5 mm from the limbus, and the tendon is approximately 3.7 mm long[5] (Table 10-2). The insertion line lies vertically such that the horizontal plane of the eye approximately bisects it (Figure 10-10, *A*).

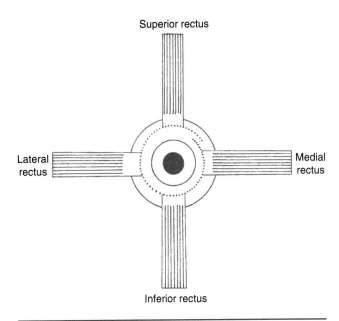

FIGURE 10-9
Insertions of rectus muscles forming spiral of Tillaux.

Table 10-2   Rectus Muscle Tendon of Insertion Measurements*

Muscle	Tendon Length	Distance from Limbus	Tendon Width
Medial rectus	3.7	5.5	10.3
Lateral rectus	8.8	6.9	9.2
Superior rectus	5.8	7.7	10.8
Inferior rectus	5.5	6.5	9.8

*All measurements in millimeters (mm).
Modified from Eggers HM: Functional anatomy of the extraocular muscles. In Tasman W, Jaeger EA, editors: *Duane's foundations of clinical ophthalmology*, Philadelphia, 1994, Lippincott.

The superior oblique muscle, ophthalmic artery, and nasociliary nerve lie above the medial rectus. Fascial expansions from the sheath of the muscle run to the medial wall of the orbit and form the well-developed medial check ligament (see Figure 8-18). The medial rectus is innervated by the inferior division of cranial nerve III, the oculomotor nerve, which enters the muscle on its lateral surface.

LATERAL RECTUS MUSCLE

The **lateral rectus muscle** has its *origin* on both limbs of the common tendinous ring and the spina recti lateralis, a prominence on the greater wing of the sphenoid bone. The lateral rectus muscle parallels the lateral orbital wall until it passes through a connective tissue pulley just posterior to the equator of the globe; at this point it follows the curve of the globe to its insertion.[34,35]

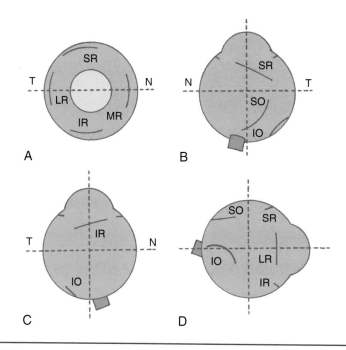

FIGURE 10-10

Insertions of extraocular muscles. Globe viewed from **A,** in front; **B,** above; **C,** below; and **D,** lateral side. *LR,* Lateral rectus; *MR,* medial rectus; *SR,* superior rectus; *IR,* inferior rectus; *SO,* superior oblique; *IO,* inferior oblique; *N,* nasal; *T,* temporal.

The *insertion* parallels that of the medial rectus and is approximately 6.9 mm from the limbus, and the length of the tendon is approximately 8.8 mm.[5]

The lacrimal artery and nerve run along the superior border of the lateral rectus muscle. The ciliary ganglion, the abducens nerve, and the ophthalmic artery lie medial to the lateral rectus between it and the optic nerve. Fascial expansions from the muscle sheath attach to the lateral wall of the orbit and form the lateral check ligament (see Figure 8-18). The lateral rectus is innervated by cranial nerve VI, the abducens nerve, which enters on the medial side of the muscle.

SUPERIOR RECTUS MUSCLE

The **superior rectus muscle** has its *origin* on the superior part of the common tendinous ring and the sheath of the optic nerve.[30] The muscle passes forward beneath the levator muscle; the sheaths enclosing these two muscles are connected to each other, allowing coordination of eye movement with eyelid position and resulting in elevation of the eyelid with upward gaze. An additional band of this tissue connects to the superior conjunctival fornix. The superior rectus muscle parallels the roof of the orbit until it passes through a connective tissue pulley just posterior to the equator of the globe; at this point it follows the curve of the globe to its insertion.[34,35]

The *insertion* of the superior rectus is approximately 7.7 mm from the limbus[5] and is curved slightly, with the convex side forward. The line of the insertion is oblique, with the nasal side closer to the limbus than the temporal side (see Figure 10-10, *B*). The tendon length is approximately 5.8 mm.[5] A line drawn from the origin to the insertion along the muscle will form an angle of approximately 23 degrees with the sagittal axis.

The frontal nerve runs above the superior rectus and levator muscles, and the nasociliary nerve and the ophthalmic artery lie below. The tendon of insertion for the superior oblique muscle runs below the anterior part of the superior rectus muscle (see Figure 10-7).

The superior rectus is innervated by the superior division of the oculomotor nerve, which enters the muscle on its inferior face. Branches pass either through the muscle or around it to innervate the levator.

INFERIOR RECTUS MUSCLE

The **inferior rectus muscle** has its *origin* on the lower limb of the tendinous ring; its *insertion* is about 6.5 mm from the limbus in an arc, convex side forward, with the nasal side nearer the limbus; the tendon length is approximately 5.5 mm.[5] The inferior rectus approximately parallels the superior rectus, making an angle of 23 degrees with the sagittal axis.

The inferior rectus muscle parallels the orbital floor until it passes through a connective tissue pulley just posterior to the equator of the globe; at this point it follows the curve of the globe to its insertion,[34] which is parallel to the insertions of the superior rectus (see Figure 10-10, C).

Below the inferior rectus lies the floor of the orbit and above it is the inferior division of the oculomotor nerve. Anteriorly, the inferior oblique muscle comes between the inferior rectus and the orbital floor (see Figure 10-7). The sheaths of these two inferior muscles unite to contribute to the suspensory ligament of Lockwood (see Figure 8-17). The capsulopalpebral fascia, an anterior extension from the sheath of the inferior rectus muscle and the suspensory ligament, inserts into the inferior edge of the tarsal plate, allowing coordination of eye movements with eyelid position and ensuring lowering of the lid on downward gaze.[36] The inferior rectus is innervated by the inferior division of cranial nerve III, the oculomotor nerve, which enters the muscle on its superior surface.

SUPERIOR OBLIQUE MUSCLE

The **superior oblique muscle** has its *origin* on the lesser wing of the sphenoid bone, medial to the optic canal near the frontoethmoid suture.[17] The muscle courses forward and passes through the **trochlea,** a U-shaped piece of cartilage attached to the orbital plate of the frontal bone (see Figure 10-7). The tendon of insertion actually begins approximately 1 cm posterior to the trochlea. Normally, no connective adhesions exist between these two structures, allowing the tendon to slide easily through the trochlea.[1]

The superior oblique muscle is the longest and thinnest of the extraocular muscles because of its long (2.5 cm) tendon of insertion.[30] The tendon of insertion changes direction as it passes through the trochlea to run in a posterior direction and lies inferior to the superior rectus muscle. The *insertion* of the superior oblique muscle attaches in the superoposterior lateral aspect of the globe[37] and is fan shaped, concave forward, and oblique (see Figure 10-10, B).

The trochlea is considered the *physiologic* or *effective origin* of the superior oblique muscle in determining muscle action because it acts as a pulley and changes the direction of muscle pull. In considering the action of the superior oblique, a line is drawn from the trochlea to the insertion rather than from the anatomic origin to the insertion. A line drawn from the physiologic origin to the insertion makes an angle of approximately 55 degrees with the sagittal axis.[37] The superior oblique muscle lies above the medial rectus, with the nasociliary nerve and the ophthalmic artery lying between them. Innervation is by the trochlear

Table 10-3 Extraocular Muscle Innervation

Muscle	Nerve
Medial rectus	Inferior division of oculomotor (CN III)
Lateral rectus	Abducens (CN VI)
Superior rectus	Superior division of oculomotor (CN III)
Inferior rectus	Inferior division of oculomotor (CN III)
Superior oblique	Trochlear (CN IV)
Inferior oblique	Inferior division of oculomotor (CN III)

CN, Cranial nerve.

nerve, cranial nerve IV, which enters the posterior area of the muscle.

INFERIOR OBLIQUE MUSCLE

The **inferior oblique muscle** has its *origin* on the maxillary bone just posterior to the inferior medial orbital rim and lateral to the nasolacrimal canal.[38] The inferior oblique is the only extraocular muscle to have its anatomic origin in the anterior orbit. The muscle runs from the medial corner of the orbit to the lateral aspect of the globe, its length approximately paralleling the tendon of insertion of the superior oblique muscle.

The *insertion* of the inferior oblique is on the posterior portion of the globe on the lateral side, mostly inferior, lying just outer to the macular area (see Figure 10-10, D).[1,30] The insertion is curved concave downward, the tendon of insertion is quite short, just 1 mm in length. The muscle makes an angle of approximately 51 degrees with the sagittal axis.[34] Above the inferior oblique are the inferior rectus and globe, and below it lies the floor of the orbit. The inferior oblique is innervated by the inferior division of the oculomotor nerve, which enters the muscle on its upper surface.

Table 10-3 lists the motor innervation of the extraocular muscles.

FIBERS OF THE EXTRAOCULAR MUSCLES

The fibers of the extraocular muscles have a layered organization. The *global layer* is adjacent to the globe and consists of fibers of various diameters.[39] This group of fibers extends the full length of the muscle and is attached at the origin and insertion through well-defined tendons.[18,40] The global layer inserts into the sclera and causes movement of the globe.[41] The outer *orbital layer* is adjacent to orbital bone, consists of smaller-diameter fibers, and is more vascularized than the global layer.[39,42] These fibers end before the muscle tendon and have insertions into the muscle sheath. The orbital layer of the oblique muscles may encircle the global layer.[18,39,40] The orbital layer inserts into connective tissue muscle pulleys that can influence the rotational axis of the muscle.[18,41]

The orbital layer fibers make up 40% to 60% of the fibers within an extraocular muscle.[40]

Fibers of extraocular muscles can be divided into types having some of the usual characteristics of striated muscle. All of these types are involved in all muscle contractions. Orbital fibers with a high number of mitochondria and that are singly innervated have small myofibrils, allowing for rapid access of Ca^{2+} to contractile fibers. These are generally fast twitch and fatigue resistant fibers resulting in rapid contraction.[18] Orbital fibers that are multiply innervated have several nerve terminals along the length of a single fiber, and they include both fast twitch and slowly contracting fibers.[18]

Among the global fibers that are singly innervated, the red fibers (having high amount of myoglobulin) may be fast twitch and fatigue resistant; the white fibers (lesser amount of myoglobulin) are fast twitch and may be fatigable.[18] Global fibers that are multiply innervated are associated with the myotendinous cylinder or palisade endings; they are large myofibrils and appear to be slow and tonic.[18]

ORBITAL CONNECTIVE TISSUE STRUCTURES

Connective tissue sleeves or pulleys can be identified using detailed magnetic resonance imaging (MRI); the pulleys that couple the rectus muscles to the orbital walls and Tenon's capsule were the first to be visualized.[34,35,43-45] Pulleys along the inferior oblique and superior oblique muscle paths have subsequently been identified.[18,40] Although not as prominent as the pulley of the superior oblique muscle, and only consisting of soft tissue,[40] the pulleys encircle each extraocular muscle like a sleeve and can affect the mechanisms of muscle positioning. Smooth muscle-connective tissue struts attach the pulleys to the periorbita of the orbital wall and may help to refine coordination of binocular eye movements.[35,41,44,46] The smooth muscle of the pulley is richly innervated by sympathetic and parasympathetic nerves, suggesting both excitatory and inhibitory capabilities.[18,46] The smooth muscle either regulates the stiffness of the connective tissue or moves the pulleys to alter the pulling direction.[41] The pulleys reduce sideslip of the extraocular muscles during globe rotation and help to determine the effective direction of pull.[43] Pulley displacement can clinically mimic muscle dysfunction, and orbital imaging may be needed to distinguish it accurately from a palsy. The pulley for the medial rectus is the most fully developed.[47]

Dense connective tissue septa between the extraocular muscle sheaths and between the sheaths and the orbital bones form a highly organized network that contributes to the framework supporting the globe within the orbit. The horizontal rectus muscles are anchored to the periorbita at the anterior orbital walls through the medial and lateral check ligaments. The medial check ligament is attached to the bones of the medial orbital wall, and the lateral check ligament is attached to the lateral tubercle on the zygomatic bone of the lateral wall; both ligaments are posterior to the orbital septum. The medial check ligament is better developed than the lateral.[32] Traditionally, these ligaments were described as "brakes" that limit the extent of movement of the globe; that is, in abduction the medial check ligament stops lateral movement of the globe when extension of the medial rectus muscle starts to exert pull on the relatively inelastic ligament.

The connective tissue septa that connect muscle to muscle and periodically connect individual muscles to the orbital walls along a significant portion of the muscle length have been identified in dissection studies.[45,48,49] These intermuscular septa include those joining (1) lateral rectus, inferior rectus, and medial rectus; (2) medial rectus and superior rectus; (3) lateral rectus and superior rectus; (4) medial rectus to superior oblique and to orbital roof and floor; (5) medial rectus to periorbita of ethmoid; (6) superior oblique to frontoethmoid angle; (7) inferior rectus to orbital floor; (8) lateral rectus to lateral wall; (9) levator to adjacent periorbita[32]; and (10) superior oblique to orbital roof[45] (Figure 10-11).

The presence and orientation of these septa vary from front to back. Figure 10-12 shows a representation of the septa at midorbit. The considerable amount of attachment between muscle and bone helps to stabilize the muscle path and can limit eye movement.[18,45]

ISOLATED AGONIST MODEL

One of the earliest models developed to explain eye movement is the isolated agonist model described by Duane.[50] This straightforward model has been used widely in the clinical evaluation of extraocular muscles and can be used to describe the movement around the axes that occurs with contraction of each muscle. However, it is important to remember that *during eye movements, all six extraocular muscles are in some state of contraction or relaxation,* and it is strictly hypothetical to discuss the movement of the eye as if only one muscle contracts. In each of these descriptions the eye begins in primary position.

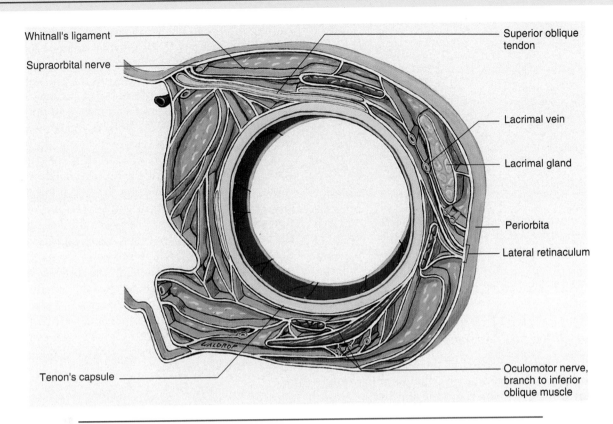

FIGURE 10-11
Connective tissue system in cross section through anterior orbit at level of Whitnall's ligament. (From Dutton JJ: *Atlas of clinical and surgical orbital anatomy*, Philadelphia, 1994, Saunders.)

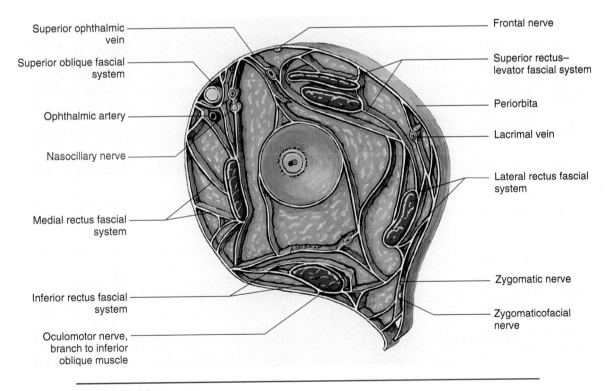

FIGURE 10-12
Connective tissue system in cross section at midorbit. (From Dutton JJ: *Atlas of clinical and surgical orbital anatomy*, Philadelphia, 1994, Saunders.)

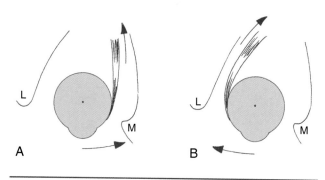

FIGURE 10-13
A, Adduction on contraction of medial rectus muscle with eye in primary position. **B,** Abduction on contraction of lateral rectus muscle with eye in primary position. *L,* Lateral; *M,* medial.

MOVEMENTS FROM PRIMARY POSITION

Horizontal Rectus Muscles

The medial rectus lies parallel to the sagittal axis and perpendicular to the vertical axis; therefore it has only one action, which is rotation around the vertical axis in a nasal direction–adduction. The lateral rectus also lies parallel to the sagittal axis and perpendicular to the vertical axis; contraction causes rotation in a temporal direction–abduction (Figure 10-13).

Vertical Rectus Muscles

The action of the superior rectus is more complex than that of the medial and lateral rectus muscles because it lies at an angle to each of the axes; with the insertion above the origin and on the anterior globe, movement around the horizontal axis causes elevation. The muscle insertion is lateral to the origin, so movement around the vertical axis causes adduction; the oblique insertion on the superior surface of the globe causes intorsion on contraction (Figure 10-14, *A*). The primary action of the superior rectus is said to be elevation; adduction and intorsion are secondary actions.

The primary action of the inferior rectus is depression because the insertion is below the origin and on the anterior of the globe. Secondary actions are adduction, because the insertion is lateral to the origin, and extorsion, which results from the oblique insertion on the inferior surface of the globe (Figure 10-14, *B*).

Oblique Muscles

The primary action of the superior oblique muscle is intorsion.[5,17,51-53] This action results from the oblique insertion on the posterosuperior lateral aspect of the globe (Table 10-4); contraction rotates the eye around the sagittal axis,

causing intorsion. The secondary actions are depression and abduction.[5,17,51-53] Depression occurs because the insertion is posterior and inferior to the physiologic origin; contraction of the muscle pulls the back of the eye up, and the anterior pole moves down. Because the insertion is lateral to the trochlea, contraction of the superior oblique pulls the back of the globe medially, thus moving the anterior pole laterally (Figure 10-15, *A*, page 194).

The primary action of the inferior oblique—extorsion—occurs because the muscle wraps around the lower portion of the globe and the insertion is superior and lateral to the origin. Secondary actions are elevation and abduction.[5,17,51-53] Because the insertion is on the posterior eye and above the origin, contraction pulls the back of the eye down, elevating the front. Abduction occurs because the insertion on the back of the eye is pulled toward the medial side; thus the anterior pole is moved laterally in abduction (Figure 10-15, *B*).

Some authors offer the contrasting view that the primary action of the superior oblique is depression, that of the inferior oblique is elevation, and the torsional actions are secondary.[54]

MOVEMENTS FROM SECONDARY POSITIONS

As the position of the globe changes, the relationship between the muscle origin and insertion changes relative to the axes, and contraction of a muscle has a different effect than when the eye is in primary position. If the eye is elevated, contraction of the horizontal rectus muscles no longer causes strictly adduction or abduction, but also causes a slight elevation; if the eye is depressed, contraction causes further depression.[55]

Vertical Rectus Muscles

With the eye abducted approximately 23 degrees from primary position, the vertical rectus muscles *parallel* the sagittal axis, and lie *perpendicular* to the horizontal axis; thus only vertical movement will occur. In this position, contraction of the superior rectus will cause only elevation, and contraction of the inferior rectus will cause only depression[50] (Figure 10-16, *B*, page 195).

As the eye adducts, it approaches a position where the plane of the vertical rectus muscles is at a right angle to the sagittal axis; this occurs at approximately 67 degrees of adduction (which may be physically impossible because of the connective tissue constraints of the orbit). If the muscle plane of the vertical rectus muscles is at a *right angle* to the sagittal axis, and thus *parallel* to the horizontal axis, contraction of the superior or inferior rectus muscle will not cause vertical movement[50] (Figure 10-16, *A*).

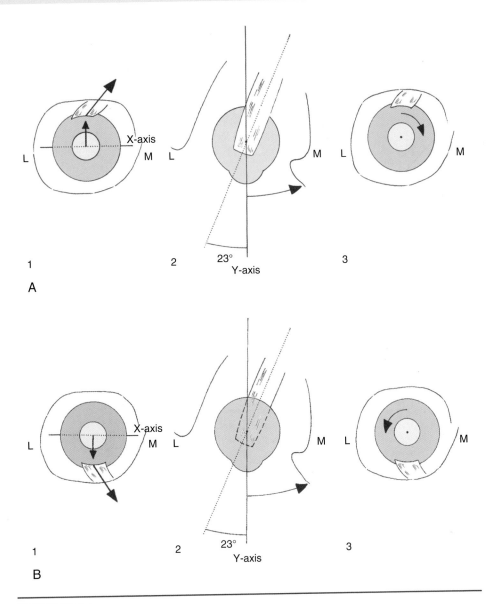

FIGURE 10-14

A, Globe movement around each of Fick's axes on contraction of superior rectus muscle, with eye in primary position. *1,* Elevation, movement around the *x*-axis; *2,* adduction, movement around *z*-axis; *3,* intorsion, movement around *y*-axis. **B,** Globe movement around each of Fick's axes on contraction of inferior rectus muscle, with eye in primary position. *1,* Depression, movement around *x*-axis; *2,* adduction, movement around *z*-axis; *3,* extorsion, movement around *y*-axis. *L,* Lateral; *M,* medial.

Oblique Muscles

As the eye adducts 51 to 55 degrees, the plane of the oblique muscles becomes *parallel* to the sagittal axis and *perpendicular* to the horizontal axis. In this position the superior oblique will cause only depression, and the inferior oblique will cause only elevation. When the eye is abducted 35 to 39 degrees, the plane of the oblique muscles makes a *right angle with* the sagittal axis and *parallels* the horizontal axis, and the obliques cannot cause vertical movement[50] (Figure 10-17).

This analysis is used in the clinical assessment of extraocular muscle function. As the eye increases in abduction, the elevating and depressing abilities of the vertical rectus muscles increase as the elevating and depressing abilities of the oblique muscles decrease. As the eye increasingly moves into adduction, the elevating and depressing abilities of the oblique muscles increase as the elevating and depressing abilities of the vertical rectus muscles decrease.

Table 10-4   Origin, Insertion, and Action of the Extraocular Muscles

Muscle	Origin	Insertion	Primary Action	Secondary Action
Medial rectus	Common ring tendon and optic nerve sheath	Anterior globe	Adduction	None
Lateral rectus	Common ring tendon and greater wing of sphenoid	Anterior globe	Abduction	None
Superior rectus	Common ring tendon and optic nerve sheath	Superior, anterior globe	Elevation	Adduction, intorsion
Inferior rectus	Common ring tendon	Inferior, anterior globe	Depression	Adduction, extorsion
Superior oblique	Anatomic: lesser wing of sphenoid Physiologic: trochlea	Superior, posterior, lateral globe	Intorsion	Depression, abduction
Inferior oblique	Medial maxillary bone	Inferior, posterior, lateral globe	Extorsion	Elevation, abduction

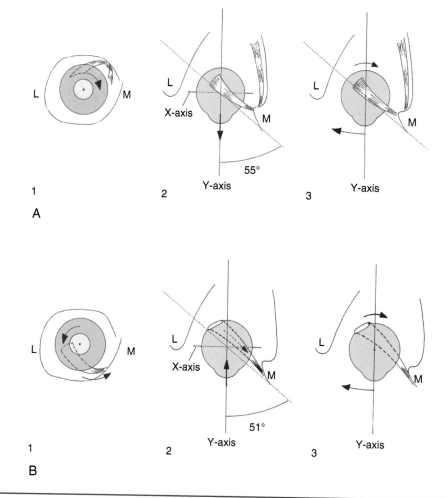

FIGURE 10-15

A, Globe movement around each of Fick's axes on contraction of superior oblique muscle, with eye in primary position. *1,* Intorsion, movement around *y*-axis; *2,* depression, movement around *x*-axis; *3,* abduction, movement around *z*-axis. **B,** Globe movement around each of Fick's axes on contraction of inferior oblique muscle, with eye in primary position. *1,* Extorsion, movement around *y*-axis; *2,* elevation, movement around *x*-axis; *3,* abduction, movement around *z*-axis. *L,* Lateral; *M,* medial.

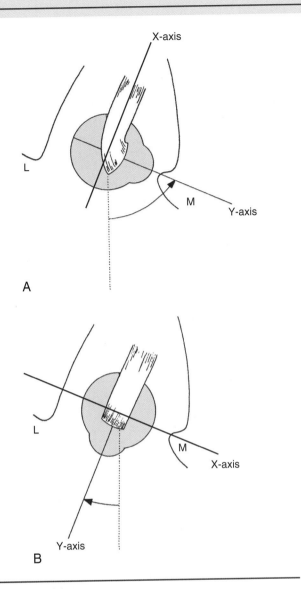

FIGURE 10-16
Relationship between line of muscle movement and Fick's axes when eye is in a secondary position. **A,** When eye is adducted 67 degrees (putting plane of muscle parallel to *x*-axis), contraction of superior rectus muscle cannot cause elevation. **B,** When eye is abducted 23 degrees (putting plane of muscle perpendicular to *x*-axis), contraction of superior rectus muscle causes only elevation. *L,* Lateral; *M,* medial.

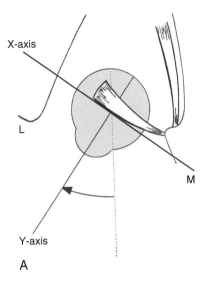

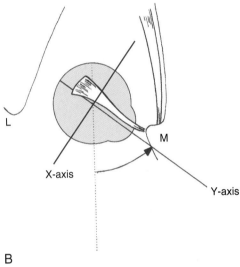

FIGURE 10-17
Relationship between line of muscle movement and Fick's axes when eye is in a secondary position. **A,** When eye is abducted 35 degrees (putting plane of muscle parallel to *x*-axis), contraction of superior oblique muscle cannot cause depression. **B,** When eye is adducted 55 degrees (putting plane of muscle perpendicular to *x*-axis), contraction of superior oblique muscle almost exclusively causes depression. *L,* Lateral; *M,* medial.

AGONIST AND ANTAGONIST MUSCLES

In any position of gaze, innervation of all extraocular muscles is controlled carefully by the central nervous system, and each muscle is in some stage of contraction or relaxation. No single muscle acts alone; muscles work together as agonists, antagonists, or synergists. In all these movements, fine motor control should provide for smooth, continuous movements. According to

Sherrington's law of reciprocal innervation, contraction of a muscle is accompanied by a simultaneous and proportional relaxation of the antagonist.[56] In adduction the increased contraction of the medial rectus muscle is accompanied by the increased relaxation of the antagonist, the lateral rectus muscle.

When the superior rectus muscle and the inferior oblique muscle contract at the same time, the adduction action of the superior rectus and the abduction action of the inferior oblique, as well as the intorsion of the superior rectus and the extorsion of the inferior oblique, will counteract each other. The resultant eye movement is elevation; the muscles are synergists in elevation. Jampel demonstrated this by stimulating the superior rectus and inferior oblique muscles simultaneously and noting that the eye moved directly up.[57]

When the superior oblique and inferior rectus muscles were stimulated simultaneously, the eye moved directly downward.[57] The superior oblique and the inferior rectus are synergists in depression. The superior oblique is the antagonist for the inferior oblique in vertical movements and torsional movements but is synergistic for abduction.

In primary position the muscles are in a balanced state, each exerting contraction sufficient to keep the eye centered in the palpebral fissure. If one muscle is inactive, the eye will be deviated from primary position in the direction of the pull of the antagonist of the dysfunctional muscle. If the medial rectus muscle is paralyzed, the eye, in primary position, will be positioned temporally because of the unopposed action of the lateral rectus muscle.

Clinical Comment: Extraocular Muscle Assessment

Assessment of eye position and movements can be an important tool in determining the integrity of the extraocular muscles and associated nerves. The practitioner first notes the position of each eye while directing the patient to fixate on a target straight ahead. An eye that is deviated toward the nose would indicate an underactive lateral rectus muscle; the medial rectus is unopposed by the lateral rectus. Figure 10-18, A, shows the direction of pull of each muscle when the eye is in primary position.

Ocular motility testing provides further information on the contractile abilities of the muscles. Evaluation of horizontal eye movement is straightforward. If the eye cannot adduct, the problem lies with the medial rectus; if the eye cannot move into the abducted position, the problem lies with the lateral rectus muscle.

With the more complex movements of the other muscles, the most reliable way to determine a dysfunctional muscle is to put the eye into a position in which one muscle is the primary actor. In the adducted position the oblique muscles are the primary elevator and depressor; in the abducted position the vertical rectus muscles are the primary elevator and depressor. This arrangement can be represented by the "H" diagrams in Figure 10-18, B. Thus when doing ocular motility testing, it is important to move the eyes to such a position as to isolate the vertical abilities of these muscles. The usual manner of performing ocular motility testing follows:

1. *Using a small target, usually a bead, the patient is instructed to follow the target.*
2. *The horizontal ability is determined first by moving the bead to the far right and to the far left, noting any inability of either eye to follow.*

3. *In left gaze the bead is elevated to determine the ability of the left superior rectus (left eye is abducted) and the right inferior oblique (right eye is adducted). The bead is depressed to determine the ability of the left inferior rectus and the right superior oblique muscles.*
4. *In right gaze the bead is elevated to determine the ability of the right superior rectus (right eye is abducted) and the left inferior oblique (left eye is adducted). The bead is depressed to determine the ability of the right inferior rectus and the left superior oblique muscles.*

The extensive network of connective tissue septa and fibroelastic pulley system associated with the extraocular muscle may affect eye movement, and MRI may be an additional tool to determine the extent of muscle involvement once a strabismic condition is diagnosed.

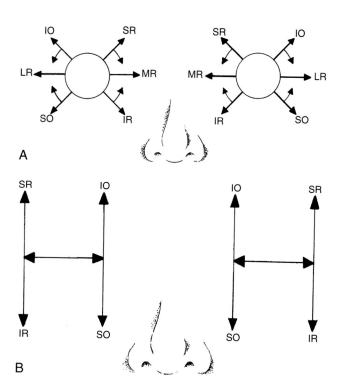

FIGURE 10-18

A, Direction of eye movement on contraction of each muscle, with eye in primary position. For example, if superior rectus muscle contracts, eye will move up and in and intort. Curved arrows represent torsional movements. **B,** Muscles that cause vertical movement when eye is either adducted or abducted. In adduction, for example, the muscle that causes elevation is the inferior oblique, and the muscle causing depression is the superior oblique. *IO,* Inferior oblique; *IR,* inferior rectus; *LR,* lateral rectus; *MR,* medial rectus; *SO,* superior oblique; *SR,* superior rectus.

Clinical Comment: Strabismus

> The patient is diagnosed with strabismus when movement is not coordinated between the two eyes and the visual axes are not straight when the patient is asked to look in the primary position. This condition can be congenital or acquired. In congenital forms of strabismus, suppression is often used as an adaptation response to prevent diplopia. Suppression must be overcome to retrain the muscle to achieve binocular vision even if the treatment includes surgery. In acquired dysfunction the causative factor must be determined.

Clinical Comment: Strabismus Surgery

> Surgical correction for strabismus can be complicated because of the extensive connective tissue network linking extraocular muscles to each other and to the orbital bones. This may be one of the reasons why a patient reverts to presurgery strabismic posture.[58] The realization that there is connection between the muscle sheath and the connective tissue sheath of the globe, not just at the point of the tendon insertion, should be a consideration in muscle resection surgery.[58]

Clinical Comment: Brown Superior Oblique Sheath Syndrome

> Inability to elevate the eye in the adducted position is usually caused by a dysfunctional inferior oblique muscle. However, such a limitation could also be caused by an immobile superior oblique muscle (Figure 10-19). Using electromyography, Brown[59] determined that a patient with an inability to elevate the eye in adduction had a functional inferior oblique muscle, but that the movement of the superior oblique through the trochlea was restricted. The superior oblique could not lengthen when the inferior oblique contracted.[59] In congenital Brown's syndrome, the cause could be a short or anchored tendon; in acquired Brown's syndrome the cause could be an accumulation of fluid or tissue between the trochlea and the tendon.[51,60]

Clinical Comment: Long-Standing Immobility

> In assessing ocular motility and determining the damaged muscle, it may be difficult to determine the dysfunctional muscle, especially if the injury is long term. As a muscle becomes inactive, it can become immobile and can neither contract nor stretch, in effect influencing the abilities of the other extraocular muscles to move the eye.

Clinical Comment: Hyperthyroidism (Graves' Disease)

> Enlargement of the extraocular muscles produced by Graves' disease is caused by chronic inflammatory infiltration of the muscles with glycoprotein and mucopolysaccharide deposition, resulting in proptosis.[1] In addition, restricted ocular motility is evident. However, evaluation of the restricted movement may not depict the correct dysfunctional muscle because fibrosis of the muscles can occur, limiting muscle activity. For example, if the medial rectus is fibrotic, eye movement may be restricted in the lateral direction because the medial rectus is unable to elongate and acts as a check on lateral movement. Restriction may appear to be impairment of the lateral rectus but may actually be caused by the fibrotic medial rectus muscle.

Clinical Comment: Forced Duction Test

> *A FORCED DUCTION TEST* can be performed if a fibrotic muscle is suspected. With the patient under topical anesthesia, the practitioner grasps the conjunctiva near the limbus and attempts to move the eye in a direction opposite from the suspected restriction. Resistance will be met if the cause is fibrosis, but if the muscle is paralyzed, the eye can be moved. For instance, if the lateral rectus is suspect, the practitioner would attempt to move the eye medially. If the lateral rectus is fibrotic, resistance to movement occurs; if it is paralyzed, the eye can be moved with the forceps.[52]

YOKE MUSCLES

Yoke muscles are those muscles of the two eyes acting together to cause binocular movements (Figure 10-20). *Hering's law of equal innervation* states that the innervation to the muscles of the two eyes is equal and simultaneous. Thus the movements of the two eyes are normally symmetric.[61] In dextroversion, equal and simultaneous innervation is supplied to the yoke muscles—the right lateral rectus and left medial rectus; in convergence, equal and simultaneous innervation is supplied to the yoke muscles—the right medial rectus and left medial rectus.

PAIRED ANTAGONIST MODEL

A model by Boeder[55] analyzes the actions of the extraocular muscles as antagonist pairs. Figure 10-21 shows the path that the anterior pole of the eye traces with contraction of these pairs. The vertical pair of muscles have primary actions of elevation and depression, and secondary actions of adduction and torsion.

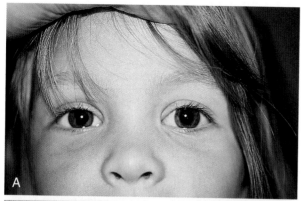
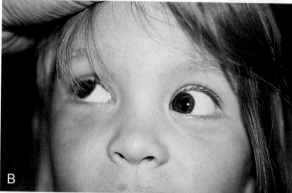
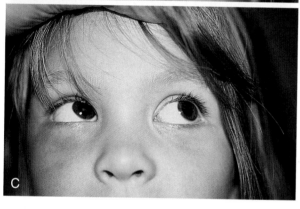

FIGURE 10-19

Brown's syndrome of left eye. A, Eyes straight in primary position. **B,** Limited elevation in adduction. **C,** Normal elevation in abduction. Positive forced duction test on elevating globe in adduction (not shown). (From Kanski JJ, Nischal KK: *Ophthalmology: clinical signs and differential diagnosis,* St Louis, 1999, Mosby.)

Adduction increases with medial movement, as do the torsional effects. In abduction, both muscles must relax.[55]

The primary actions of the paired obliques are intorsion and extorsion. The oblique muscle tendons insert obliquely into the globe, and the torsional effects do not diminish with horizontal movement because the insertion does not act as a unit. In adduction the medial fibers of the superior oblique tendon exert greater contractile force, and in abduction the lateral fibers are shortened.[61] In adduction the lateral fibers of the inferior oblique tendon are shortened, and in abduction the medial fibers contract.[57]

The contraction of one muscle is associated with lengthening of its antagonist. This state of relaxation or extension is considered an activity equivalent to contraction. In all positions of gaze, all muscles are in some state of activity. An analysis of the change of length of each muscle during a simple horizontal excursion shows that as the medial rectus shortens, the lateral rectus lengthens, and vice versa. The vertical rectus muscles behave as one, both shortening in adduction and lengthening in abduction. The obliques cocontract in abduction, but in adduction the superior oblique lengthens and the inferior oblique shortens[55] (Figure 10-22).

COMPLEXITY OF THE OBLIQUE MUSCLES

Some controversy exists over the horizontal abilities of the inferior oblique muscle. The relationship of the muscle plane of the inferior oblique with the vertical axis determines whether the inferior oblique is an adductor or an abductor. If the muscle plane lies in front of the vertical axis, the inferior oblique will aid in adduction. With increasing lateral movement of the eye, however, a point will be reached at which the inferior oblique plane is put behind the vertical axis, causing the inferior oblique then to aid in abduction.[37] Animal studies in which the muscles are stimulated directly either singularly or collectively seem to support this view.[57,62] When the superior oblique and inferior oblique were stimulated simultaneously, no ocular movement occurred; in some positions, these two muscles appeared to be complete antagonists, and abduction did not occur. These observations do not change the model used clinically. In adduction the obliques are responsible for elevation and depression, and in abduction the vertical recti are responsible for elevation and depression.

INNERVATION AND BLOOD SUPPLY

INNERVATION

The medial rectus, inferior rectus, and inferior oblique muscles are innervated by the inferior division of the oculomotor nerve. The superior rectus muscle is innervated by the superior division of the oculomotor nerve. The lateral rectus muscle is supplied by the abducens nerve. The superior oblique muscle is innervated by the trochlear nerve (see Table 10-3 and Figure 10-8).

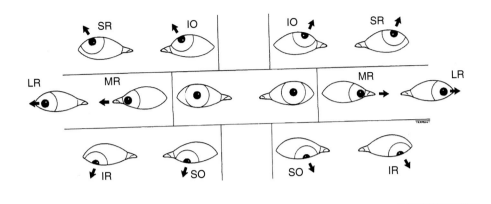

FIGURE 10-20
Six cardinal positions of gaze and yoke muscles. *IO,* Inferior oblique; *IR,* inferior rectus; *LR,* lateral rectus; *MR,* medial rectus; *SO,* superior oblique; *SR,* superior rectus. (From Kanski JJ: *Clinical ophthalmology,* ed 3, Oxford, UK, 1995, Butterworth-Heinemann, p 429.)

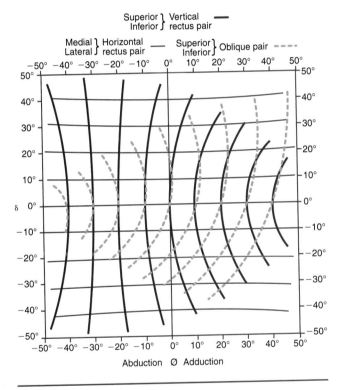

FIGURE 10-21
Traces of line of fixation with activity of each of three muscle pairs in various positions of gaze. (From Boeder P: The cooperation of extraocular muscles, *Am J Ophthalmol* 51:469, 1961.)

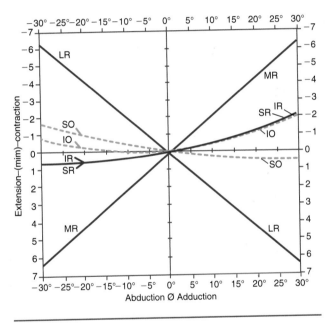

FIGURE 10-22
Changes in muscle length of all extraocular muscles occurring in a horizontal rotation. *IO,* Inferior oblique; *IR,* inferior rectus; *LR,* lateral rectus; *MR,* medial rectus; *SO,* superior oblique; *SR,* superior rectus. (From Boeder P: The cooperation of extraocular muscles, *Am J Ophthalmol* 51:469, 1961.)

BLOOD SUPPLY

The extraocular muscles are supplied by two muscular branches from the ophthalmic artery: The superior (lateral) branch supplies the superior and lateral rectus and the superior oblique muscles, and the inferior (medial) branch supplies the inferior and medial rectus and the inferior oblique muscles.[1,63] Other arteries make various contributions to the extraocular muscle blood supply, including the lacrimal, supraorbital, and infraorbital arteries. These vessels and the muscles they supply are described in Chapter 11 (see Table 11-2).

AGING CHANGES IN THE EXTRAOCULAR MUSCLES

Both horizontal rectus muscles are displaced inferiorly with age, with the medial rectus displaced more than the lateral rectus. This may be the cause of a constant partial depression and may contribute to the impaired ability to elevate the eyes often observed in elderly persons, predisposing them to an incomitant (nonconcomitant) strabismus.[47] The superior rectus and inferior rectus muscles do not change locations.[47]

Other age-related changes in extraocular muscles include a greater variety in fiber sizes, increased connective tissue in the muscle, increased adipose tissue in the bundles, deposits of lipofuscin, and degenerative changes.[64]

REFERENCES

1. Doxanas MT, Anderson RL: *Clinical orbital anatomy*, Baltimore, 1984, Williams & Wilkins, p 116.
2. Honda H, Asakura S: Calcium-triggered movement of regulated actin in vitro. A fluorescence microscopy study, *J Mol Biol* 205(4):677, 1989.
3. Bagni MA, Cecchi G, Colomo F, et al: Tension and stiffness of frog muscle fibres at full filament overlap, *J Muscle Res Cell Motil* 11:371, 1990.
4. Smith DA: The theory for sliding filament models for muscle contraction. III. Dynamics of the five-state model, *J Theor Biol* 146(4):433, 1990.
5. Eggers HM: Functional anatomy of the extraocular muscles. In Tasman W, Jaeger EA, editors: *Duane's foundations of clinical ophthalmology*, vol 1, Philadelphia, 1994, Lippincott.
6. Guyton AC: *Textbook of medical physiology*, ed 8, Philadelphia, 1991, Saunders, p 76.
7. Wirtschafter JD: Neuroanatomy of the ocular muscles. In Reeh MJ, Wobig JL, Wirtschafter JD, editors: *Ophthalmic anatomy*, San Francisco, 1981, American Academy of Ophthalmology, p 267.
8. Karatas M: Internuclear and supranuclear disorders of eye movements: clinical features and causes, *Eur J Neurol* 16:1265–1277, 2009.
9. Namba T, Nakamura T, Grob D: Motor nerve endings in human extraocular muscle, *Neurology* 18:403, 1968.
10. Hess A: Further morphological observations of "en plaque" and "en grappe" nerve endings on mammalian extrafusal muscle fibers with the cholinesterase technique, *Rev Can Biol* 21:241, 1962.
11. Brandt DE, Leeson CR: Structural differences of fast and slow fibers in human extraocular muscle, *Am J Ophthalmol* 62:478, 1966.
12. Breinin GM: The structure and function of extraocular muscle: an appraisal of the duality concept, *Am J Ophthalmol* 71:1, 1971.
13. Peachy L: The structure of the extraocular muscle fibers of mammals. In Bach-y-Rita P, Collins CC, Hyde JE, editors: *The control of eye movements*, New York, 1971, Academic Press, p 47.
14. Scott AB, Collins CC: Division of labor in human extraocular muscle, *Arch Ophthalmol* 90:319, 1973.
15. Montagnani S, De Rosa P: Morphofunctional features of human extrinsic ocular muscles, *Doc Ophthalmol* 72(2):119, 1989.
16. Porter JD: Extraocular muscle: cellular adaptations for a diverse functional repertoire, *Ann N Y Acad Sci* 956:7, 2002.
17. Burde RM, Feldon SE: The extraocular muscles. In Hart WM Jr, editor: *Adler's physiology of the eye*, ed 9, St Louis, 1992, Mosby, p 101.
18. Porter JD, Andrade FH, Baker RS: The extraocular muscles. In Kaufman PL, Alm A, editors: *Adler's physiology of the eye*, ed 10, St Louis, 2003, Mosby, p 787.
19. Ruskell GL: Extraocular muscle proprioceptors and proprioception, *Prog Retin Eye Res* 18(3):269, 1999.
20. Weir CR, Knox PC, Dutton GN: Does extraocular proprioception influence oculomotor control? *Br J Ophthalmol* 84:1071–1074, 2000.
21. Richmond FJR, Johnston WSW, Baker RS, et al: Palisade endings in human extraocular muscles, *Invest Ophthalmol Vis Sci* 25:471–476, 1984.
22. Alpern M: Movements of the eyes. In Dawson H, editor: *The eye*, New York, 1962, Academic Press.
23. Walls GL: The evolutionary history of eye movements, *Vis Res* 2:69, 1962.
24. Linwong M, Herman SJ: Cycloduction of the eyes with head tilt, *Arch Ophthalmol* 85:570, 1971.
25. Jampel RS: Ocular torsion and the function of the vertical extraocular muscles, *Am J Ophthalmol* 77:292, 1975.
26. Duke-Elder S: *Textbook of ophthalmology, vol 4*, St Louis, 1949, Mosby.
27. Diamond SG, Markham CH: Ocular counterrolling as an indicator of vestibular otolith function, *Neurology* 33:1460, 1983.
28. Collewijin H, Van der Steer J, Ferman L, et al: Human ocular counterroll: assessment of static and dynamic properties from electromagnetic scleral coil recordings, *Exp Brain Res* 59:185, 1985.
29. Ott D, Eckmiller R: Ocular torsion measured by TV and scanning laser ophthalmoscopy during horizontal pursuit in humans and monkeys, *Invest Ophthalmol Vis Sci* 30(12):2512, 1989.
30. Warwick R: *Eugene Wolff's anatomy of the eye and orbit*, ed 7, Philadelphia, 1976, Saunders, p 248.
31. Burton H: Somatic sensations from the eye. In Hart WM Jr, editor: *Adler's physiology of the eye*, ed 9, St Louis, 1992, Mosby, p 185.
32. Koornneef L: Orbital connective tissue. In Jakobiec FA, editor: *Ocular anatomy, embryology, and teratology*, Philadelphia, 1982, Harper & Row, p 835.
33. DeGottrau P, Gajisin S: Anatomic, histologic, and morphometric studies of the ocular rectus muscles and their relation to the eye globe and Tenon's capsule, *Klin Monatsbl Augenheilkd* 200(5):515, 1992:(abstract).
34. Porter JD, Poukens V, Baker RS, et al: Structure-function correlations in the human medial rectus extraocular muscle pulleys, *Invest Ophthalmol Vis Sci* 37:468, 1996.
35. Demer JL, Miller JM, Poukens V: Surgical implications of the rectus extraocular muscle pulleys, *J Pediatr Ophthalmol Strabismus* 33(4):208, 1996.
36. Wobig JL: The eyelids. In Reeh MJ, Wobig JL, Wirtschafter JD, editors: *Ophthalmic anatomy*, San Francisco, 1981, American Academy of Ophthalmology, p 38.
37. Krewson WE: Comparison of the oblique extraocular muscles, *Arch Ophthalmol* 32:204, 1944.
38. Wobig JL: The extrinsic ocular muscles. In Reeh MJ, Wobig JL, Wirtschafter JD, editors: *Ophthalmic anatomy*, San Francisco, 1981, American Academy of Ophthalmology, p 33.
39. Wasicky R, Ziya-Ghazvini F, Blumer R, et al: Muscle fiber types of human extraocular muscles: a histochemical and immunohistochemical study, *Invest Ophthalmol Vis Sci* 41(5):980, 2000.
40. Kono R, Poukens V, Demer JL: Superior oblique muscle layers in monkeys and humans, *Invest Ophthalmol Vis Sci* 46:2790–2799, 2005.
41. Demer JL, Oh SY, Poukens V: Evidence for active control of rectus extraocular muscle pulleys, *Invest Ophthalmol Vis Sci* 41:1280, 2000.
42. Oh SY, Poukens V, Cohen MS, et al: Structure-function correlation of laminar vascularity in human rectus extraocular muscles, *Invest Ophthalmol Vis Sci* 42:17, 2001.
43. Clark RA, Miller JM, Demer JL: Three-dimensional location of human rectus pulleys by path inflections in secondary gaze positions, *Invest Ophthalmol Vis Sci* 41:3787, 2000.
44. Clark RA, Miller JM, Demer JL: Location and stability of rectus muscle pulleys. Muscle paths as a function of gaze, *Invest Ophthalmol Vis Sci* 38:227, 1997.
45. Ettl A, Kramer J, Daxer A, et al: High-resolution magnetic resonance imaging of the normal extraocular musculature, *Eye* 11:793, 1997.

46. Demer JL, Poukens V, Miller JM, et al: Innervation of extraocular pulley smooth muscle in monkeys and humans, *Invest Ophthalmol Vis Sci* 38(9):1774, 1997.

47. Clark RA, Demer JL: Effect of aging on human rectus extraocular muscle paths demonstrated by magnetic resonance imaging, *Am J Ophthalmol* 134:872, 2002.

48. Miller JM: Functional anatomy of normal human rectus muscles, *Vis Res* 29(2):223, 1989.

49. Miller JM, Demer JL, Rosenbaum AL: Effects of transposition surgery on rectus muscle paths by magnetic resonance imaging, *Ophthalmology* 100(4):475, 1993.

50. Duane A: The monocular movements, *Arch Ophthalmol* 8:531, 1936.

51. Leigh RJ, Zee DS: *The neurology of eye movements*, Philadelphia, 1983, Davis, pp 145, 170.

52. Von Noorden GK, Maumenee AE: *Atlas of strabismus*, ed 2, St Louis, 1973, Mosby, pp 6, 112.

53. Kanski JJ: *Clinical ophthalmology*, ed 3, Oxford, England, 1994, Butterworth-Heinemann, p 428.

54. Bron AJ, Tripathi RC, Tripathi BJ: *Wolff's anatomy of the eye and orbit*, ed 8, London, 1997, Chapman & Hall.

55. Boeder P: The cooperation of extraocular muscles, *Am J Ophthalmol* 51:469, 1969.

56. Sherrington CS: Experimental note on two movements of the eyes, *J Physiol (Lond)* 17:27, 1984.

57. Jampel RS: The fundamental principle of the action of the oblique ocular muscles, *Am J Ophthalmol* 69:623, 1970.

58. Hakim OM, Gruber El-Hag Y, Maher H: Persistence of eye movement following disinsertion of extraocular muscle, *J AAPOS* 12:62–65, 2008.

59. Brown HW: Congenital structural muscle anomalies. In Allen ED, editor: *Strabismus ophthalmic symposium*, St Louis, 1950, Mosby, p 250.

60. Helveston EM, Merriam WW, Ellis FD, et al: The trochlea. A study of the anatomy and physiology, *Ophthalmology* 89:124, 1982.

61. Hering E: *Theory of binocular vision*, New York, 1977, Plenum.

62. Jampel RS: The action of the superior oblique muscle. An experimental study in the monkey, *Arch Ophthalmol* 75:535, 1966.

63. Hayreh SS: The ophthalmic artery: III. Branches, *Br J Ophthalmol* 46:212, 1962.

64. McKelvie P, Friling R, Davey K, et al: Changes as the result of ageing in extraocular muscles: a post-mortem study, *Aust N Z J Ophthalmol* 27:420, 1999.

Circulation to the head and neck is supplied by the common carotid artery, which divides into two vessels: the internal carotid and the external carotid. The internal carotid artery supplies the structures within the cranium, including the eye and related structures. The external carotid artery supplies the superficial areas of the head and neck, and provides a small portion of the circulation to ocular adnexa.

INTERNAL CAROTID ARTERY

The **internal carotid** artery runs upward through the neck and enters the skull through the carotid canal, located in the petrous portion of the temporal bone just superior to the jugular fossa. Within the anterior portion of the canal, only thin bone separates the artery from the cochlea and the trigeminal ganglion. The internal carotid artery leaves the canal and immediately enters the cavernous sinus, where it runs forward along the medial wall beside the sphenoid bone; it then exits through the roof of the sinus. Within the sinus, the abducens nerve is closely adherent to the lateral border of the internal carotid.[1] Throughout its pathway—up the neck, into the skull, and through the cavernous sinus—the internal carotid is surrounded by a plexus of sympathetic nerves from the superior cervical ganglion. The second and third cranial nerves accompany the vessel as it leaves the sinus; the optic nerve lies medial and the oculomotor nerve lies lateral to the internal carotid. The ophthalmic artery branches from the internal carotid artery just as it emerges from the cavernous sinus medial to the anterior clinoid process of the sphenoid bone. It is usually the first major branch from the internal carotid artery.[2]

Clinical Comment: Sclerosis of the Internal Carotid Artery

Compression of the optic nerve caused by sclerosis of the internal carotid artery was found in some postmortem studies, with pathologic changes such as atrophy, evident in the optic nerve. Visual field defects may be caused by this compression and should be one of the differential diagnoses when optic nerve head atrophy accompanies a field defect.[3]

OPHTHALMIC ARTERY

The **ophthalmic artery** enters the orbit within the dural sheath of the optic nerve and passes through the optic canal, below and lateral to the nerve[2] (Figure 11-1). A network of sympathetic nerves surrounds the vessel.[4] Once in the orbit the ophthalmic artery emerges from the meningeal sheath, runs inferolateral to the optic nerve for a short distance, and then crosses either above or below the nerve. Together with the nasociliary nerve, the ophthalmic artery runs toward the medial wall of the orbit.[5] The artery continues forward between the medial rectus and superior oblique muscles, giving off branches to various areas. Just posterior to the superior medial orbital margin, it divides into its terminal branches, the supratrochlear and dorsonasal arteries. In general, the intraorbital arteries are located in the adipose compartments and perforate the connective tissue septa as they pass between sections.[6] The ophthalmic artery is the main blood supply to the globe and adnexa but is supplemented by a few branches from the external carotid supply.

Throughout its rather tortuous course, many branches from the ophthalmic artery emerge: (1) central retinal artery, (2) lacrimal artery, (3) ciliary arteries (usually two, sometimes three), (4) ethmoid arteries (usually two), (5) supraorbital artery, (6) muscular arteries (usually two), (7) medial palpebral arteries (superior and inferior), (8) supratrochlear artery, and (9) dorsonasal artery.

Marked variability is evident in the order of the origin of the branches of the ophthalmic artery, and the sequence appears to correlate with whether the artery crosses above or below the optic nerve. The most common patterns of distribution are shown in Table 11-1.[7] Many anatomic variations can occur in the branches and their courses; those most often reported are included here.

CENTRAL RETINAL ARTERY

One of the first branches of the ophthalmic artery, the **central retinal artery,** is among the smallest branches. The central retinal artery leaves the ophthalmic artery as it lies below the optic nerve (see Figure 11-1). The artery runs forward a short distance before entering

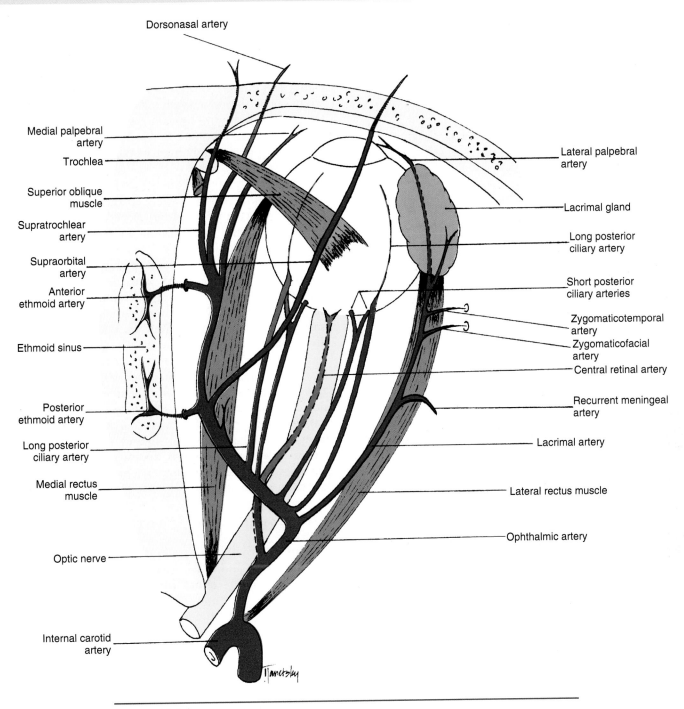

FIGURE 11-1
Orbit viewed from above, illustrating branches of ophthalmic artery.

the meningeal sheath of the nerve about 10 to 12 mm behind the globe (Figure 11-2). While within the optic nerve, the central retinal artery provides branches to the nerve and pia mater.[7] (Often, these branches are called collateral branches.) As the central retinal artery runs forward within the optic nerve, a sympathetic nerve plexus (the nerve of Tiedemann) surrounds the artery.[8]

The central retinal artery passes through the lamina cribrosa and enters the optic disc just nasal to center, branching superiorly and inferiorly. These branches divide into nasal and temporal branches, then continue to branch dichotomously within the retinal nerve fiber layer. The retinal blood vessels are discussed in Chapter 4.

Table 11-1   Order of Origin of Branches of Ophthalmic Artery

Order of Origin	SEQUENCE OF BRANCHES WHEN OPHTHALMIC ARTERY:	
	Crosses Above Optic Nerve	**Crosses Below Optic Nerve**
1	Central retinal and medial posterior ciliary	Lateral posterior ciliary
2	Lateral posterior ciliary	Central retinal
3	Lacrimal	Medial muscular
4	Muscular to superior rectus and levator	Medial posterior ciliary
5	Posterior ethmoid and supraorbital, jointly or separately	Lacrimal
6	Medial posterior ciliary	Muscular to superior rectus and levator
7	Medial muscular	Posterior ethmoid and supraorbital, jointly or separately
8	Muscular to superior oblique and medial rectus, jointly or separately	Muscular to superior oblique and medial rectus, jointly or separately
9	To areolar tissue	Anterior ethmoid
10	Anterior ethmoid	To areolar tissue
11	Medial palpebral or inferior medial palpebral	Medial palpebral or inferior medial palpebral
12	Superior medial palpebral	Superior medial palpebral
Terminal	Dorsonasal and supratrochlear	Dorsonasal and supratrochlear

Modified from Hayreh SS: The ophthalmic artery. III. Branches, *Br J Ophthalmol* 46:212, 1962.

Clinical Comment: Retinal Venous Branch Occlusion

The branches of the central retinal artery and vein are joined in a common connective tissue sheath at the point where the vessels cross each other. Generally, the artery crosses over the vein and, in such disease processes as arteriosclerosis, may compress the vein at the crossing, causing at first a deflection of the vessel, which in time may progress to a venous occlusion. Restriction of flow in the vein results in retinal edema and hemorrhage in the area surrounding the occlusion.

LACRIMAL ARTERY

One of the largest branches, the **lacrimal artery,** leaves the ophthalmic artery just after it enters the orbit (see Figure 11-1); rarely, it branches before the ophthalmic artery enters the optic canal.[9] The lacrimal artery and the lacrimal nerve run forward along the upper border of the lateral rectus muscle. Within the orbit the lacrimal artery may supply branches to the lateral rectus muscle.

A recurrent meningeal artery (see Figure 11-1) might branch from the lacrimal artery and course back, leaving the orbit through the lateral aspect of the superior orbital fissure and then forming an anastomosis with the middle meningeal artery, a branch from the external carotid artery circulation.[10] Other branches, the **zygomaticotemporal artery** and the **zygomaticofacial artery,** exit the orbit through foramina of the same name within the zygomatic bone (see Figure 11-1) and anastomose with branches from the external carotid in the temporal fossa and on the face.[7]

The lacrimal artery continues forward to supply the lacrimal gland. Terminal branches pass through the gland, pierce the orbital septum, and enter the lateral side of the upper and lower eyelids to form the **lateral palpebral arteries.** These anastomose with branches from the medial palpebral arteries and form vessel arches called the **palpebral arcades.** Other terminal branches from the lacrimal artery enter the conjunctiva and form a capillary network.

POSTERIOR CILIARY ARTERIES

The **posterior ciliary arteries** are branches of the ophthalmic artery, and much variation can occur in their distribution.[11] The **short posterior ciliary arteries** arise as 1, 2, or 3 branches that then form 10 to 20 branches. They enter the sclera in a ring around the optic nerve and form the arterial network within the choroidal stroma (Figure 11-3). Other branches from the short posterior ciliary arteries anastomose to form the **circle of Zinn (Zinn-Haller)** (see Figure 11-2), which encircles the optic nerve at the level of the choroid.[12,13] The most superficial nerve fibers that occupy the surface of the optic disc are supplied by capillaries from the retinal vasculature with no apparent direct choroidal supply.[13-15] The peripapillary network, formed by branches from the short posterior ciliary arteries and from the circle of Zinn, supplies the remaining prelaminar region of the optic nerve.[14-17] These vessels do not anastomose with the peripapillary choriocapillaris.[14] The laminar region is supplied by the short posterior ciliary arteries either directly or as branches from the circle of Zinn.[14-18]

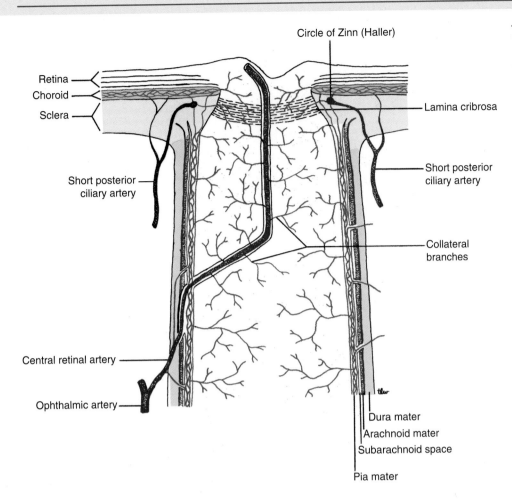

Circle of Zinn (Haller)

Retina

Choroid

Sclera

Short posterior ciliary artery

Central retinal artery

Ophthalmic artery

Lamina cribrosa

Short posterior ciliary artery

Collateral branches

Dura mater
Arachnoid mater
Subarachnoid space
Pia mater

FIGURE 11-2
Longitudinal section of the optic nerve.

Clinical Comment: Anterior Ischemic Optic Neuropathy

ANTERIOR ISCHEMIC OPTIC NEUROPATHY (AION) results from nonperfusion or hypoperfusion of the ciliary blood supply to the optic nerve head.[14] The oval that forms the circle of Zinn can be divided into superior and inferior portions by the entry points of the medial and lateral short ciliary arteries forming it. This may be the anatomic basis for the altitudinal visual field loss that characterizes nonarteritic AION. The inferior field is more often affected, but there is no adequate explanation for the preferential involvement of the superior part of the ring of vessels.[19]

Clinical Comment: Cilioretinal Artery

A CILIORETINAL ARTERY may arise either from the vessels entering the choroid or from the circle of Zinn; thus this vessel, located within the retina, arises from the ciliary circulation and not from the retinal supply. Various studies report a cilioretinal artery occurring in 15% to 50% of the population and usually entering the retina from the temporal side of the optic disc to supply the macular area[20,21] (Figure 11-4). If occlusion of the central retinal artery occurs, the direct blood supply to the macular area will be maintained in those individuals with such a cilioretinal artery.

Two long branches of the posterior ciliary arteries enter the sclera: one lateral and one medial to the ring of short ciliary arteries. These are the **long posterior ciliary arteries,** which run between the sclera and the choroid to the anterior globe (Figure 11-5). Here the arteries enter the ciliary body and branch superiorly and inferiorly.[14] These branches anastomose with each other and with the anterior ciliary arteries to form a circular blood vessel, the **major arterial circle of the iris** (Figure 11-6). This circular artery is located in the ciliary stroma near the iris root and is the source of the radial vessels found in the iris. Before forming the major circle, branches from the long posterior ciliary arteries supply the ciliary body and the anterior choroid, where they form a network that anastomoses with the choroidal vessels from the short posterior ciliary arteries (see Figure 11-3).

Clinical Comment: Fluorescein Angiography

Sodium fluorescein dye can be injected into the systemic circulation to examine the choroidal and retinal circulation for abnormalities (Figure 11-7). Two to five

continued on page 207

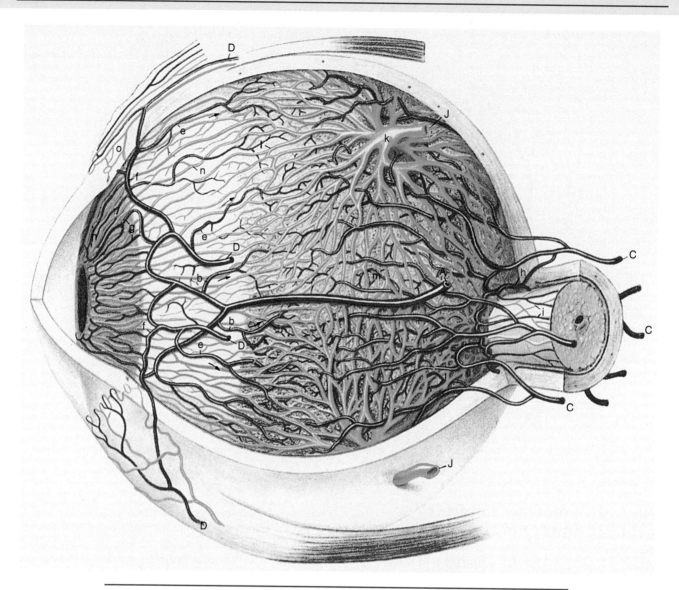

FIGURE 11-3

Uveal blood vessels. Blood supply of the eye is derived from ophthalmic artery. Except for central retinal artery, which supplies the inner retina, almost the entire blood supply of the eye comes from the uveal vessels. There are two long posterior ciliary arteries: one enters the uvea nasally and one enters temporally along the horizontal meridian of the eye near optic nerve (A). These two arteries give off three to five branches (b) at the ora serrata, which pass directly back to form anterior choriocapillaris. These capillaries nourish retina from the equator forward. Short posterior ciliary arteries enter choroid around optic nerve (C). They divide rather rapidly to form posterior choriocapillaris, which nourishes retina as far anteriorly as the equator (choriocapillaris not shown). This system of capillaries is continuous with those derived from long posterior ciliary arteries. Anterior ciliary arteries (D) pass forward with rectus muscles, then pierce sclera to enter ciliary body. Before joining major circle of iris, these arteries give off 8 to 12 branches (e) that pass back through ciliary muscle to join anterior choriocapillaris. Major circle of iris (f) lies in pars plicata and sends branches posteriorly into ciliary body as well as forward into iris (g). Circle of Zinn (h) is formed by pial branches (i) as well as branches from short posterior ciliary arteries. Circle of Zinn lies in sclera and furnishes part of blood supply to optic nerve and disc. Vortex veins exit from eye through posterior sclera (j) after forming an ampulla (k) near internal sclera. Venous branches that join anterior and posterior part of vortex system are meridionally oriented and are fairly straight (l), whereas those joining vortices on medial and lateral sides are oriented circularly about the eye (m). Venous return from iris and ciliary body (n) is mainly posterior into vortex system, but some veins cross anterior sclera and limbus (o) to enter episcleral system of veins. (From Hogan MJ, Alvarado JA, Weddell JE: *Histology of the human eye*, Philadelphia, 1971, Saunders.)

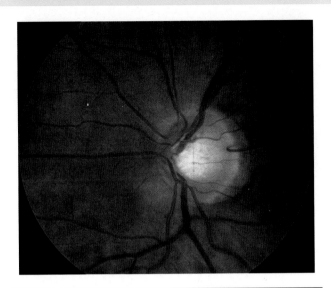

FIGURE 11-4
Fundus photograph of the right eye. A cilioretinal artery can be seen looping up into retina at temporal edge of optic disc. (Courtesy Family Vision Center, Pacific University, Forest Grove, Ore.)

cc of the dye is injected into a vein in the arm. Serial black and white photos are taken of the fundus through filters that enhance the image. This documents the movement of the blood through the choroidal and retinal vasculature. The dye enters the skull through the internal carotid artery, passes into the ophthalmic artery, and then to the posterior ciliary arteries, which fill before the central retinal artery. Within 10 seconds of injection the choroidal flush can be seen; the dye can leak out of the fenestrated choriocapillaris easily but should not seep into the retina because of the blood-retinal barrier of zonula occludens in the RPE. Ten to 12 seconds after injection, the retinal arterioles fill and the capillaries are filled in the next second; another 1 to 2 seconds and the veins fill, and the dye starts to exit the ocular tissue. Defects in the RPE can be seen if the dye leaks into the retina before the retinal vessels fill. Abnormal retinal vasculature such as neovascularization and capillary leakage will be evident.

ETHMOID ARTERIES

As the ophthalmic artery courses near the medial wall, two branches arise and enter the ethmoid bone (see Figure 11-1). The **posterior ethmoid artery** passes through the posterior ethmoid canal to supply the posterior ethmoid sinus and the sphenoid sinus; it sends branches into the nasal cavity to supply the upper part of the nasal mucosa. The **anterior ethmoid artery** generally is larger and passes through the anterior ethmoid canal and supplies the anterior and middle ethmoid sinuses, the sphenoid sinus, the frontal sinus, the nasal cavity, and the skin of the nose.

SUPRAORBITAL ARTERY

The **supraorbital artery** arises from the ophthalmic artery as it lies medial to the optic nerve (see Figure 11-1). The supraorbital artery runs upward to a position above the superior extraocular muscles, turns anteriorly, and runs with the supraorbital nerve between the periorbita of the orbital roof and the levator muscle. It passes through the supraorbital notch or foramen, often dividing into two branches to supply the skin and the muscles of the forehead and scalp (see Figure 11-8). Terminal branches anastomose with the artery from the opposite side, with the supratrochlear artery, and with the anterior temporal artery from the external carotid. While the supraorbital artery is in the orbit, it sends branches to the superior rectus, superior oblique, and levator muscles and to the periorbita.

MUSCULAR ARTERIES

Much variation occurs in the vessels supplying the muscles, and in an individual, any combination of the vessels named here might be present. In one common presentation, the muscular arteries come from the ophthalmic artery as two branches, the lateral (or superior) and the medial (or inferior). The **lateral (superior) branch** supplies the lateral rectus, superior rectus, superior oblique, and levator muscles.[7-9] The **medial (inferior) branch** supplies the medial rectus, inferior rectus, and inferior oblique muscles.[7-9] Additional branches supplying the muscles may come from other sources. The lacrimal artery supplies the lateral and superior rectus muscles. The supraorbital artery supplies the superior rectus, superior oblique, and levator muscles. The infraorbital artery supplies the inferior rectus and inferior oblique muscles (Table 11-2).

ANTERIOR CILIARY ARTERIES

The **anterior ciliary arteries** branch from the vessels supplying the rectus muscles. These arteries exit the muscles near the muscle insertions, run forward along the tendons a short distance, then loop inward to pierce the sclera just outer to the limbus (see Figure 11-3). An accumulation of pigment may be evident at the point at which the artery enters the sclera. Before entering the sclera, the anterior ciliary arteries send branches into the conjunctiva, forming a network of vessels in the limbal conjunctiva (see Figure 11-6). Other branches enter the episclera to form a network of vessels before entering the uvea. The anterior ciliary arteries then enter the ciliary body and anastomose with the branches of the long posterior ciliary arteries, forming the **major circle of the iris** (see Figure 11-3).

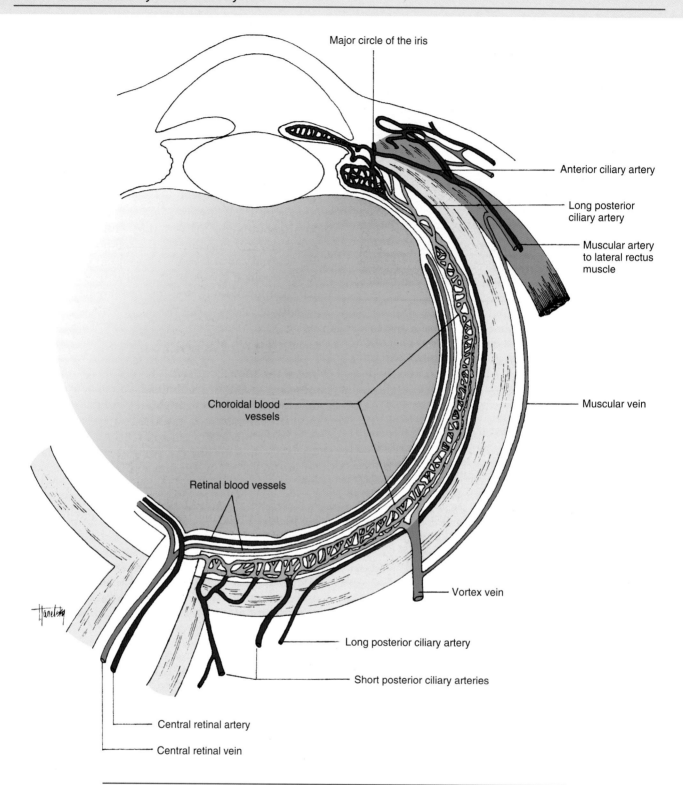

FIGURE 11-5
Horizontal section of the eye showing ciliary circulation. Short posterior ciliary arteries supply choroidal vassels, long posterior ciliary artery passes through suprachoroidal space to anterior globe to anastomose with anterior ciliary artery. (From Vaughan D, Asbury T: *General ophthalmology*, East Norwalk, Conn, 1980, Appleton & Lange.)

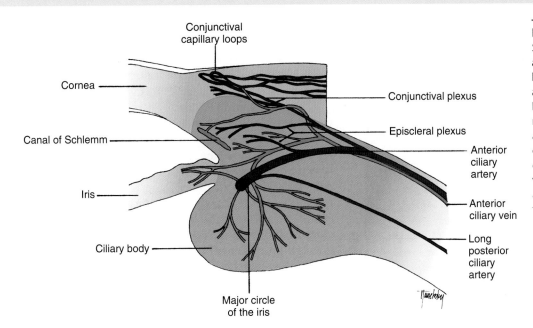

Conjunctival capillary loops

Cornea

Canal of Schlemm

Iris

Ciliary body

Conjunctival plexus

Episcleral plexus

Anterior ciliary artery

Anterior ciliary vein

Long posterior ciliary artery

Major circle of the iris

FIGURE 11-6
Section through ciliary body and limbal area, showing branches of anterior ciliary artery. Anterior ciliary artery has entered globe from rectus muscle blood supply and sends branches into ciliary body, episclera, and conjunctiva; anastomosis with long posterior ciliary artery forms major circle of the iris.

Generally, two anterior ciliary arteries emanate from each of the rectus muscles, with the exception of the lateral rectus, which provides only one such artery.

Clinical Comment: "Red Eye"

Inflammations generate an increase of the blood flow to the affected area, causing hyperemia. In cases of a "red eye," an understanding of the organization of the blood supply in the limbal area can help in differentiating a less serious presentation, such as conjunctivitis, from a more serious situation, such as uveitis. In conjunctivitis *and mild corneal involvement, the superficial blood vessels are injected, giving the conjunctiva a bright-red color that often increases toward the fornix. The vessels move with conjunctival movement and can be blanched with a topical vasoconstrictor. In* uveitis *the deeper scleral and episcleral vessels are injected, giving the circumlimbal area a purplish or rose-pink color.[22] These vessels do not move with the conjunctiva and are not blanched with a topical vasoconstrictor.*

MEDIAL PALPEBRAL ARTERIES

Two **medial palpebral arteries** branch either directly from the ophthalmic artery or from the dorsonasal artery near the trochlea of the superior oblique muscle. The medial palpebral arteries pierce the orbital septum on either side of the medial palpebral ligament and enter the superior and inferior eyelids (see Figure 11-8). These branches run through the eyelid and form arches between the orbicularis muscle and the tarsal plate. They anastomose with branches from the lacrimal artery and form the vessels known as the **palpebral arcades**. Usually, two arcades occur in each lid: the *marginal arcade*, which runs near the marginal edge of the tarsal plate, and the *peripheral*

arcade, which runs near the peripheral edge of the tarsal plate. These provide the blood supply for the eyelid structures. Additional branches from the medial palpebral arteries supply the structures in the medial canthus.

SUPRATROCHLEAR ARTERY

One of the terminal branches of the ophthalmic artery, the **supratrochlear artery**, pierces the orbital septum at the superior, medial corner of the orbit[5] (see Figure 11-8). It passes with the supratrochlear nerve upward to supply the skin of the forehead and scalp and the muscles of the forehead. The supratrochlear artery forms anastomoses with the supraorbital artery, the opposite supratrochlear artery, and the anterior temporal artery of the external carotid supply.

DORSONASAL ARTERY

The other terminal branch of the ophthalmic artery, the **dorsonasal artery (dorsal nasal artery)**, also leaves the orbit by piercing the orbital septum below the trochlea above the medial palpebral ligament.[5] It sends vessels to supply the lacrimal sac, then runs alongside the nose to anastomose with the angular artery from the external carotid supply.

PHYSIOLOGY OF OCULAR CIRCULATION

The endothelial cells that line blood vessels secrete substances that modulate vascular tone and vessel caliber. Blood flow is strongly dependent on endothelial-derived

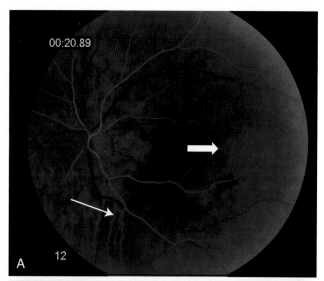

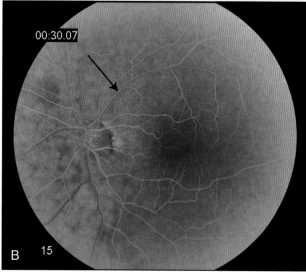

FIGURE 11-7
Fluorescein angiography in a 68-year old white male with internal carotid artery stenosis. (Note the delay in dye passage into the vessels.) **A,** Photo taken 20 seconds after injection; choroidal vessels fill first and then the CRA. The thin arrow indicates a choroidal vessel and the thick arrow shows the choroidal flush as dye seeps out of choriocapillaris but is prevented from entering retina by the tight junction of RPE. **B,** Photo taken 30 seconds after injection, dye has filled retinal capillaries and can now be seen along the walls of the retinal veins *(arrow)* as it exits the eye. (Courtesy Densie Good win, O.D., Pacific University Family Vision Center, Forest Grove, Ore.)

vasoactive substances such as nitric oxide, which causes vasodilation and endothelin-1, a vasoconstrictor.[23,24] The choroidal blood flow is largely dependent on vasoactive autonomic innervation, and sympathetic stimulation causes vasoconstriction but the effect of parasympathetic stimulation is less clear.[23] Retinal vessels lack autonomic innervation and are autoregulated,

and blood flow remains stable with transient increases in blood pressure.[23] Retinal vessel walls have "pacemaker" mechanisms that regulate vessel wall tension, constriction and dilation, are influenced by changes in the environment in the surrounding tissue, responding to levels of O_2 and CO_2, as well as pH changes. Some investigators believe that choroidal vessels exhibit some autoregulation.[25]

Although blood flow through the choroidal vessels is extremely high compared with flow through retinal vessels (2000 ml/min/100 g tissue versus 60 ml/min/100 g tissue), oxygen extraction from the choriocapillaris is low.[24] The high choroidal flow rate provides high oxygen tension enhancing oxygen diffusion through Bruch's membrane and the RPE to mitochondria in the photoreceptor inner segment. The high choroidal blood flow can also act to stabilize temperature, protecting the retina from thermal damage.[24,25]

EXTERNAL CAROTID ARTERY

The other branch of the common carotid, the **external carotid artery,** passes upward through the tissue of the neck. Only those few branches of this artery that supply the globe and orbit are discussed.

FACIAL ARTERY

The **facial artery** arises from the external carotid near the angle of the mandible, runs along the posterior edge of the lower jaw, and curves upward over the outside of the jaw and across the cheek to the angle of the mouth. It ascends along the side of the nose and sends a terminal branch, the **angular artery,** to the medial canthus (Figure 11-9). The angular artery supplies the lacrimal sac, the medial part of the lower lid, and the skin of the cheek. Some branches pass beneath the medial canthal ligament to anastomose with the infraorbital artery, and some anastomose with the dorsonasal artery.

SUPERFICIAL TEMPORAL ARTERY

The **superficial temporal artery** is a terminal branch of the external carotid artery (see Figure 11-9). Branches of the superficial temporal artery that supply areas near the orbit are the anterior temporal, zygomatic, and transverse facial arteries.[26] The **anterior temporal artery** supplies the skin and muscles of the forehead and anastomoses with the supraorbital and supratrochlear arteries. The **zygomatic artery** extends above the zygomatic arch and supplies the orbicularis muscle. The **transverse facial artery supplies** the

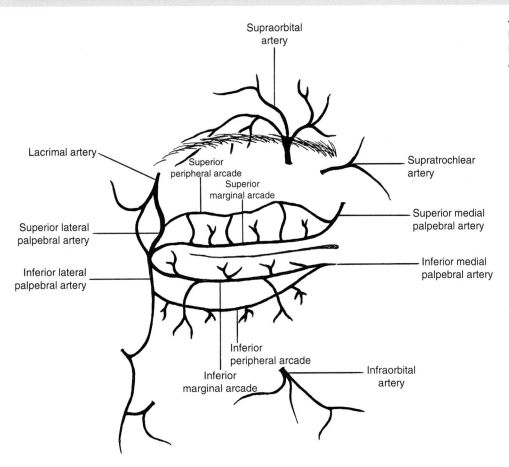

Supraorbital
artery

Lacrimal artery

Superior
peripheral arcade

Superior
marginal arcade

Superior lateral
palpebral artery

Inferior lateral
palpebral artery

Supratrochlear
artery

Superior medial
palpebral artery

Inferior medial
palpebral artery

Inferior
peripheral arcade

Inferior
marginal arcade

Infraorbital
artery

FIGURE 11-8
Lateral and medial palpebral
arteries.

skin of the cheek and anastomoses with the infraorbital artery.

Clinical Comment: Temporal Arteritis

> *TEMPORAL ARTERITIS (or giant cell arteritis) is an inflammatory condition that can affect large arteries but is found primarily in the arteries in the temporal or occipital region. The disease often is accompanied by swelling, redness, and tenderness in the temporal area. Ocular symptoms, including vision loss, may occur. Biopsy of the superficial temporal artery often is necessary to confirm the diagnosis before treatment begins.[29] The biopsy is taken from the artery as it crosses the zygomatic process and travels superiorly anterior to the ear.[28]*

MAXILLARY ARTERY

The other branch of the external carotid that supplies areas in proximity to the orbit is the **maxillary artery.** It passes through the infratemporal fossa and then upward, medial to the mandibular joint toward the maxillary bone (see Figure 11-9). Within the infratemporal fossa,

Table 11-2   Extraocular Muscle Blood Supply

Muscle	Arterial Supply
Medial rectus	Medial (inferior) muscular
Lateral rectus	Lateral (superior) muscular Lacrimal
Superior rectus	Lateral (superior) muscular Lacrimal Supraorbital
Inferior rectus	Medial (inferior) muscular Infraorbital
Superior oblique	Lateral (superior) muscular Supraorbital
Inferior oblique	Medial (inferior) muscular Infraorbital

the maxillary artery shows some variability in both its branching pattern and in its topographic relations with other structures.[29-31] It runs along the pterygopalatine fossa and enters the orbit through the inferior orbital fissure as the **infraorbital artery.** The artery then runs forward along the infraorbital *groove* in the maxillary bone, passes through the infraorbital *canal*, and exits through

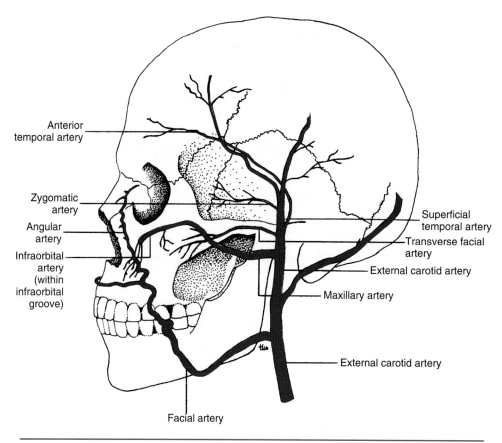

FIGURE 11-9
Branches of external carotid artery that supply ocular adnexa. (Redrawn from Clemente CD: *Anatomy: a regional atlas of the human body*, Munich, 1987, Urban and Schwarzenberg.)

the infraorbital *foramen* (see Figure 11-8). It supplies the lower eyelid and lacrimal sac, and it anastomoses with the angular artery and the dorsonasal artery.[26] While in the infraorbital canal, the infraorbital artery supplies the inferior rectus and inferior oblique muscles and sends some branches to the maxillary sinus and to the teeth of the upper jaw.

The branches from the internal and external carotid arteries that supply the ocular structures, as well as their most common anastomoses, are shown in the flow chart in Figure 11-10.

VEINS OF THE ORBIT

The veins of the orbit have no valves; thus the direction of blood flow may change and is determined by pressure gradients.[5] Over a large part of their path, the veins are embedded within the connective tissue septa that compartmentalize the orbit.[5] Unlike the parallel routes of veins and arteries in most of the body, many orbital veins follow a course that differs from the corresponding arteries.[9,32] The orbit has a single ophthalmic artery but two ophthalmic veins. The superior and inferior

ophthalmic veins primarily drain into the cavernous sinus.

SUPERIOR OPHTHALMIC VEIN

The **superior ophthalmic vein** is formed by the joining of the angular and supraorbital veins within the orbit (Figure 11-11). The supraorbital vein enters the orbit through the supraorbital notch, and the angular vein passes through the orbital septum above the medial palpebral ligament.[33]

The superior ophthalmic vein, the larger of the two ophthalmic veins, runs with the ophthalmic artery and, as it passes posteriorly, receives blood from veins that drain the superior orbital structures. It passes below the superior rectus muscle and crosses the optic nerve to the upper part of the superior orbital fissure, where it leaves the orbit to empty into the cavernous sinus.

The veins that drain into the superior ophthalmic vein are the anterior and posterior ethmoid veins, the muscular veins draining the superior and medial muscles, the lacrimal vein, the central retinal vein, and the superior vortex veins.[33]

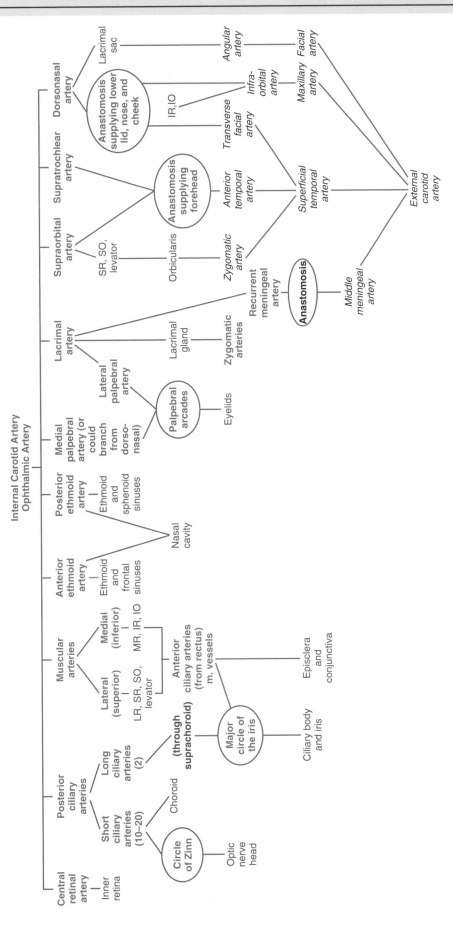

FIGURE 11-10

Flow chart of branches of internal and external carotid arteries that supply orbital structures. Blue indicates branches of internal carotid artery; purple indicates branches of external carotid artery; green indicates target structures. Circles show anastomoses *LR*, Lateral rectus; *SR*, superior rectus; *SO*, superior oblique; *MR*, medial rectus; *IR*, inferior rectus; *IO*, inferior oblique.

FIGURE 11-11
View from lateral side of orbit showing veins draining globe and orbit.

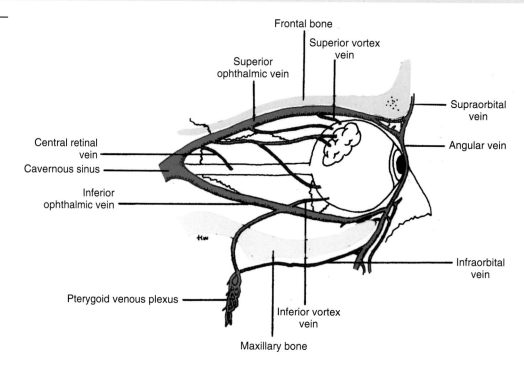

CENTRAL RETINAL VEIN

The venous branches located in the retinal tissue come together and exit the eyeball as a single **central retinal vein.** This vessel leaves the optic nerve approximately 10 to 12 mm behind the lamina cribrosa alongside the central retinal artery. It emerges from the meningeal sheath of the optic nerve and either joins the superior ophthalmic vein or exits the orbit and drains directly into the cavernous sinus.

Clinical Comment: Spontaneous Venous Pulsation

The pressure within the central retinal vein is approximately equal to the intraocular pressure (IOP) and at peak pulse pressure the vessel walls expand slightly. The increase in blood volume can be seen during ophthalmoscopy of the healthy eye as the central retinal vein can be seen to pulsate at its exit through the optic disc. The IOP can vary slightly (1 to 2 mm Hg) with this change in blood volume.[24]

Clinical Comment: Papilledema

The sheaths that surround the optic nerve are continuous with the meningeal sheaths of the brain. The subarachnoid space, located within these layers, contains cerebrospinal fluid. Thus the fluid that surrounds the optic nerve is continuous with the fluid found throughout the cranial cavity. With increased

intracranial pressure, the central retinal vein can be compressed as it crosses the subarachnoid space on its exit from the optic nerve. The central retinal artery is not affected because it has a thicker sheath and is not compressed as easily as is the vein.[34] The resultant blockage causes congestion of the retinal veins and edema of the retina. Edema of the optic nerve head (papilledema) will be evident as blurred disc margins, with hemorrhages sometimes evident as well.

VORTEX VEINS

The **vortex veins** drain the choroid, and usually one of the four or five vortex veins is located in each quadrant (see Figure 11-3). These veins exit the globe 6 mm posterior to the equator.[8] The vortex veins can be seen with an indirect ophthalmoscope and a dilated pupil.

INFERIOR OPHTHALMIC VEIN

The **inferior ophthalmic vein** begins as a plexus near the anterior floor of the orbit. It drains blood from the lower and lateral muscles, the inferior conjunctiva, the lacrimal sac, and the inferior vortex veins.[33] It may form two branches: one that empties into either the superior ophthalmic vein[22,35] or the cavernous sinus and one that empties into the pterygoid venous plexus (see Figure 11-11). The latter branch exits the orbit through the inferior orbital fissure, and the other branch passes through the superior orbital fissure either to join the superior ophthalmic vein or to empty directly into the cavernous sinus.

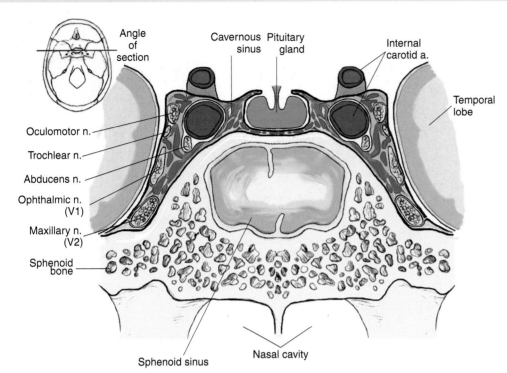

Angle of section

Cavernous sinus   Pituitary gland

Internal carotid a.

Temporal lobe

Oculomotor n.

Trochlear n.

Abducens n.

Ophthalmic n. (V1)

Maxillary n. (V2)

Sphenoid bone

Sphenoid sinus   Nasal cavity

FIGURE 11-12
Coronal section through sphenoid bone and cavernous sinus showing location of internal carotid as it passes through sinus. (From Mathers LH, Chase RA, Dolph J, et al: *Clinical anatomy principles*, St Louis, 1996, Mosby.)

ANTERIOR CILIARY VEINS

The **anterior ciliary veins** receive branches from the conjunctival capillary network and then accompany the anterior ciliary arteries, pierce the sclera, and join with the muscular veins.

INFRAORBITAL VEIN

The **infraorbital vein** is formed by several veins that drain the face. It enters the infraorbital foramen and, along with the infraorbital artery and nerve, passes posteriorly through the infraorbital canal and groove. It receives branches from some structures in the inferior part of the orbit and may communicate with the inferior ophthalmic vein. The infraorbital vein drains into the pterygoid venous plexus (see Figure 11-11).

CAVERNOUS SINUS

The **cavernous sinus** is a relatively large venous channel formed by a splitting of the dura mater on each side of the body of the sphenoid bone. The cavernous sinus extends from the medial end of the superior orbital fissure to the petrous portion of the temporal bone. The internal carotid artery and the abducens nerve are located medially within the sinus, covered by the endothelial lining of the sinus. The oculomotor, ophthalmic, and maxillary nerves are found in the lateral wall of the cavernous sinus (Figure 11-12).

The cavernous sinus drains into the superior petrosal sinus, located along the upper crest of the petrous portion of the temporal bone, and into the inferior petrosal sinus, located in the groove between the petrous portion and the occipital bone. Both drain either directly or indirectly into the internal jugular vein (Figure 11-13).

Clinical Comment: Cavernous Sinus Thrombosis

Infections of the face or orbit can be dangerous. An infected embolus that forms in a facial or orbital vein can readily pass into the cavernous sinus via an ophthalmic vein because these veins do not have valves. A cavernous sinus thrombosis can be fatal and must be treated aggressively with antibiotics.

Clinical Comment: Carotid-Cavernous Sinus Fistula

A CAROTID-CAVERNOUS SINUS FISTULA is an abnormal communication between the internal carotid artery and the cavernous sinus caused by a tear in the artery wall, either traumatic or spontaneous. The sinus communicates directly with the veins of the orbit, so arterial pressure can be transmitted to the ophthalmic veins, which may become pulsatile. If arterial pressure is reduced because of this leak, a decrease in perfusion to ocular tissue will occur.[36,37]

FIGURE 11-13
Superior view of venous sinus drainage of cranium. (From Mathers LH, Chase RA, Dolph J, et al: *Clinical anatomy principles*, St Louis, 1996, Mosby.)

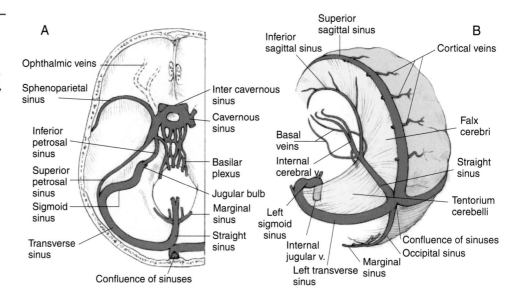

FIGURE 11-13
Superior view of venous sinus drainage of cranium. (From Mathers LH, Chase RA, Dolph J, et al: *Clinical anatomy principles*, St Louis, 1996, Mosby.)

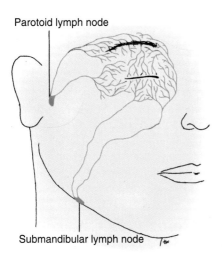

FIGURE 11-14
Lymphatic drainage of the ocular adnexa. medial lids and conjunctiva drain into submandibular lymph node, lateral lids and conjunctiva drain into parotoid lymph node.

LYMPHATIC DRAINAGE

No lymphatic vessels occur in the globe proper; lymphatics are found in the conjunctiva and the eyelids. The lymphatics that drain the medial aspects of the lids and the medial canthal structures (including the lacrimal sac) empty into the **submandibular** lymph nodes. Those that drain the lateral eyelids and the lacrimal gland empty into the **parotid lymph nodes** in the preauricular area[9,35] (Figure 11-14).

EFFECT OF AGING ON OCULAR CIRCULATION

Changes occurring with age differ between individuals. Genetic and environmental factors are contributory, but there are some generalities that can be made. The density of the choroidal and retinal capillary beds and choroidal and retinal vessel diameter all decrease with age.[38] Endothelial dysfunction can occur with age and can result in increased vascular tone, a reduction in vessel distensibility, and a decrease in tissue perfusion.[38] Because there is a coincident decrease in retinal cells, this decrease in blood flow may be a response to decreased metabolic need.[39,40]

REFERENCES

1. Nuza AB, Taner D: Anatomical variations of the intracavernous branches of the internal carotid artery with reference to the relationship of the internal carotid artery and sixth cranial nerve, *Acta Anat (Basel)* 138(3):238, 1990.
2. Hayreh SS, Dass R: The ophthalmic artery. I. Origin and intracranial and intra-canalicular course, *Br J Ophthalmol* 46:65, 1962.
3. Liu XJ: Pathological changes of the optic nerve from compression by the internal carotid artery, *Chung Hua Yen Ko Tsa Chih* 26(6):364, 1990:(abstract).
4. Erdogmus S, Govsa F: Anatomic characteristics of the ophthalmic and posterior ciliary arteries, *J Neuroophthalmol* 28:320–324, 2008.
5. Hayreh SS: The ophthalmic artery. II. Intraorbital course, *Br J Ophthalmol* 46:165, 1962.
6. Koorneef L: Orbital connective tissue. In Jakobiec FA, editor: *Ocular anatomy, embryology, and teratology*, Philadelphia, 1982, Harper & Row, p 835.

7. Hayreh SS: The ophthalmic artery. III. Branches, *Br J Ophthalmol* 46:212, 1962.
8. Warwick R: *Eugene Wolff's anatomy of the eye and orbit*, ed 7, Philadelphia, 1976, Saunders, pp 92, 146, 406.
9. Doxanas MT, Anderson RL: *Clinical orbital anatomy*, Baltimore, 1984, Williams & Wilkins, p 153.
10. Diamond MK: Homologies of the meningeal-orbital arteries of humans: a reappraisal, *J Anat* 178:223, 1991.
11. Yoshii I, Ikeda A: A new look at the blood supply of the retro-ocular space, *Anat Rec* 233:321, 1992.
12. Olver JM: Functional anatomy of the choroidal circulation: methyl methacrylate casting of human choroid, *Eye* 4:262, 1990.
13. Onda E, Cioffi GA, Bacon DR, et al: Microvasculature of the human optic nerve, *Am J Ophthalmol* 120:92, 1995.
14. Hayreh SS: The blood supply of the optic nerve head and the evaluation of it: myth and reality, *Prog Retin Eye Res* 20(5):563, 2001.
15. MacKenzie PJ, Cioffi G: Vascular anatomy of the optic nerve head, *Can J Ophthalmol* 43:308–312, 2008.
16. Hayreh SS: Blood supply of the optic nerve head and its role in optic atrophy, glaucoma, and oedema of the optic disc, *Br J Ophthalmol* 53:721, 1969.
17. Hayreh SS: Pathogenesis of cupping of the optic disc, *Br J Ophthalmol* 58:863, 1974.
18. Borchert MS: Vascular anatomy of the visual system, *Ophthalmol Clin North Am* 9(3):327, 1996.
19. Olver JM, Spalton DJ, McCartney AC: Microvascular study of the retrolaminar optic nerve in man: the possible significance in anterior ischaemic optic neuropathy, *Eye* 4:7, 1990.
20. Hayreh SS: The central artery of the retina: its role in the blood supply of the optic nerve, *Br J Ophthalmol* 47:651, 1963.
21. Justice J Jr, Lehmann RP: Cilioretinal arteries: a study based on a review of stereo fundus photographs and fluorescein angiographic findings, *Arch Ophthalmol* 94:1355, 1976.
22. Catania LJ: *Primary care of the anterior segment*, East Norwalk, Conn, 1988, Appleton & Lange, p 194.
23. Brown SM, Jampol LM: New concepts of regulation of retinal vessel tone, *Arch Ophthalmol* 114:199–204, 1996.
24. Cioffi GA: Granstam E Alm A: Ocular circulation. In Kaufman PL, Alm A, editors: *Adler's physiology of the eye*, ed 10, St Louis, 2003, Elsevier.
25. Kilgaar JF, dJensen PK: The choroid and optic nerve head. In Fischbanrg J, editor: *In The Biology of the eye*, Amsterdam, 2006, Elsevier, pp 273–290.
26. Tucker SM, Lindberg JV: Vascular anatomy of the eyelids, *Ophthalmology* 101:1118, 1994.
27. Berkow R, editor: *The Merck manual*, ed 14, Rahway, NJ, 1982, Merck, p 557.
28. Sires BS, Gausas R, Cook BE Jr, et al: Orbit. In Kaufman PL, Alm A, editors: *Adler's physiology of the eye*, ed 10, St Louis, 2003, Elsevier.
29. Morton AL, Khan A: Internal maxillary artery variability in the pterygopalatine fossa, *Otolaryngol Head Neck Surg* 104(2):204, 1991.
30. Ortug G, Moriggl B: The topography of the maxillary artery within the infratemporal fossa, *Anat Anz* 172(3):197, 1991:(abstract).
31. Pretterklieber ML, Skopakoff C, Mayr R: The human maxillary artery reinvestigated: topographical relations in the infratemporal fossa, *Acta Anat (Basel)* 142(4):281, 1991.
32. Murakami K, Murakami G, Komatsu A, et al: Gross anatomical study of veins in the orbit, *Nippon Ganka Gakkai Zasshi* 95(1):31, 1991:(abstract).
33. Cheung N, McNab AA: Venous anatomy of the orbit, *Invest Ophthalmol Vis Sci* 44(3):988, 2003.
34. Whiting AS, Johnson LN: Papilledema: clinical clues and differential diagnosis, *Am Fam Physician* 45(3):125, 1992.
35. Wobig JL: The blood vessels and lymphatics of the orbit and lid. In Wobig JL, Reeh MJ, Wirtschafter JD, editors: *Ophthalmic anatomy*, San Francisco, 1981, American Academy of Ophthalmology, p 77.
36. De Keizer R: Carotid-cavernous and orbital arteriovenous fistulas: ocular features, diagnostic and hemodynamic considerations in relation to visual impairment and morbidity, *Orbit* 22(2):121, 2003.
37. Bhatti MT, Peters KR: A red eye and then a really red eye, *Surv Ophthalmol* 48(2):224, 2003.
38. Ehrlich R, Kheradiya NS, Winston DM, et al: Age-related ocular vascular changes, *Graefes Arch Clin Exp Ophthalmol* 247:583–591, 2009.
39. Grunwald JE, Hariprasad SM, DuPont J: Effect of aging on foveolar choroidal circulation, *Arch Ophthalmol* 116:150, 1998.
40. Lam AK, Chan S, Chan H, et al: The effect of age on ocular blood supply determined by pulsatile ocular blood flow and color Doppler ultrasonography, *Optom Vis Sci* 89(4):305, 2003.

The orbital structures are innervated by cranial nerves (CNs) II, III, IV, V, VI, and VII (Table 12-1). Motor functions of the striated muscles are controlled by CN III, the oculomotor nerve; CN IV, the trochlear nerve; CN VI, the abducens nerve; and CN VII, the facial nerve. CN V, the trigeminal nerve, carries the sensory supply from the orbital structures. CN II, the optic nerve, carries visual information and is discussed in Chapter 13. This chapter discusses sensory and motor innervation of the orbit, including pathways, functions, and presenting signs of dysfunction.

THE NERVOUS SYSTEM

Information comes into the central nervous system (CNS) via afferent fibers. Afferent sensory fibers usually have specialized nerve endings that respond to such sensations as touch, pressure, temperature, and pain.

Information processing occurs within the brain or spinal cord and involves communication between different areas of the CNS through fiber tracts. A fiber tract also may be called a fasciculus, a peduncle, or a brachium. The portion of the cranial nerve from the cell body in the nucleus to the exit from the brain stem is the fascicular part of the nerve.

Efferent fibers, either somatic or autonomic, carry information from the CNS to the target structures: muscles, organs, or glands. The efferent pathway in the somatic system generally consists of a fiber that runs the distance from the CNS to the target muscle. The autonomic pathway generally has a synapse within its efferent pathway (see Chapter 14).

AFFERENT PATHWAY: ORBITAL SENSORY INNERVATION

The eye is richly supplied with sensory nerves that carry sensations of touch, pressure, warmth, cold, and pain. Sensations from the cornea, iris, conjunctiva, and sclera consist primarily of pain; even light touching of the cornea is registered as irritation or pain.[1]

TRIGEMINAL NERVE

The fibers of the trigeminal nerve (CN V) serving ocular structures are sensory and originate in the innervated structures. The description of the pathways of these nerves begins at the involved structures and follows the nerves as they join to become larger nerves, come together in the ganglion of the fifth cranial nerve, and then exit the ganglion and enter the pons. It is hoped that this presentation, although unconventional, will enable the reader to keep in mind the actual direction of the action potential, and thus the information flow, in these fibers. Figure 12-1 shows the major branches and paths of the trigeminal nerve within the orbit.

Ophthalmic Division of Trigeminal Nerve

Nasociliary Nerve

Sensory fibers from the structures of the medial canthal area—caruncle, canaliculi, lacrimal sac, medial aspect of the eyelids, and skin at the side of the nose —join to form the **infratrochlear nerve**. This nerve penetrates the orbital septum, enters the orbit below the trochlea, and runs along the upper border of the medial rectus muscle, becoming the nasociliary nerve as other branches join it (see Figure 12-1).

Sensory fibers from the skin along the center of the nose, the nasal mucosa, and the ethmoid sinuses form the **anterior ethmoid nerve;** fibers from the ethmoid sinuses and the sphenoid sinus form the **posterior ethmoid** nerve. The ethmoid nerves enter the orbit with their companion arteries through foramina within the frontoethmoid suture.[2] Both nerves join the nasociliary nerve as it runs along the medial aspect of the orbit (see Figure 12-1).

Corneal sensory innervation is dense, estimated to be 400 times as dense as other epithelial tissue innervation.[3] Three networks of nerves are formed. One is located in the corneal epithelium, another (the subepithelial plexus) is in the anterior stroma, and the third, the stromal plexus, is in the middle of the stroma[4] (Figure 12-2). No nerves are found in posterior stroma, Descemet's membrane, or endothelium. The fibers

Table 12-1   Cranial Nerves to Orbital Structures

Cranial Nerve	Origin	Destination	Function
II. Optic	Retinal ganglion cells	Lateral geniculate body	Sensory: sight
III. Oculomotor, inferior division	Midbrain	Medial rectus muscle Inferior rectus muscle Inferior oblique muscle Ciliary ganglion	Motor: adduction Depression, adduction, extorsion Elevation, abduction, extorsion Parasympathetic: motor to iris sphincter and ciliary muscle for miosis and accommodation
III: Oculomotor, superior division	Midbrain	Superior rectus muscle Superior palpebral levator muscle	Elevation, adduction, intorsion Motor: elevation of eyelid
IV: Trochlear	Midbrain	Superior oblique muscle	Motor: depression, abduction, intorsion
VI: Abducens	Pons	Lateral rectus muscle	Motor: abduction
VII: Facial	Pons	Frontalis, procerus, corrugator, and orbicularis muscles Sphenopalatine ganglion	Motor: facial expressions, closure of eyelids Parasympathetic: secretomotor to lacrimal gland for lacrimation

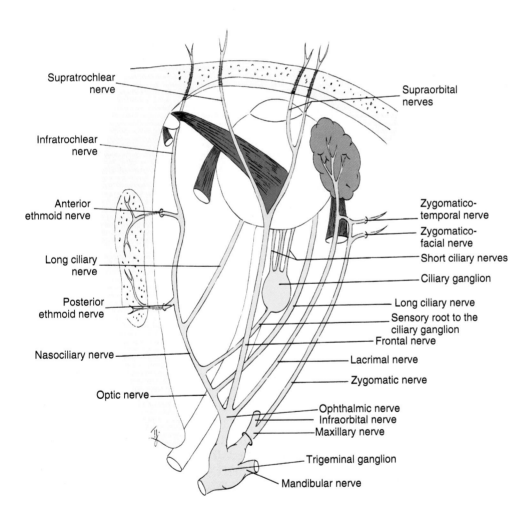

Supratrochlear nerve

Infratrochlear nerve

Anterior ethmoid nerve

Long ciliary nerve

Posterior ethmoid nerve

Nasociliary nerve

Optic nerve

Supraorbital nerves

Zygomatico-temporal nerve

Zygomatico-facial nerve

Short ciliary nerves

Ciliary ganglion

Long ciliary nerve

Sensory root to the ciliary ganglion

Frontal nerve

Lacrimal nerve

Zygomatic nerve

Ophthalmic nerve
Infraorbital nerve
Maxillary nerve

Trigeminal ganglion

Mandibular nerve

FIGURE 12-1
Orbit viewed from above showing branches of ophthalmic nerve.

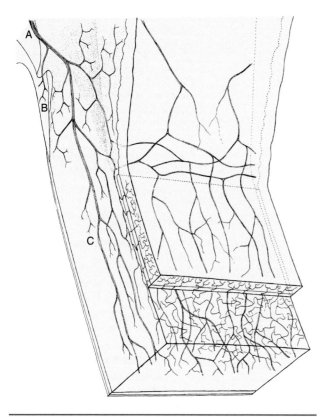

FIGURE 12-2
Innervation of limbus and cornea. Long ciliary nerve (**A**) supplies limbal region, then sends branches into cornea. Nerves also supply trabecular meshwork (**B**) and region of Schlemm canal. Note paucity of nerves in deep cornea (**C**) and their absence in region of Descemet membrane. (From Hogan MJ, Alvarado JA, Weddell JE, editors: *Histology of the human eye,* Philadelphia, 1971, Saunders.)

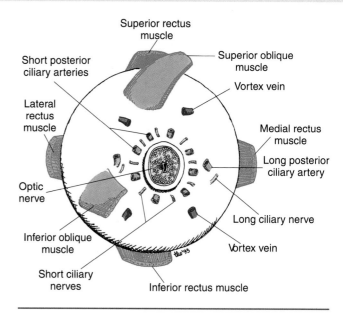

FIGURE 12-3
Posterior sclera. Posterior portion of globe showing optic nerve passing through posterior scleral foramen; long and short ciliary arteries and nerves passing through posterior apertures; and vortex veins passing through middle apertures.

Clinical Comment: (Scleral) Nerve Loops (of Axenfeld)

A slight variation can occur in the pathway of the long ciliary nerve in which the fibers loop into the sclera from the suprachoroidal space, forming a dome-shaped elevation about 2 mm from the limbus on either the nasal or the temporal side. Often this raised area is pigmented, usually blue or black, and should be differentiated from a melanoma.[8] The nerve loop may be painful when touched, a characteristic that should aid in its diagnosis.[5]

from these plexus come together in peripheral stroma and radiate out into the limbus as 70 to 80 branches; they become myelinated in the last 2 mm of the cornea.[5-7]

Some of these branches join with nerves from other anterior segment structures to form two **long ciliary nerves.** These long ciliary nerves, one on the lateral side and one on the medial side of the globe, course between the choroid and sclera to the back of the eye, where they leave the globe at points approximately 3 mm on each side of the optic nerve (Figure 12-3). (In addition to afferent fibers, the long ciliary nerves transmit sympathetic fibers to the dilator muscle of the iris.) The two long ciliary nerves then join the nasociliary nerve.

The other branches radiating from the cornea into the limbus join other sensory nerves from the anterior segment; they enter the choroid, join with the choroidal nerves, then course to the back of the eye, where they leave as 6 to 10 **short ciliary nerves** (see Figure 12-3). The short ciliary nerves exit the sclera in a ring around the optic nerve in company with the short posterior ciliary arteries and enter the ciliary ganglion (see Figure 12-1). The sensory fibers do not synapse but pass through the ganglion, leaving as the **sensory root of the ciliary ganglion,** which then joins the nasociliary nerve. (The short ciliary nerves carry sympathetic and parasympathetic fibers in addition to sensory fibers.)

Thus, the **nasociliary nerve** is formed by the joining of the infratrochlear nerve, the anterior and posterior ethmoid nerves, the long ciliary nerves, and the sensory root of the ciliary ganglion (see Figure 12-1). The nasociliary nerve exits the orbit by passing through the oculomotor foramen *within* the common tendinous ring and the superior orbital fissure into the cranial cavity.

Clinical Comment: Herpes Zoster

HERPES ZOSTER is an acute CNS infection caused by the varicella-zoster virus. Signs and symptoms include pain and rash in the distribution area supplied by the affected sensory nerves.[9] It is believed that the virus lies dormant in a sensory ganglion and, on becoming activated, migrates down the sensory pathway to the skin.[10] An eruption of herpes zoster is more common in elderly persons but may occur at any age and may be related to a delayed hypersensitivity reaction.[11] Approximately 10% of all cases affect the ophthalmic division of the trigeminal nerve.[12] Involvement of the tip of the nose often indicates that the eye will also be involved, reflecting the distribution of the nasociliary branches. This association of ocular involvement with zoster affecting the tip of the nose is the Hutchinson sign.[13]

Frontal Nerve

Sensory fibers from the skin and muscles of the forehead and upper eyelid come together and form the **supratrochlear nerve**. This nerve enters the orbit by piercing the superior medial corner of the orbital septum (Figure 12-4).

Sensory fibers from the skin and muscles of the forehead and upper eyelid form a second nerve, the **supraorbital nerve**, lateral to the supratrochlear nerve. The supraorbital nerve enters the orbit as one or two branches: one branch enters through the supraorbital notch, accompanying the supraorbital artery. The supraorbital nerve joins the supratrochlear nerve midway in the orbit and forms the **frontal nerve** (see Figure 12-1). The frontal nerve courses back through the orbit between the levator muscle and the periorbita, exiting the orbit through the superior orbital fissure *above* the common tendinous ring.

Lacrimal Nerve

Sensory fibers from the lateral aspect of the upper eyelid and temple area come together and enter the lacrimal gland; they join the sensory fibers that serve the gland itself to form the **lacrimal nerve.** The lacrimal nerve leaves the gland and runs posteriorly

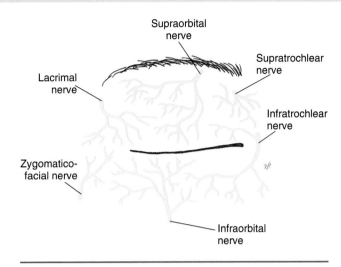

FIGURE 12-4
Sensory innervation to upper and lower eyelids.

along the upper border of the lateral rectus muscle (see Figure 12-1). It receives a branch from the zygomatic nerve containing the autonomic innervation of the lacrimal gland. The lacrimal nerve exits the orbit through the superior orbital fissure *above* the muscle cone.

Ophthalmic Nerve Formation

After exiting the orbit, the nasociliary nerve, the lacrimal nerve, and the frontal nerve join and form the **ophthalmic division of the trigeminal nerve** (see Figure 12-1). The ophthalmic nerve then enters the lateral wall of the cavernous sinus, coursing between the two dural layers.[14] While in the wall of the sinus the nerve receives sensory fibers from the oculomotor, trochlear, and abducens nerves. Some of these fibers probably carry proprioceptive information from the extraocular muscles.[15]

Maxillary Division of Trigeminal Nerve

Infraorbital Nerve

The **infraorbital nerve**, formed by sensory fibers from the cheek, upper lip, and lower eyelid, enters the maxillary bone through the infraorbital *foramen* (Figure 12-5). It runs posteriorly through the infraorbital *canal* and *groove*; while it is in the maxillary bone, branches join from the upper teeth and maxillary sinus. As the nerve leaves the infraorbital groove it exits the orbit through the inferior orbital fissure and joins other fibers in forming the maxillary nerve.

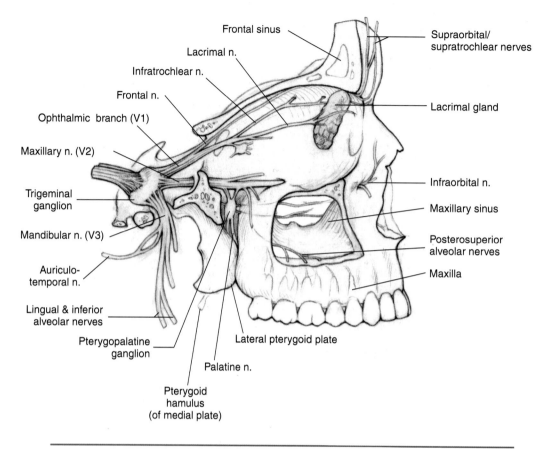

FIGURE 12-5
Three divisions of trigeminal nerve. (From Mathers LH, Chase RA, Dolph J, et al: *Clinical anatomy principles*, St Louis, 1996, Mosby.)

Clinical Comment: Referred Pain

> *REFERRED PAIN is pain felt in an area remote from the actual site of involvement; however, the two areas usually are connected by a sensory nerve network. Frequently, the pathways of the trigeminal nerve are involved in referred pain. A common example is a momentary severe bilateral frontal headache sometimes experienced when an individual eats ice cream.[5] An abscessed tooth can cause pain described by a patient as ocular pain and should be suspected when no orbital cause for the pain can be found. This situation likely occurs because the overload of sensation carried by the infraorbital nerve from the upper teeth is interpreted by the brain as coming from another area also served by the trigeminal nerve.*

Zygomatic Nerve

Sensory fibers from the lateral aspect of the forehead enter the orbit through a foramen in the zygomatic bone as the zygomaticotemporal nerve. Fibers from the lateral aspect of the cheek and lower eyelid enter the orbit through a foramen in the zygomatic bone as the zygomaticofacial nerve.[13] These two nerves join to become the **zygomatic nerve** and course along the lateral orbital wall, exiting the orbit through the inferior orbital fissure and joining with the maxillary nerve (see Figure 12-1).

Maxillary Nerve Formation

Having been formed by the joining of the infraorbital nerve, the zygomatic nerve, and nerves from the roof of the mouth, upper teeth and gums, and mucous membranes of the cheek, the **maxillary nerve** traverses the area between the maxilla and the sphenoid bone. As it passes near the pterygopalatine fossa, it receives some autonomic fibers from the pterygopalatine ganglion (see Figure 12-5). (These autonomic fibers are destined for the lacrimal gland and are discussed in Chapter 14.) The maxillary nerve enters the skull through the foramen rotundum.

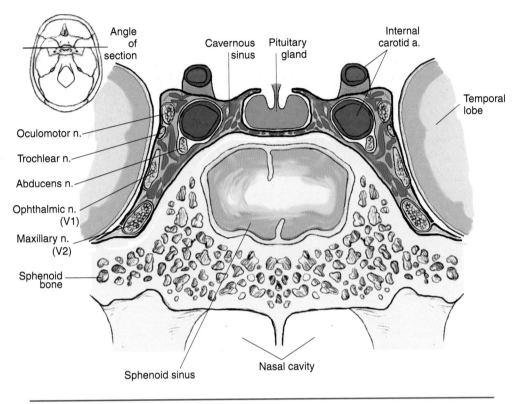

FIGURE 12-6
Detailed cross section of cavernous sinus. (From Mathers LH, Chase RA, Dolph J, et al: *Clinical anatomy principles*, St Louis, 1996, Mosby.)

Mandibular Division of Trigeminal Nerve

The mandibular nerve innervates the lower face and contains both sensory and motor fibers. It enters the skull via the foramen ovale.

TRIGEMINAL NERVE FORMATION

As the ophthalmic and maxillary divisions enter the skull, they run posteriorly within the lateral wall of the cavernous sinus (Figure 12-6).[16,17] The mandibular division lies just below the cavernous sinus. The sensory fibers from the three divisions enter the **trigeminal ganglion (gasserian ganglion, semilunar ganglion),** where they synapse. The ganglion, flattened and semilunar in shape, is located lateral to the internal carotid artery and the posterior portion of the cavernous sinus. The motor fibers of the mandibular division, which innervate the

muscles of mastication, pass along the lower edge of the ganglion.[18] Only the sensory fibers synapse within the ganglion.

The fibers leave the trigeminal ganglion and enter the lateral aspect of the pons as either the sensory root or the motor root of the **trigeminal nerve.** The sensory root carries information from the structures of the face and head, including all orbital structures. After entering the brain stem, these fibers form an ascending and a descending tract, both terminating in sensory nuclei of the trigeminal nerve (Figure 12-7). The ascending tract terminates in the **principal sensory nucleus** in the pons; it registers the sensations of touch and pressure.[1] The descending tract, which carries pain and temperature sensations, courses through the pons and medulla to the **elongated nucleus of the spinal tract**.[1] The tract extends into the second cervical segment of the spinal cord.[19] Information from the trigeminal nuclei is relayed to the thalamus.

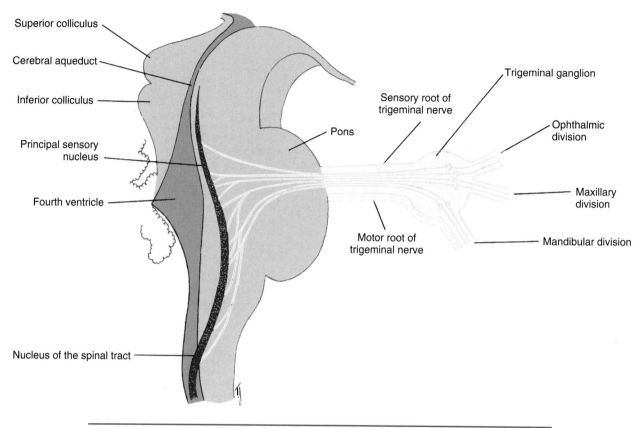

FIGURE 12-7
Sagittal section through brain stem showing divisions, ganglion, motor, and sensory roots, and nuclei of cranial nerve V.

Clinical Comment: Oculocardiac Reflex

THE OCULOCARDIAC REFLEX consists of bradycardia (slowed heartbeat), nausea, and faintness and can be elicited by pressure on the globe or stretch on the extraocular muscles (e.g., during ocular surgery).[20-22] Fibers from the trigeminal spinal nucleus project into the reticular formation near the vagus nerve nuclei and can activate vagus synapses, precipitating this reflex. The motor aspect of the reflex can be blocked by retrobulbar anesthesia or intravenous or intramuscular atropine.[1,13,23,24]

EFFERENT PATHWAY: MOTOR NERVES

The cranial nerves that supply striated muscles of the orbit and adnexa are the oculomotor nerve, the trochlear nerve, the abducens nerve, and the facial nerve.

OCULOMOTOR NERVE: CRANIAL NERVE III

The **oculomotor nerve** innervates the superior rectus, medial rectus, inferior rectus, inferior oblique, and superior palpebral levator muscles. It also provides a route along which the autonomic fibers travel to innervate the iris sphincter muscle, the ciliary muscle, and the smooth muscles of the eyelid.

Oculomotor Nucleus

The **oculomotor nucleus** is located in the midbrain, at the level of the superior colliculus, ventral to the cerebral aqueduct, and dorsal to the medial longitudinal fasciculus (Figure 12-8).[28] It extends in a column from the posterior edge of the floor of the third ventricle to the trochlear nucleus.[2,13]

A definitive area or subnucleus within the oculomotor nucleus controls each muscle. The proposed

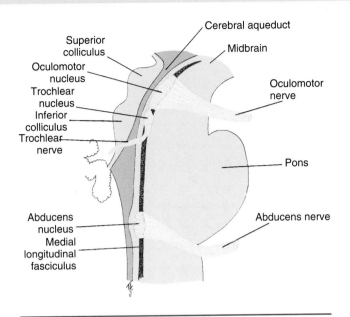

Cerebral aqueduct
Superior colliculus
Midbrain
Oculomotor nucleus
Oculomotor nerve
Trochlear nucleus
Inferior colliculus
Trochlear nerve
Pons
Abducens nucleus
Medial longitudinal fasciculus
Abducens nerve

FIGURE 12-8
Sagittal section through brainstem showing trigeminal, oculomotor, trochlear, abducens, and facial nuclei.

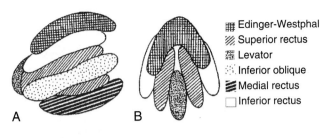

Edinger-Westphal
Superior rectus
Levator
Inferior oblique
Medial rectus
Inferior rectus

A   B

FIGURE 12-9
Oculomotor nerve nuclei. **A,** Lateral view. **B,** Dorsal view.

arrangement of the subnuclei are postulated primarily on the basis of animal models.[23,25-27] The nucleus for the medial rectus is located toward the lower border of the oculomotor nucleus; the inferior rectus nucleus lies toward the upper border, with the nucleus for the inferior oblique between. The nucleus of the superior rectus lies in the medial and caudal two thirds of the oculomotor nucleus. Each of these subnuclei are found in the right and left oculomotor nucleus. The nucleus for the levator muscle is single and is located centrally in the caudal area (Figure 12-9).

Fibers to the inferior rectus, inferior oblique, and medial rectus muscles supply the *ipsilateral eye;* fibers innervating the superior rectus muscle decussate and supply the *contralateral eye.* The decussating fibers pass through the opposite superior rectus nucleus; thus damage to the right oculomotor nucleus might have bilateral superior rectus muscle involvement.[27-30] The centrally placed caudal nucleus provides innervation for *both* levator muscles.

An autonomic nucleus, the accessory third nerve nucleus (Edinger-Westphal nucleus), supplies parasympathetic innervation to the ciliary and iris sphincter muscles. It is located in the rostral, ventral portion of the oculomotor nucleus[30,31] (see Figure 12-9).

Oculomotor Nerve Pathway

Fibers from each of the individual nuclei join, forming the fascicular part of the nerve that passes through the red nucleus and the decussating fibers of the superior cerebellar peduncle.[32] These fibers emerge just medial to the cerebral peduncles and within the interpeduncular

fossa on the anterior aspect of the midbrain as the **oculomotor nerve**. The nerve passes between the superior cerebellar and posterior cerebral arteries as it runs forward, lateral to, and slightly inferior to the posterior communicating artery of the circle of Willis (Figure 12-10). The nerve pierces the roof of the cavernous sinus and runs within the two dural layers of its lateral wall above the trochlear nerve[2,14,16] (see Figure 12-6). While in the cavernous sinus, the oculomotor nerve sends small sensory branches (likely proprioceptive) to the ophthalmic nerve and receives sympathetic fibers from the plexus around the internal carotid artery.[2,19]

The oculomotor nerve exits the sinus and enters the orbit through the superior orbital fissure, having divided into superior and inferior divisions; both divisions are located *within* the oculomotor foramen. The superior branch runs medially above the optic nerve and enters the superior rectus on its inferior surface; additional fibers either pierce the muscle or pass around its border to innervate the levator[14,33] (Figure 12-11).

The inferior branch runs below the optic nerve and divides into three branches. One branch enters the medial rectus on its lateral surface, and one enters the inferior rectus on its upper surface (see Figure 12-11). The third branch gives off parasympathetic fibers that form the parasympathetic root extending to the ciliary ganglion; then it runs along the lateral border of the inferior rectus, crossing it to enter the inferior oblique muscle near its midpoint.[5,14,34,35]

TROCHLEAR NERVE: CRANIAL NERVE IV

The **trochlear nerve** innervates the superior oblique muscle.

Trochlear Nucleus

The **trochlear nucleus** is located in the midbrain, at the level of the inferior colliculus, anterior to the cerebral aqueduct, dorsal to the medial longitudinal

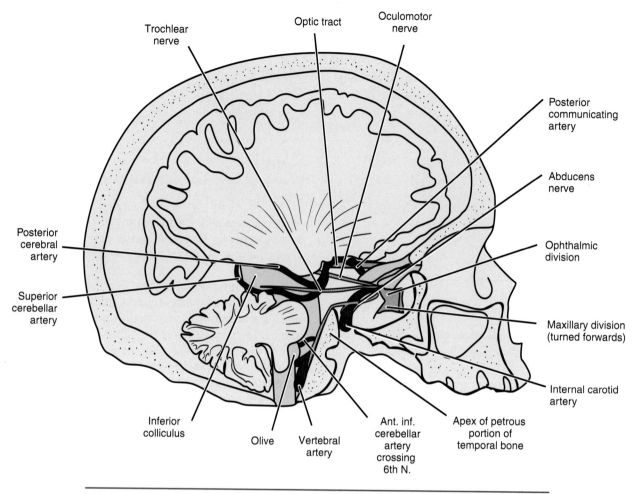

FIGURE 12-10

Sagittal section through brain showing relationships among cranial nerves III, IV, and VI and neighboring blood vessels.

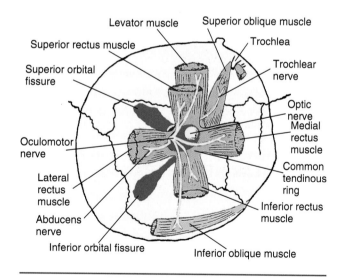

FIGURE 12-11

Orbital apex with the globe removed, showing the origin of the rectus muscles at the annulus of Zinn and the relationship between superior orbital fissure and common tendinous ring.

fasciculus, and below the oculomotor nucleus[32] (see Figure 12-8). The fibers travel dorsally and decussate. CN IV is the only cranial nerve to cross; thus the trochlear nucleus innervates the *contralateral* superior oblique muscle.

Trochlear Nerve Pathway

Of the cranial nerves, the **trochlear nerve** is the only one that leaves the dorsal aspect of the CNS. It is the most slender of the cranial nerves, and its attachment is very delicate. (The small diameter of the nerve probably reflects the fact that it supplies only one muscle, the most slender of the extraocular muscles.) As the trochlear nerve emerges from the dorsal midbrain immediately below the inferior colliculus, it decussates and curves around the cerebral peduncle at the upper border of the pons, approximately paralleling the superior cerebellar and posterior cerebral arteries. It passes between these two vessels and runs forward lateral to the oculomotor nerve (see Figure 12-10).

The trochlear nerve enters the wall of the cavernous sinus and lies between the oculomotor nerve and the ophthalmic division of the trigeminal nerve (see Figure 12-6).[5,16] While in the sinus, the trochlear nerve sends sensory fibers (likely proprioceptive) to the ophthalmic nerve. It enters the orbit through the superior orbital fissure *above* the common tendinous ring, outside the muscle cone (see Figure 12-11). The trochlear nerve runs with the frontal nerve to the medial side of the orbit above the levator and superior rectus muscles and enters the upper surface of the superior oblique muscle.[10]

ABDUCENS NERVE: CRANIAL NERVE VI

The **abducens** nerve innervates the lateral rectus muscle.

Abducens Nucleus

The **abducens nucleus** is located near the inferior dorsal midline of the pons beside the floor of the fourth ventricle (see Figure 12-8). The fibers from the nucleus pass through the pons and lie adjacent to the corticospinal tract for part of their path[32]; they exit in the groove between the pons and the medulla oblongata. The abducens nucleus also contains *internuclear neurons* that communicate with the nucleus for the *contralateral* medial rectus muscle in the oculomotor complex via the medial longitudinal fasciculus.[36] This is the pathway for conjugate horizontal eye movements. This pathway receives information from higher CNS centers, including the paramedial pontine reticular formation, the cerebellum, and the vestibular nucleus. Thus coordinated movement of the ipsilateral lateral rectus muscle and the contralateral medial rectus muscle results in conjugate horizontal eye movement.[36]

Abducens Nerve Pathway

In its long, tortuous, intracranial course, the **abducens nerve** runs along the occipital bone at the base of the skull and up along the posterior slope of the petrous portion of the temporal bone, makes a sharp bend over the petrous ridge (see Figure 12-10), and enters the cavernous sinus.[5,13,37] Within the sinus it lies near the lateral wall of the internal carotid artery[6,38] (see Figure 12-6). Small sympathetic branches leave the internal carotid plexus and travel with the abducens nerve. The abducens carries these autonomic fibers and sensory fibers, which are possibly proprioceptive, to the ophthalmic division of the trigeminal nerve.[38] The abducens nerve enters the orbit through the superior orbital fissure *within* the common tendinous ring and innervates the lateral rectus muscle on the medial surface (see Figure 12-11).

SUPERIOR ORBITAL FISSURE

The trochlear, frontal, and lacrimal nerves as well as the superior ophthalmic vein are located in the superior orbital fissure *above* the muscle cone. The superior and inferior divisions of the oculomotor nerve, the abducens nerve, and the nasociliary nerve are located *within* the superior orbital fissure and the common tendinous ring. The inferior ophthalmic vein lies *below* the fissure and the tendinous ring (see Figure 8-15).

CONTROL OF EYE MOVEMENTS

Communication among areas of the CNS is necessary to produce controlled and coordinated eye movements. The **corticonuclear tract** contains fibers that travel from the cerebral hemispheres to the nuclei of CNs III, IV, and VI; the **tectobulbar tract** connects the superior colliculus to the CN III, IV, and VI nuclei. The **medial longitudinal fasciculus** extends from the midbrain into the spinal cord and connects the vestibular nucleus, the oculomotor nucleus, the abducens nucleus, and the trochlear nucleus, providing a connection between eye movement control and the vestibular apparatus (see Figure 12-8).

FACIAL NERVE: CRANIAL NERVE VII

The **facial nerve** has two roots: the large motor root innervates the facial muscles, and the smaller root contains sensory and parasympathetic fibers. The sensory fibers carry taste sensations from the tongue. The parasympathetic nerves supply secretomotor fibers to various glands of the face; those supplying the lacrimal gland are discussed in Chapter 14.

Facial Nucleus

The **motor nucleus of the facial nerve** is located in the reticular formation of the pons. The upper segment of the nucleus supplies the frontalis, procerus, corrugator superciliaris, and orbicularis muscles, and the lower segment supplies the remaining facial muscles.[39,40]

Facial Nerve Pathway

The fibers leave the facial nucleus, arch around the abducens nucleus, and emerge as the **facial nerve** from the brain stem at the lower border of the pons. The facial nerve enters the internal acoustic foramen in the petrous portion of the temporal bone and runs through a canal in the bone. While in the temporal bone, parasympathetic

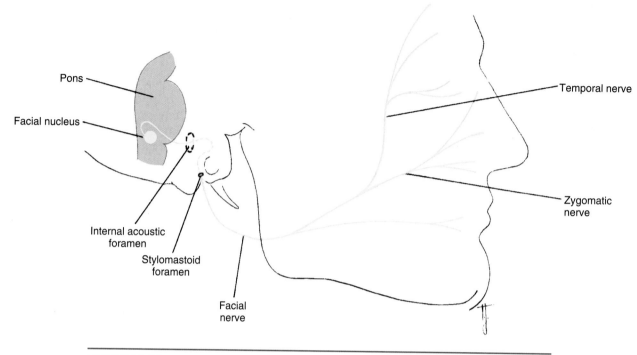

Pons

Facial nucleus

Temporal nerve

Zygomatic nerve

Internal acoustic foramen

Stylomastoid foramen

Facial nerve

FIGURE 12-12
Facial nerve pathway. Motor pathway of facial nerve to facial muscles of orbit.

fibers en route to the lacrimal gland are given off as the greater petrosal nerve.[39,40] The motor fibers of the facial nerve emerge through the stylomastoid foramen, pass below the external auditory canal, travel over the mandibular ramus, and divide into several branches (Figure 12-12). The upper two — the temporal and zygomatic branches — supply the frontalis, procerus, corrugator, and orbicularis muscles.

The following Clinical Comments discuss damage to the cranial nerves, specifically the oculomotor, trochlear, and abducens nerves, caused by involvement of adjacent cranial and orbital structures and the resulting clinical presentation.

Clinical Comment: Cranial Nerve Damage

Injury to sensory cranial nerve fibers results in anesthesia, a loss of sensation in the innervated area. Injury to a cranial motor nerve causes either a partial loss (paresis) or a total loss (paralysis) of muscle function. Paresis or paralysis of an extraocular muscle can result in diplopia if the involvement is acquired; in congenital involvement, diplopia usually is

not a complaint because the brain has learned to disregard the double image, resulting in suppression.

Nerve fibers can be ischemic, damaged by a compromised blood supply caused by vascular diseases (e.g., hypertension, atherosclerosis, diabetes mellitus) or by space-occupying lesions (e.g., aneurysms, hemorrhages, tumors) that exert pressure on the nerve fibers. The location of the involvement will influence the presenting signs and symptoms.

In some studies of isolated extraocular muscle nerve paralysis, the sixth cranial nerve is reported to be affected most often, and the fourth cranial nerve affected least often.[41-43] The tortuosity and length of the abducens nerve make it susceptible to compression and stretching injuries and may explain why it is damaged so frequently.[16]

A number of clinical signs and symptoms accompany damage to the motor nerves that innervate the extraocular muscles. Muscle paresis or paralysis will be evident in testing ocular motility (as described in Chapter 10). In acquired extraocular muscle impairment, a patient often attempts to minimize diplopia by carrying the head in a compensatory position. If a horizontal deviation is present, the head will be turned to the right or left. With a vertical deviation, the head is raised or lowered, and if a torsional deviation occurs the head is tilted toward the shoulder usually away from the involved side.[35] With right superior oblique involvement the head may be turned to the left, positioned down, and tilted toward the left shoulder[44,45] (Figure 12-13).

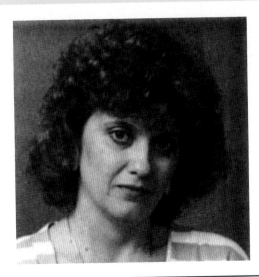

FIGURE 12-13
Patient tilts head toward the left shoulder and turns head to the left and down, resulting from right superior oblique dysfunction. (From Eskridge JB: Evaluation and diagnosis of incomitant ocular deviations, *J Am Optom Assoc* 60[5]:378, 1989.)

Clinical Comment: Oculomotor Damage

MIDBRAIN INVOLVEMENT

A lesion in the midbrain can affect the entire oculomotor nucleus or selectively affect only some subnuclei; however, such selective damage is unusual.[28] If the lesion affects the entire oculomotor nucleus, the muscles involved are the ipsilateral medial rectus, inferior rectus, and inferior oblique, contralateral superior rectus, and both levators. The ipsilateral superior rectus might be involved as well because the decussating fibers pass through the contralateral superior rectus nucleus.[28,32] Dilation of the pupil may also be present. The trochlear nucleus is near the oculomotor nucleus, and if it too is involved, the contralateral superior oblique muscle will be affected. The clinical presentation would show the ipsilateral eye positioned out in primary position and only able to move in as far as the midline. The contralateral eye would be unable to elevate in abduction and unable to depress in adduction.

INTRACRANIAL INVOLVEMENT

The oculomotor nerve lies near several blood vessels in its intracranial path and frequently is affected by an aneurysm of the posterior communicating artery.[46] An aneurysm of the superior cerebellar artery or the posterior cerebral artery could also impinge on the nerve, damaging fibers.

Once the oculomotor nerve exits the midbrain, all its fibers supply the ipsilateral eye, and the dysfunction is unilateral. Damage to the nerve results in ptosis because of levator muscle paralysis; in primary position, the eye is positioned out because of the unopposed action of the superior oblique and lateral rectus muscles (Figure 12-14, A and B). (Because the superior oblique muscle is unaffected, the eye also should be positioned down, but clinically this is not always evident.[47]) The eye cannot adduct (Figure 12-14, D) and,

in the abducted position, cannot move up or down (Figure 12-14, E and F).[2] If injury involves the cerebral peduncles, a contralateral hemiparesis will be present.[48] In paralysis of the iris sphincter and ciliary muscle, the pupil will be dilated, and accommodation will not occur.

Incomplete lesions of the oculomotor nerve are possible. In external ophthalmoplegia, the extraocular muscles are paralyzed and the intrinsic muscles (those to the iris sphincter and the ciliary muscle) are spared; in internal ophthalmoplegia the internal muscles are paralyzed and the extraocular muscles are spared. As the oculomotor nerve exits the midbrain, the parasympathetic fibers are superficial, and as the nerve nears the orbit, the parasympathetic fibers move into the center of the nerve and therefore are better protected in compressive lesions. The parasympathetic fibers are often spared in ischemic lesions, accounting for normal pupillary responses usually seen with diabetic ophthalmoplegia.[28,49-51] Third nerve palsies that include a dilated pupil are highly suspicious of a compressive lesion.

CAVERNOUS SINUS INVOLVEMENT

The lateral wall of the cavernous sinus contains the oculomotor nerve as well as the trochlear, ophthalmic, and maxillary nerves. A lesion that affects all these nerves would leave only the lateral rectus muscle still functioning. The eye would be positioned out in primary gaze and could move only from the lateral position to the midline. Anesthesia of the facial areas served by the ophthalmic and maxillary nerves would be present in addition to the impaired ocular motility.

ORBITAL INVOLVEMENT

Both divisions of the oculomotor nerve are located within the muscle cone, together with the abducens and nasociliary nerves. A retrobulbar tumor or inflammation involving these nerves would leave only the superior oblique muscle functional. In primary position, the eye would be positioned downward and outward slightly and would be fairly immobile. Corneal sensitivity could be decreased because of nasociliary nerve involvement.

ABERRANT REGENERATION OF THE OCULOMOTOR NERVE

After injury, the brain may attempt to repair a nerve, and some attempts may be misdirected, eliciting an unusual clinical presentation. Lid elevation might occur with downward gaze or adduction.[32] Some cases even can involve pupil responses; fibers going to the inferior oblique may sprout branches that also innervate the sphincter, causing pupillary constriction on elevation. Fibers innervating the medial rectus may send sprouts that innervate the sphincter, causing miosis with adduction or convergence.

Clinical Comment: Trochlear Damage

When the superior oblique muscle is affected by trochlear nerve damage, the eye is elevated in primary gaze and is unable to move down in the adducted position. The head may be tilted toward the opposite shoulder to compensate for the unopposed extortion of the inferior oblique muscle[5]

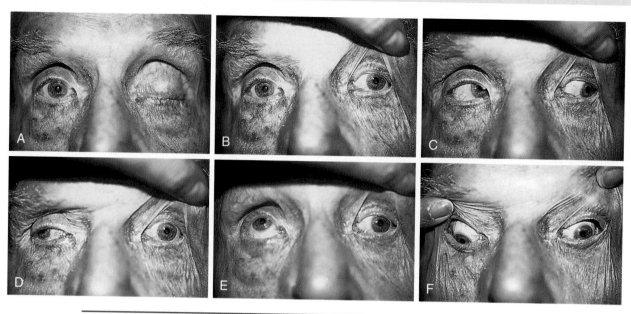

FIGURE 12-14
Third nerve palsy, left eye OS. **A,** Lid ptosis. **B,** Primary gaze, eye positioned out.
C, Normal abduction. **D,** Unable to adduct. **E,** Unable to elevate. **F,** Unable to depress.
(From Kanski JJ: *Clinical ophthalmology: a systematic approach,* ed 5, Oxford, UK, 2003,
Butterworth-Heinemann.)

(see Figure 12-13). Under the age of 10 years, palsies involving the trochlear nerve are usually congenital, and between 21 and 40 years of age the usual cause is trauma; otherwise the palsy may be idiopathic.[52-54]

MIDBRAIN INVOLVEMENT
Damage to the trochlear nucleus will affect the contralateral superior oblique muscle. Because of the proximity of the oculomotor nucleus, a lesion could affect both cranial nerve nuclei, resulting in the clinical presentation just discussed.

INTRACRANIAL INVOLVEMENT
For the most part, the trochlear nerve follows the same path as the oculomotor nerve and is susceptible to the same injuries. Damage to the trochlear nerve affects the ipsilateral superior oblique muscle, causing the eye to be elevated in primary gaze and unable to move down in the adducted position (Figure 12-15).

CAVERNOUS SINUS INVOLVEMENT
A lesion in the lateral wall of the cavernous sinus could affect the trochlear nerve. It could also affect the oculomotor, ophthalmic, and maxillary nerves, causing the previously described clinical presentation.

ORBITAL INVOLVEMENT
The trochlear nerve lies above the muscle cone near the frontal nerve, and injury affecting both nerves could impair the superior oblique muscle, limiting depression in the adducted position. Decreased sensitivity of the areas of the skin and scalp innervated by the branches of the frontal nerve might be observed.

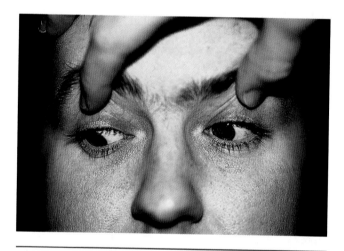

FIGURE 12-15
Fourth nerve palsy OS, limitation in downgaze when adducted.
(From Kanski JJ: *Clinical ophthalmology: a systematic approach,*
ed 5, Oxford, UK, 2003, Butterworth-Heinemann.)

Clinical Comment: Abducens Damage

Damage to the abducens nerve results in paralysis of the lateral rectus muscle; because of the unopposed action by the medial rectus muscle, a convergent strabismus is evident.[55] *The eye will be unable to abduct (Figure 12-16). The patient might try to compensate for the diplopia by turning the face toward the paralyzed side.*[5]

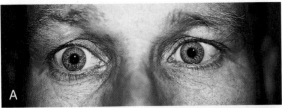

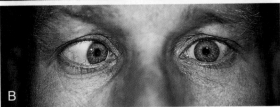

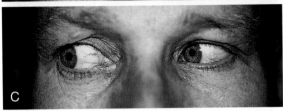

FIGURE 12-16
Sixth nerve palsy OS. **A,** Primary position, left eye positioned in. **B,** Unable to abduct; **C,** Normal adduction. (From Kanski JJ: *Clinical ophthalmology: a systematic approach,* ed 5, Oxford, UK, 2003, Butterworth-Heinemann.)

PONS INVOLVEMENT
Both the abducens and facial nuclei are located in the pons, and the fasciculus of the facial nucleus arches around the abducens nucleus. Damage here could affect the lateral rectus and the muscles of the forehead and the orbicularis. Symptoms might include the inability to abduct the eye and lagophthalmos. The abducens nucleus also contains the internuclear neurons, so the patient may have a restriction when attempting to turn both eyes toward the side of the lesion. The contralateral medial rectus muscle may not be activated in this lateral gaze, but the patient will be able to converge.

INTRACRANIAL INVOLVEMENT
The course of the abducens nerve renders it particularly susceptible to increased intracranial pressure, which causes the brain stem to be displaced posteriorly, stretching the nerve over the bony prominence of the temporal bone.[13,37,41] Fractures of the base of the skull and aneurysms of the basilar and carotid arteries can affect the abducens nerve.

CAVERNOUS SINUS INVOLVEMENT
The abducens nerve is located near the internal carotid artery within the cavernous sinus. Often, it is the first nerve affected with an aneurysm of this vessel. A lateral rectus muscle palsy with Horner's syndrome on the same side, suggesting sympathetic involvement, is indicative of cavernous sinus and internal carotid artery involvement.

ORBITAL INVOLVEMENT
The abducens nerve is located within the muscle cone. It accompanies the two divisions of the oculomotor nerve and the nasociliary nerve (with the resultant clinical presentation described earlier).

REFERENCES

1. Burton H: Somatic sensations from the eye. In Hart WM Jr, editor: *Adler's physiology of the eye,* ed 9, St Louis, 1992, Mosby, p 71.
2. Warwick R: *Eugene Wolff's anatomy of the eye and orbit,* ed 7, Philadelphia, 1976, Saunders, p 275.
3. Ehlers N, Hjortdal J: The cornea. In Fischbarg J, editor: *The biology of the eye,* vol 10, 2006, Elsevier, pp 83–111.
4. Oliveira-Soto L, Efron N: Morphology of corneal nerves using confocal microscopy, *Cornea* 20(4):374, 2001.
5. Wirtschafter JD: The peripheral courses of the third, fourth, fifth, sixth, and seventh cranial nerves. In Reeh MJ, Wobig JL, Wirtschafter JD, editors: *Ophthalmic anatomy,* San Francisco, 1981, American Academy of Ophthalmology, p 234.
6. Müller LJ, Pels E, Vrensen GF: Ultrastructural organization of human corneal nerves, *Invest Ophthalmol Vis Sci* 37(4):476, 1996.
7. Müller LJ, Pels E, Vrensen GF, et al: Architecture of human corneal nerves, *Invest Ophthalmol Vis Sci* 38(5):985, 1997.
8. Catania LJ: *Primary care of the anterior segment,* East Norwalk, Conn, 1988, Appleton & Lange, p 74.
9. Berkow R, editor: *The Merck manual,* ed 14, Rahway, NJ, 1982, Merck, p 187.
10. Bartlett JD, Jaanus SD: *Clinical ocular pharmacology,* ed 2, Boston, 1989, Butterworth-Heinemann, p 544.
11. Schlaegel TF: Uveitis associated with viral infections. In Duane TD, Jaeger EA, editors: *Clinical ophthalmology,* Philadelphia, 1982, Harper & Row.
12. Kanski JJ: *Clinical ophthalmology,* ed 3, London, 1994, Butterworth-Heinemann, p 111.
13. Doxanas MT, Anderson RL: *Clinical orbital anatomy,* Baltimore, 1984, Williams & Wilkins, p 131.
14. Iaconetta G, de Notaris M, Cavallo LM, et al: The oculomotor nerve: microanatomical and endoscopic study, *Neurosurgery* 66:593–601, 2010.
15. Feldon SE, Burde RM: The oculomotor system. In Hart WM Jr, editor: *Adler's physiology of the eye,* ed 9, St Louis, 1992, Mosby.
16. Umansky J, Nathan H: The lateral wall of the cavernous sinus: with special reference to the nerves related to it, *J Neurosurg* 56:228, 1982.
17. Nuza AB, Taner D: Anatomical variations of the intracavernous branches of the internal carotid artery with reference to the relationship of the internal carotid artery and sixth cranial nerve. A microsurgical study, *Acta Anat* 138:238, 1990.
18. Beck RW, Smith CH: Trigeminal nerve. In Tasman W, Jaeger EA, editors: *Duane's foundations of clinical ophthalmology,* vol 1, Philadelphia, 1994, Lippincott.
19. Warwick R, Williams PL, editors: *Gray's anatomy,* ed 35, Philadelphia, 1973, Saunders, pp 1001–1006.
20. Stott DG: Reflex bradycardia in facial surgery, *Br J Plast Surg* 42(5):595, 1989.
21. Eustis HS, Eiswirth CC, Smith DR: Vagal responses to adjustable sutures in strabismus correction, *Am J Ophthalmol* 114(3):307, 1992.
22. Hampl KF, Marsch SC, Schneider M, et al: Vasovagal heart block following cataract surgery under local anesthesia, *Ophthalmic Surg* 24(6):422, 1993.
23. Chong JL, Tan SH: Oculocardiac reflex in strabismus surgery—a study of singapore patients under general anesthesia, *Singapore Med J* 31(1):38, 1990.
24. Grover VK, Bhardwaj N, Shobana N, et al: Oculocardiac reflex during retinal surgery using peribulbar block and nitrous narcotic anesthesia, *Ophthalmic Surg Lasers* 29(3):207, 1998:(abstract).
25. Warwick R: Representation of the extraocular muscles in the oculomotor nucleus of the monkey, *J Comp Neurol* 98:449, 1953.

26. Warwick R: Oculomotor organization. In Bender MB, editor: *The oculomotor system*, New York, 1964, Harper & Row, p 173.

27. Castro O, Johnson LN, Mamourian AC: Isolated inferior oblique paresis from brain stem infarction, *Arch Neurol* 47:235, 1990.

28. Brazis PW: Localization of lesions of the oculomotor nerve: recent concepts, *Mayo Clin Proc* 66(10):1029, 1991.

29. Bienfans DC: Crossing axons in the third nerve nucleus, *Invest Ophthalmol* 12:927, 1975.

30. Marinkovic S, Marinkovic Z, Filipovic B: The oculomotor nuclear complex in humans: microanatomy and clinical significance, *Neurology* 38(2):135, 1989.

31. Jampel RS, Mindel J: The nucleus for accommodation in the midbrain of the macaque, *Invest Ophthalmol* 6:40, 1967.

32. Brazis PW: Isolated palsies of cranial nerves III, IV, and VI, *Semin Neurol* 29:14–28, 2009.

33. Sacks JG: Peripheral innervation of the extraocular muscles, *Am J Ophthalmol* 95:520, 1983.

34. Krewson W: Comparison of the oblique extraocular muscles, *Arch Ophthalmol* 32:204, 1944.

35. Reeh MJ, Wobig JL, Wirtschafter JD: *Ophthalmic anatomy*, San Francisco, 1981, American Academy of Ophthalmology, p 75.

36. Müri RM, Chermann JF, Cohen L, et al: Ocular motor consequences of damage to the abducens area in humans, *J Neuroophthalmol* 16(3):191, 1996.

37. Umansky F, Valarezo A, Elidan J: The microsurgical anatomy of the abducens nerve in its intracranial course, *J Neurosurg* 75(2):294, 1991.

38. Romero FR, Ramos JG, Chaddad-Neto F, et al: Microsurgical anatomy and injuries of the abducens nerve, *Arq Neuropsiquiatr* 67:96–101, 2009.

39. Monkhouse WS: The anatomy of the facial nerve, *Ear Nose Throat J* 69:677, 1990.

40. Proctor B: The anatomy of the facial nerve, *Otolaryngol Clin North Am* 24:479, 1991.

41. Chi SL, Bhatti MT: The diagnostic dilemma of neuro-imaging in acute isolated sixth nerve palsy, *Curr Opin Ophthalmol* 20:423–426, 2009.

42. Rush JA, Younge BR: Paralysis of cranial nerves III, IV, and VI, *Arch Ophthalmol* 99:76, 1981.

43. Tiffin PA, MacEwen CJ, Craig EA, et al: Acquired palsy of the oculomotor, trochlear, and abducens nerves, *Eye* 10:377, 1996.

44. Eskridge JB: Evaluation and diagnosis of incomitant ocular deviations, *J Am Optom Assoc* 60(5):375, 1989.

45. Rubin MM: Trochlear nerve palsy simulating an orbital blowout fracture, *J Oral Maxillofac Surg* 50:1238, 1992.

46. Troost BT, Glaser JS: Aneurysms, arteriovenous communications and related vascular malformations. In Glaser JS, editor: *Neuro-ophthalmology*, Hagerstown, Md, 1978, Harper & Row, p 319.

47. Jampel RS: Ocular torsion and the function of the vertical extraocular muscles, *Am J Ophthalmol* 79:292, 1975.

48. Adams ME, Linn J, Yousry I: Pathology of the ocular motor nerves III, IV, and VI, *Neuroimaging Clin North Am* 18:261–282, 2008.

49. Goldstein JE, Cogan DG: Diabetic ophthalmoplegia with special reference to the pupil, *Arch Ophthalmol* 64:592, 1960.

50. Gray LG: A clinical guide to third nerve palsy, *Opt J Rev Optom* 1:86, 1994.

51. Ing EB, Leavitt JA, Younge BR: Incidence of pupillary involvement in ischemic oculomotor nerve palsies, *Ann Ophthalmol* 32(2):90, 2000.

52. Burger LJ, Kalvin NH, Smith JL: Acquired lesions of the fourth cranial nerve, *Brain* 93:567, 1970.

53. Young BR, Sutla F: Analysis of trochlear nerve palsies: diagnosis, etiology, and treatment, *Mayo Clin Proc* 52:11, 1977.

54. Gunderson CA, Maxow ML, Avilla CW: Epidemiology of CN IV palsies, *Am J Orthop* 51:99, 2001.

55. Galetta SL, Smith JL: Chronic isolated sixth nerve palsies, *Arch Neurol* 46:79, 1989.

The visual pathway consists of the series of cells and synapses that carry visual information from the environment to the brain for processing. It includes the retina, optic nerve, optic chiasm, optic tract, lateral geniculate nucleus (LGN), optic radiations, and striate cortex (Figure 13-1). The first cell in the pathway—a special sensory cell, the photoreceptor—converts light energy into a neuronal signal that is passed to the bipolar cell and the amacrine cell and then to the ganglion cell; all these cells and synapses lie within the retina. The axons of the ganglion cells exit the retina via the optic nerve, with the nasal fibers from each eye crossing in the optic chiasm and terminating in the opposite side of the brain. The optic tract carries these fibers from the chiasm to the LGN, where the next synapse occurs. The fibers leave the LGN as the optic radiations that terminate in the visual cortex of the occipital lobe. From various points in this pathway, information about the visual environment is transferred to related neurologic centers and to visual association areas.

This chapter discusses the structures of the visual pathway and orientation of the fibers within each structure, then briefly reviews characteristic field defects associated with specific locations in the visual pathway. Most of the current knowledge of the visual pathway is based on degeneration studies using laboratory animals, particularly monkeys and cats.[1-3] This type of investigation is based on the finding that damage to a neuron causes the cell and its processes to degenerate. After a small area of nerve tissue is damaged, researchers make serial sections of the tissue through which the neuronal processes are believed to pass. By examining these sections under the microscope, they identify the pathway by determining the location of the degenerating processes. In some studies, small lesions were made in the retina, and the degeneration was followed through the optic nerve, chiasm, and tract into the LGN.[1,3] In other studies, lesions were made in the striate cortex, and the degeneration was followed through the optic radiations toward the LGN.[2] Whenever possible, reference to studies on the human pathway are cited.

ANATOMY OF VISUAL PATHWAY STRUCTURES

The anatomy of the retina and optic disc are discussed in Chapter 4.

OPTIC NERVE

The retinal nerve fibers make a 90-degree turn at the optic disc and exit as the **optic nerve**. This nerve consists of visual fibers, 90% of which will terminate in the LGN. Approximately 10% project to areas controlling pupil responses or the circadian rhythm.[4] Various counts of the optic nerve fibers range from 1 million to 2.22 million, with their size ranging from small-diameter macular fibers to larger-caliber extramacular fibers.[1,2,5-7]

The nerve is 5 to 6 cm long and can be divided into four segments on the basis of location: intraocular (0.7 to 1 mm), intraorbital (30 mm), intracanalicular (6 to 10 mm), and intracranial (10 to 16 mm).[6,8,9]

The intraocular section of the optic nerve can be divided into *prelaminar* and *laminar* sections on the basis of association with the lamina cribrosa. In the prelaminar optic nerve, a glial tissue network provides structural support for the delicate nerve fibers; sheaths of astrocytes bundle the nerve fibers into fascicles, containing approximately 1000 fibers each.[8] The optic nerve fibers are separated from the retinal layers by a ring of glial tissue, the *intermediary tissue (of Kuhnt)*. The continuation of this glial tissue, the *border tissue (of Jacoby)*, separates the choroid from the optic nerve fibers, and a ring of collagenous tissue of scleral derivation, the *marginal (or border) tissue (of Elschnig)*, lies outer to the glial sheaths.[8] Tight junctions within the glial border tissue may prevent leakage from adjacent choriocapillaris into the optic nerve head.[10] These layers are shown in Figure 13-2.

The intraorbital (postlaminar) length exceeds the distance from the globe to the apex of the orbit, giving the nerve a slight sine wave-shaped curve, allowing for full eye excursions without stretching the nerve.[6,11] Within the orbit, the nerve is surrounded by the rectus muscles; the sheaths of the superior and medial rectus muscles are adherent to the sheath of the optic nerve (which explains the pain associated with eye movements in optic neuritis).[8]

The optic nerve is surrounded by three meningeal sheaths continuous with the meningeal coverings of the cranial contents. The outermost sheath, the dura mater, is tough, dense connective tissue containing numerous elastic fibers.[8] Next to it, the thin collagenous membrane of the arachnoid sends a fine network of trabeculae through the subarachnoid space and connects to the

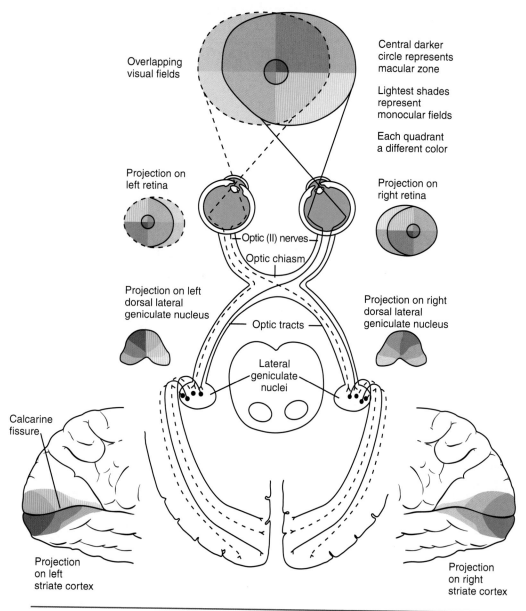

Overlapping visual fields

Central darker circle represents macular zone

Lightest shades represent monocular fields

Each quadrant a different color

Projection on left retina

Projection on right retina

Optic (II) nerves

Optic chiasm

Projection on left dorsal lateral geniculate nucleus

Projection on right dorsal lateral geniculate nucleus

Optic tracts

Lateral geniculate nuclei

Calcarine fissure

Projection on left striate cortex

Projection on right striate cortex

FIGURE 13-1
The visual pathway.

innermost layer, the pia mater. The subarachnoid space around the optic nerve is continuous with the intracranial subarachnoid space and contains cerebrospinal fluid. The loose, vascular connective tissue of the pia mater branches, sending blood vessels and connective tissue septa into the nerve (see Figure 13-2). All three of these layers fuse and become continuous with the sclera and with the periorbita.[8] Of these sheaths, only the pia continues along the intracranial optic nerve.[10]

As the unmyelinated retinal fibers pass through the scleral perforations of the lamina cribrosa, they become myelinated by oligodendrocytes because no Schwann cells exist in the central nervous system. It is postulated that the lamina cribrosa is a barrier to oligodendrocytes

because these cells are not located in retinal tissue and myelination does not normally occur in the retina.[10] The sheath of connective tissue branching from and continuous with the pia mater meningeal covering is added to the glial sheath of each fascicle posterior to the lamina (Figure 13-3). These additional tissues double the diameter of the optic nerve as it leaves the eye; the nerve is approximately 1.5 mm in diameter at the level of the retina and 3 mm after its exit from the globe. The septa that separate the fiber fascicles end near the chiasm.[8] Astrocytes present in the optic nerve probably function similar to Müller cells of the retina; they provide structure, store glycogen, and regulate the extracellular concentration of certain ions.[10]

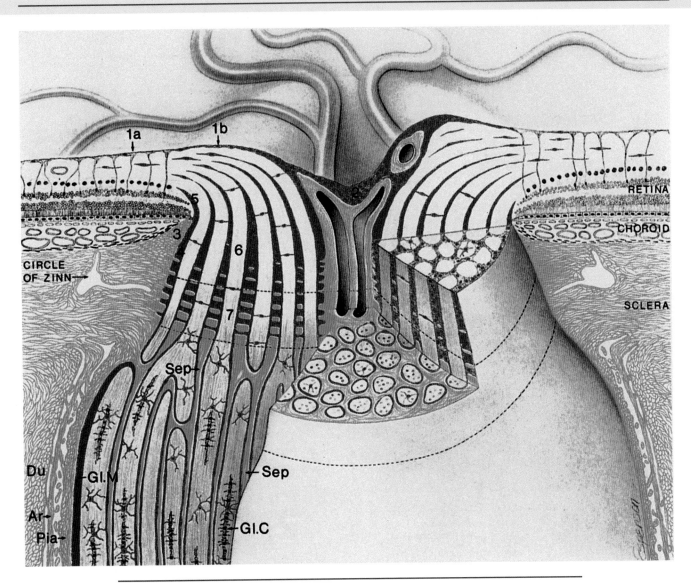

FIGURE 13-2

Intraocular and part of orbital optic nerve. Where retina terminates at optic disc edge, Müller cells (*1a*) are in continuity with astrocytes, forming internal limiting membrane of Elschnig (*1b*). In some specimens this membrane is thickened in central portion of disc, forming central meniscus of Kuhnt (*2*). At posterior termination of choroid on temporal side, border tissue of Elschnig (*3*) lies between astrocytes surrounding optic nerve canal (*4*) and stroma of choroid. On nasal side, choroidal stroma is directly adjacent to these astrocytes, known as border tissue of Jacoby, which is continuous with similar glial lining—intermediary tissue of Kuhnt (*5*)—at termination of retina. Nerve fibers of retina are segregated into about 1000 bundles, or fascicles, by astrocytes (*6*). On reaching lamina cribrosa (*upper dotted line*), nerve fascicles (*7*) and surrounding astrocytes are separated by connective tissue (drawn in blue). This connective tissue is cribriform plate, an extension of scleral collagen and elastic fibers through the optic nerve. External choroid also sends connective tissue to anterior part of lamina. At external part of lamina cribrosa (*lower dotted line*), nerve fibers become myelinated, and columns of oligodendrocytes (*Gl.C*) (black and white cells) and a few astrocytes (red-colored cells) are present in nerve fascicles. Astrocytes surrounding fascicles form thinner layer here than in laminar and prelaminar portion. Bundles continue to be separated by connective tissue (septal tissue, derived from pia mater) all the way to optic chiasm (*Sep*). Mantle of astrocytes (*Gl.M*), are continuous anteriorly with border tissue of Jacoby, surrounding the optic nerve along its orbital course (*Du*, dura; *Ar*, arachnoid; *Pia*, pia mater). Central retinal vessels are surrounded by a perivascular connective tissue throughout its course in optic nerve. This central supporting connective tissue strand blends with connective tissue of cribriform plate in lamina cribrosa. (From Anderson D, Hoyt W: Ultrastructure of interorbital portion of human and monkey optic nerve, *Arch Ophthalmol* 82:506, 1969.)

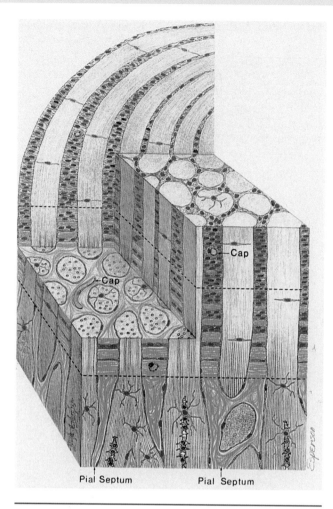

FIGURE 13-3

Prelaminar, laminar, and postlaminar optic nerve. Nerve bundles are drawn in black and white, astrocytes in red, oligodendrocytes in black and white, and connective tissue in blue. In prelaminar region, nerves coming from retina become segregated into bundles invested with tubelike layer of astrocytes, which are oriented, with their processes, perpendicular to nerve bundles. Capillaries (*Cap*) course within astrocyte tubes. As laminar cribrosa is reached (*upper dotted line*), nerve fascicles are separated by layer of astrocytes, which is covered by mantle of connective tissue containing collagen, elastic fibers, fibroblasts, and capillaries. In posterior lamina cribrosa (*lower dotted line*), nerves become myelinated, and columns of oligodendrocytes and a few astrocytes are found in fascicles. Astrocytes separating nerve fascicles in laminar and postlaminar regions form thinner layer than in prelaminar portion. Connective tissue of lamina cribrosa is continuous with pial septa. (From Anderson D: Ultrastructure of human and monkey lamina cribrosa and optic nerve head, *Arch Ophthalmol* 82:800, 1969.)

The anterior perforated substance, the root of the olfactory tract, and the anterior cerebral artery lie superior to the optic nerve in its intracranial path. The sphenoid sinus is medial, with only a thin plate of bone separating it from the nerve.[8] The internal carotid artery

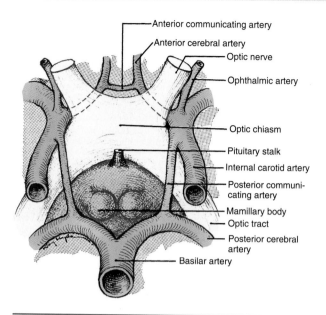

FIGURE 13-4

Relationship of optic chiasm to vessels of circle of Willis. (From Harrington DO: *The visual fields*, ed 5, St Louis, 1981, Mosby.)

is below and then lateral to the nerve, and the ophthalmic artery enters the dural sheath of the optic nerve as it passes through the optic canal.

OPTIC CHIASM

The **optic chiasm** is roughly rectangular, approximately 15 mm in its horizontal diameter, 8 mm anterior to posterior, and 4 mm high.[6,9,12] As with the optic nerve, the optic chiasm is surrounded by the meningeal sheaths and cerebrospinal fluid.

The chiasm lies within the circle of Willis, a circle of blood vessels that is a common location for aneurysms.[6] The circle of Willis is an anastomotic group of anterior and posterior arteries that join the anterior circulation of the internal carotid arteries with the posterior circulation of the basilar artery (Figure 13-4). The internal carotid arteries supply the anterior cranial regions, including most of the cerebral hemispheres and orbital and ocular structures. The vertebral branches of the basilar artery supply the posterior regions, including the brainstem, occipital lobes, and inferomedial temporal lobes, thus supplying most of the ocular motor centers and the cortical visual areas.[13] If the circle is complete, the anterior cerebral arteries are joined via the anterior communicating artery, and each internal carotid artery is joined to the ipsilateral posterior cerebral artery by a posterior communicating artery. The anterior cerebral and anterior communicating arteries are anterior to the chiasm, and an internal carotid artery lies on each lateral side of the chiasm.

Above the optic chiasm is the floor of the third ventricle, and approximately 1 cm below the chiasm is the

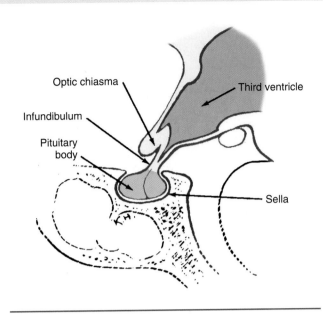

FIGURE 13-5
Sagittal section through optic chiasm showing its relationship to third ventricle, pituitary body, pituitary stalk, sella turcica, and sphenoid sinus. (From Harrington DO: *The visual fields*, ed 5, St Louis, 1981, Mosby.)

pituitary gland (Figure 13-5). The position of the optic chiasm above the sella turcica (the fossa in which the pituitary gland sits) can vary from being directly above it (in 75% of the population) to a position referred to as *prefixed* (if the optic nerves are short and the gland lies below the posterior part of the chiasm) or *postfixed* (if the optic nerves are long and the gland is situated toward the anterior of the chiasm).[12] The chiasm is anteriorly displaced in approximately 10% of individuals and posteriorly displaced in 15%.[10]

Posterior to the optic chiasm, the visual pathway continues into both the right and the left sides of the brain (the structures on only one side are described here).

OPTIC TRACT

The **optic tract** is a cylindric, slightly flattened band of fibers approximately 3.5 mm high and 5.1 mm long that runs from the posterolateral corner of the optic chiasm to the LGN.[9] Most of the fibers (which are still the axons of retinal ganglion cells) terminate in the LGN. Fibers from the retinal ganglion cells may branch so that the same cell sends fibers to various target structures or some axons may be destined for a specific structure. The afferent fibers of the pupillomotor reflex leave the optic tract before reaching the LGN and pass by way of the superior brachium to the pretectal nucleus in the midbrain. Other fibers project to areas in the hypothalamus involved with the circadian rhythm, and others terminate in the superior colliculus. The rather poorly defined accessory

optic system, including the nucleus of the optic tract, is involved in the optokinetic nystagmus response and receives information generated by retinal ganglion cells.[4]

The optic tract lies along the upper anterior and then the lateral surface of the cerebral peduncle and is parallel to the posterior cerebral artery. The globus pallidus is above, the internal capsule is medial, and the hippocampus is below the optic tract.[8]

LATERAL GENICULATE NUCLEUS

Information from all the sensory systems except the olfactory pass through the thalamus before being transferred to the cerebral cortex; visual information is processed in the LGN and then is relayed to higher cortical centers.[14] The **lateral geniculate nucleus (LGN, lateral geniculate body)** is located on the dorsolateral aspect of the thalamus and resembles an asymmetric cone, the rounded apex of which is oriented laterally. The retinal axons terminate here. Most of the fibers that leave the LGN project to the visual cortex.

The LGN is a layered structure; the layers are piled on each other, with the larger ones draping over smaller ones, and some layers becoming fragmented and irregular. The cells within a layer are all of the same type, and three types have been identified according to size. Magnocellular layers contain large cells, parvocellular layers contain medium-sized cells, and koniocellular layers contain small cells. The number of layers present depends on the location of the plane through the structure. In the classic textbook presentation of the LGN, six layers are seen. Two *magnocellular layers* are located inferiorly and numbered 1 and 2, and four *parvocellular layers* are above them and numbered 3, 4, 5, and 6 (Figure 13-6). Below each of these six layers lies a *koniocellular layer* (Figure 13-7). The retinal ganglion cells that project to each of these layers differ in a number of their characteristics.[15]

The LGN is not a simple relay station; it also receives input from cortical and subcortical centers and reciprocal innervation from the visual cortex and is a center of complex processing.[6,16] It regulates the flow of visual information, ensuring that the most important information is sent to the cortex.[17] The optic tract enters the LGN anteriorly; the internal capsule is lateral, the medial geniculate nucleus is medial, and the inferior horn of the lateral ventricle is posterolateral to the LGN.[8] The axons leave the LGN as the optic radiations.

OPTIC RADIATIONS (GENICULOCALCARINE TRACT)

The **optic radiations** spread out fanwise as they leave the LGN, deep in the white matter of the cerebral hemispheres, sweeping laterally and inferiorly around the

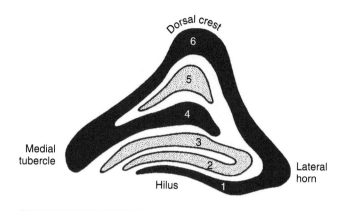

FIGURE 13-6

Laminae in right lateral geniculate nucleus. Crossed retinal projections terminate in laminae *1, 4,* and *6.* Uncrossed projections terminate in laminae *2, 3,* and *5.* Selective partial involvement of one or more of these laminae will produce asymmetric homonymous visual field defects, depending on the extent of laminar damage. (From Harrington DO: *The visual fields,* ed 5, St Louis, 1981, Mosby.)

anterior tip of the temporal horn of the lateral ventricle (Figure 13-8). Some fibers loop into the temporal lobe en route to the occipital lobe. The fibers within the parietal lobe pass lateral to the occipital horn of the lateral ventricle before terminating in the striate cortex.[8,18]

PRIMARY VISUAL CORTEX (STRIATE CORTEX)

The **primary visual cortex (Brodmann area 17** or, according to more recent nomenclature, **V1),** is located almost entirely on the medial surface of the occipital lobe; just a small portion (perhaps 1 cm long) extends around the posterior pole onto the lateral surface. The visual cortex also is called the **striate cortex** because a white myelinated fiber layer, the white stria of Gennari, is characteristic of this area.[6] The **calcarine fissure** extends from the parieto-occipital sulcus to the posterior pole, dividing the visual cortex into an upper portion (the **cuneus gyrus**) and a lower part (the **lingual gyrus**) (Figure 13-9); most of the primary visual cortex is buried in the tissue within the calcarine fissure.[19]

The primary visual cortex has a thickness of about 2 mm and is organized into horizontal layers and vertical columns. Layer I, the most superficial layer, contains a few scattered neurons. Layer II contains neurons that send axons only to deeper cortical layers. Layer III contains neurons that communicate with both near and far cortical locations. Layer IV contains the stria of Gennari and is subdivided into strata, one of which receives information from the magnocellular layers and another that receives information from the parvocellular layers.[20,21]

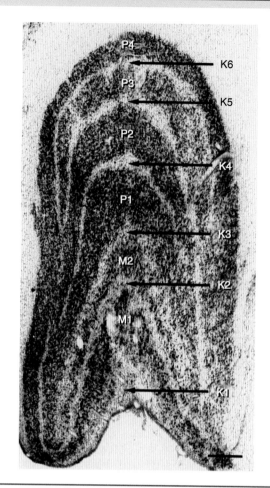

FIGURE 13-7

Coronal section through lateral geniculate nucleus of macaque monkey showing parvocellular (*P*), magnocellular (*M*), and koniocellular (*K*) layers. At this plane there are four P layers, two M layers, and six K layers. (From Casagrande VA, Ichida JM: The lateral geniculate nucleus. In Kaufman PL, Alm A, editors: *Adler's physiology of the eye,* ed 10, St Louis, 2003, Elsevier.)

Layer IV sends axons to more superficial visual cortex, as well as other visual cortical areas. Layer V sends axons to the superior colliculus and other areas in the brainstem. Layer VI sends projections back to the LGN.[17]

Certain cortical regions are active during motion stimulation, whereas others are active during color vision.[22] The magnocellular areas probably mediate movement detection and low-spatial-frequency contrast sensitivity, and the parvocellular areas likely mediate color and high-spatial-frequency contrast sensitivity, although this generalization oversimplifies the properties.[23-26]

Cells are also distributed in a vertical organization, according to the eye of origin, forming alternating parallel ocular dominance columns.[21,27,28] These columns are lacking in the area of the cortex that represents the physiologic blind spot because this region receives information exclusively from one eye.[14] A second system of columns, specific for stimulus orientation, responds on

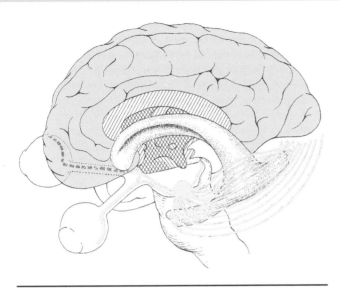

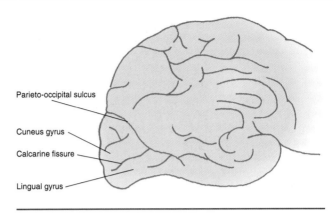

FIGURE 13-9
Medial surface of cerebral cortex showing striate cortex of occipital lobe.

FIGURE 13-8
The visual pathway from retina to calcarine fissure of occipital lobe. Cutaway view from gross dissections shows distribution of visual fibers in optic radiation. (From Harrington DO: *The visual fields*, ed 5, St Louis, 1981, Mosby.)

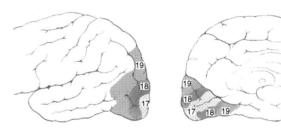

FIGURE 13-10
Visual area, or striate cortex, in occipital lobe. Lateral and medial views show Brodmann areas *17* (striate area), *18* (parastriate area), and *19* (peristriate area). Area 17 is sharply delineated cortical termination of visual pathway. (From Harrington DO: *The visual fields*, ed 5, St Louis, 1981, Mosby.)

the basis of the direction of a light slit or edge.[21] Contour analysis and binocular vision are two functions of the visual cortex, and such processing is a function of both its horizontal and its vertical organization. The cells within the striate cortex are activated only by input from the LGN, although other cortical areas have input into the striate cortex.[16,29,30] The striate cortex communicates with the superior colliculus and the frontal eye fields.

The **superior colliculus,** which has a complete retinotopic map of the contralateral field of vision, also receives communication from fibers exiting the posterior optic tract. It does not analyze sensory information for perception but is important for visual orientation, foveation, and the control of saccadic eye movements with input from the frontal eye fields.[14,31] The **frontal eye fields,** in the frontal lobe, receive fibers from the striate cortex that contribute to the control of conjugate eye movements. Both voluntary and reflex ocular movements are mediated in this area, as are pupillary responses to near objects (see Chapter 14).[8]

The striate cortex combines and analyzes the visual information relayed from the LGN and transmits this information to the higher visual association areas (the **extrastriate cortex**), which provide further interpretation.[14] These areas surround the striate cortex and are located on the lateral aspects of the occipital cortex. Historically called **Brodmann areas 18 and 19** (Figure 13-10), these areas now are known to contain several distinct cortical areas (designated **V2, V3, V4, and V5**) in which visual processing occurs. A study involving the macaque monkey has identified 32 such areas associated with visual processing.[14] The visual and visual

association areas in one hemisphere are connected to the corresponding areas in the other hemisphere through the posterior portion of the corpus callosum.[6] Magnetic resonance imaging (MRI) techniques that are sensitive to changes in blood flow and oxygenation occurring with neuronal activity can be used to study the human visual system in vivo. Innovative studies are attempting (1) to identify the areas of visual cortex and associated visual areas activated during visual stimulation and visual processing, (2) to detect the storage areas for learned visual patterns, and (3) to establish the pathway of activation in the cortex for recall and recognition of a visual pattern.[32-38]

BLOOD SUPPLY TO THE VISUAL PATHWAY

The structures of the visual pathway have an extensive blood supply. Figure 13-11 shows many of the involved vessels. The outer retinal layers receive nutrition from the choroid, whereas the inner retina is supplied by the

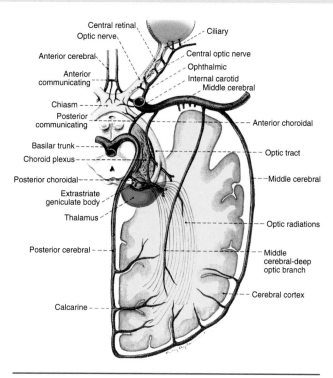

FIGURE 13-11
Vascular supply of visual pathway from retina to occipital cortex. (From Harrington DO: *The visual fields*, ed 5, St Louis, 1981, Mosby.)

central retinal artery. The circle of Zinn, the anastomotic ring of branches of the short ciliary arteries, and peripapillary vessels supply the optic disc.[6] Capillaries within the optic nerve are composed of nonfenestrated endothelium joined by zonula occludens, thus the vessels perfusing the nerve head are part of the blood-brain barrier.[10,39] Pial vessels supply the optic nerve throughout its length; the intraorbital portion is supplied by branches from the ophthalmic artery, and the intracranial optic nerve is nourished by branches of the ophthalmic, anterior cerebral, anterior communicating, and internal carotid arteries.[6,8]

The blood supply to the optic chiasm is rich and anastomotic, with arterioles from the circle of Willis forming capillary beds at two levels.[40,41] The superior network is supplied by the anterior cerebral and anterior communicating arteries, whereas the inferior network is supplied by the internal carotid, posterior cerebral, and posterior communicating arteries.[6,8,12,13] The anterior choroidal artery, a branch of the internal carotid, is a primary supplier of the optic tract, although small branches from the middle cerebral artery also contribute.[6,8,12,42,43] The blood supply to the LGN is derived from the anterior choroidal artery and the lateral choroidal and posterior choroidal branches of the posterior cerebral artery.[8,42,44]

The optic radiations can be divided into three sections: (1) the anterior radiations, which pass laterally over the inferior horn of the ventricle, are supplied by the anterior choroidal artery and the middle cerebral artery; (2) the middle group of fibers passing lateral to the ventricle is supplied by the deep optic branch of the middle cerebral artery; and (3) branches of the posterior cerebral artery, including the calcarine branch, supply the posterior radiations as they spread out in the occipital lobe. Branches from the middle cerebral artery also contribute.[6,8,12] The calcarine branch of the posterior cerebral artery is the major blood supply for the striate cortex, often supplemented by the posterior temporal or parietooccipital branch of the posterior cerebral artery or the occipital branch of the middle cerebral artery.[6,8,12,45]

FIBER ORIENTATION AND VISUAL FIELDS

With the eye looking straight ahead and fixating on an object, one is able to detect other objects around the point of regard, although the details may not be discernible. This entire visible area is termed the visual field. Information from the visual field is taken in by the retina and processed through the afferent visual sensory pathway. The location and orderly arrangement of the fibers throughout this pathway have been extensively studied. Damage in this afferent visual pathway will cause a defect in the visual field. Knowledge of the fiber patterns in the pathway can help to identify the location of the lesion on the basis of the resultant visual field defect.

RETINA

The axons of the retinal ganglion cells form characteristic patterns in the nerve fiber layer. The group of fibers that course from the macular area to the optic disc is called the **papillomacular bundle**. The superior and inferior temporal fibers, separated at the 180th meridian by the **horizontal retinal raphe**, must arch superiorly and inferiorly around the macular area, forming characteristic *arcuate* patterns in their course to the optic disc; the temporal retinal vessels usually do not cross the horizontal raphe either. The nasal fibers can travel directly to the optic disc and are described as *radiating* (Figure 13-12). Nasal and temporal fibers are separated by a theoretic vertical line passing through the center of the fovea. The long nerve fibers, from the peripheral retina, are more vitread in location than are the short peripapillary fibers, with extensive intermingling in the prelaminar optic nerve.[46]

OPTIC DISC

All of the axons in the nerve fiber layer come together at the optic disc, creating a specific pattern. The nasal fibers radiate directly to the *nasal* side of the disc, whereas the papillomacular bundle courses directly to the *temporal*

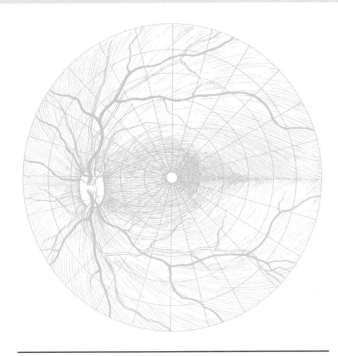

FIGURE 13-12
Nerve fiber pattern of retina in its relationship to retinal vascular tree. (From Harrington DO: *The visual fields*, ed 5, St Louis, 1981, Mosby.)

side of the disc.[46-48] The fibers from the superior temporal retina arch around the papillomacular bundle to enter the *superior pole* of the disc; fibers from the inferior temporal retina curve below the papillomacular bundle to the *inferior pole*.[48] The macular fibers take up approximately one third of the disc, although the macular area encompasses only one twentieth of the retinal area.[1,8] The temporal fibers occupy approximately one third of the disc, as do the nasal fibers (Figure 13-13, *A*). The boundaries between each set of fibers are not always clear-cut in all parts of the pathway. The fibers from the peripheral retina are more superficial than those coming from the central retina.[48]

OPTIC NERVE

Near the lamina cribrosa, the fibers have the same orientation as they do in the disc, but within a short distance the macular fibers move to the center of the nerve.[3,8] The rest of the fibers take up their logical positions: superior temporal fibers in the superior temporal optic nerve, inferior temporal fibers in the inferior temporal nerve, superior nasal fibers in the superior nasal nerve, and inferior nasal fibers in the inferior nasal optic nerve (Figure 13-13, *B*).

OPTIC CHIASM

In the optic chiasm the nasal fibers cross *(decussate)*; the ratio of crossed to uncrossed fibers in the chiasm is approximately 53 to 47.[49] The crossing pattern

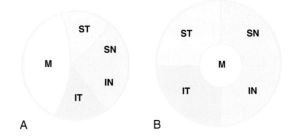

FIGURE 13-13
A, Surface of optic disc showing orientation of nerve fibers as they enter disc. **B,** Coronal section showing orientation of nerve fibers in optic nerve proximal to chiasm. (Right disc and nerve viewed from front.) *ST,* Superior temporal; *SN,* superior nasal; *IT,* inferior temporal; *IN,* inferior nasal; *M,* macular.

depends on processes that occur during embryologic development, with certain molecular guides directing the path taken by nerve fibers. The inferior nasal retinal fibers are inferior in the anterior chiasm; they cross to the other side, and many loop into the terminal part of the *opposite* optic nerve before turning to run back through the chiasm into the *contralateral* optic tract[1] (Figure 13-14). These anterior loops **(anterior knees of Wilbrand)** bring fibers from the opposite eye into the posterior optic nerve.[50] Some investigators believe that these "knees" are artifacts and suggest that the fibers shift into such a location after loss from fiber degeneration.[51]

The superior nasal fibers enter the superior chiasm, where they cross and then leave the chiasm in the *contralateral* optic tract; some of these fibers loop posteriorly into the optic tract on the same side before crossing. The fibers were historically called the **posterior knees of Wilbrand**[1,8] (see Figure 13-14). The fibers from the temporal retina course directly back through the chiasm into the optic tract. The nasal macular fibers also cross and are spread throughout most of the chiasm.[51]

A small number of fibers have been identified that exit the posterior of the chiasm and enter the suprachiasmatic nucleus in the hypothalamus and have a role in synchronization of circadian rhythm.[52-54]

OPTIC TRACT

As the fibers leave the chiasm in the optic tract, the crossed and uncrossed fibers intermingle. The superior fibers (the fibers from both the *ipsilateral* superior temporal retina and the *contralateral* superior nasal retina) move to the medial side of the tract. The fibers from the inferior retina (*ipsilateral* inferior temporal retinal fibers and *contralateral* inferior nasal retinal fibers) occupy the lateral area of the tract.[1,3] Figure 13-15 shows the regrouping that occurs as the fibers pass through the chiasm and into the optic tract. The macular fibers, crossed

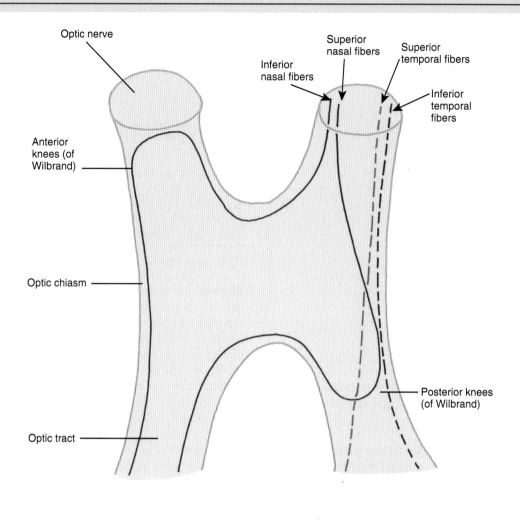

FIGURE 13-14
Fiber orientation through optic chiasm. Temporal fibers (*dotted lines*) pass through chiasm and exit in ipsilateral optic tract. Nasal fibers (*solid lines*) cross in chiasm to exit in contralateral optic tract.

and uncrossed, are located between these two groups[1] (Figure 13-16).

LATERAL GENICULATE NUCLEUS

Fibers from the superior retinal quadrants terminate in the *medial* aspect of the LGN, whereas fibers from the inferior retinal quadrants terminate in the *lateral* aspect.[8] A dorsal wedge, composing two thirds to three fourths of the LGN, represents the macula.[3,55,56] Based on animal study mapping, each of the magnocellular and parvocellular layers receives input from just one eye: Layers 1, 4, and 6 receive fibers from the *contralateral nasal retina*, whereas layers 2, 3, and 5 receive *ipsilateral temporal retinal fibers*[49] (Figure 13-17). Most of the structure, including the wedge representing the macula, contains all layers, although in the far medial and lateral aspects, some of the layers merge.[6,55]

The anatomic structure of the human LGN is similar to that of the monkey, so detailed maps of the monkey LGN have been applied to the human structure.[57] Each layer of the LGN contains a retinotopic map or representation of the *contralateral hemifield* of vision. A **retinotopic map** is a "point-to-point localization" of the retina.[14] These maps are stacked on one another, such that if a line (called a line of projection) were passed through all six layers, perpendicular to the surface, the intercepted cells all would be carrying information about the same point in the visual field. This alignment is so precise that there is a gap in each contralateral layer along the line of projection that corresponds to the location of the optic disc.[15] Thus the fibers that carry information from the same site in the visual field of each eye terminate in adjacent layers of the LGN, right next to one another[8] (see Figure 13-17). The fibers course through the posterior limb of the internal capsule as they leave the LGN to form the optic radiations.

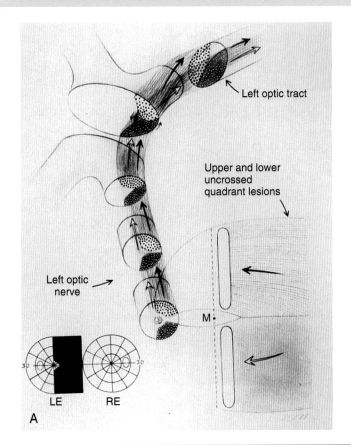

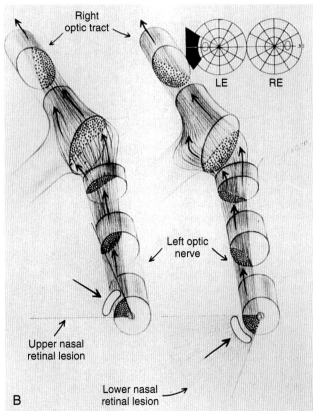

FIGURE 13-15
A, Course of uncrossed retinal ganglion cell axons through optic nerve, chiasm, and tract of monkey. Left retina is represented below on right. Vertical white bars are lesions made by photocoagulator; macula (*M*) has not been damaged. Hypothetic visual field defect produced by these lesions is shown in lower left. **B,** Course of crossed retinal ganglion cell axons. Photocoagulator lesions in left retina are indicated by white crescents in retinal diagrams at bottom of figure; hypothetic visual field defects produced by these lesions are shown at upper right. *LE,* Left eye; *RE,* right eye. (From Hoyt WF, Luis O: Visual fiber anatomy in the infrageniculate pathway of the primate: uncrossed and crossed retinal quadrant fiber projections studied with the Nauta silver stain, *Arch Ophthalmol* 68:428, 1962.)

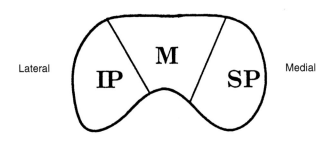

FIGURE 13-16
Coronal section showing orientation of nerve fibers in optic tract. *IP,* Inferior peripheral; *M,* macular; *SP,* superior peripheral.

OPTIC RADIATIONS

The fibers leaving the *lateral* aspect of the LGN, representing *inferior* retina, follow an indirect route to the occipital lobe. They pass into the temporal lobe and loop around the tip of the temporal horn of the lateral ventricle, forming **Meyer loops**; these fibers form the inferior radiations[8,18] (Figure 13-18). Fibers from the *medial* aspect of the LGN, representing *superior* retina, lie superiorly as they pass through the parietal lobe. The fibers from the macula are generally situated between superior and inferior fibers.

STRIATE CORTEX

The superior radiations terminate in the area of the striate cortex above the calcarine fissure, called the **cuneus gyrus**; the inferior radiations terminate in the region below the calcarine fissure—the **lingual gyrus**. Thus the cuneus gyrus receives projections from the *superior retina* and the lingual gyrus from the *inferior retina*. Only one third of the striate cortex is on the surface of the occipital lobe; the majority is buried within

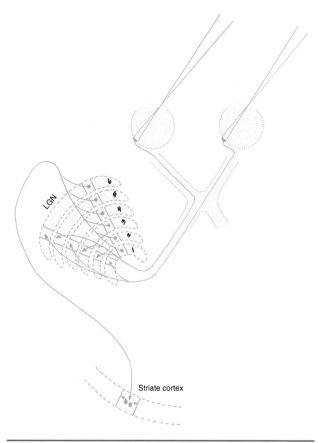

FIGURE 13-17
Retinotopic map representation in lateral geniculate nucleus (or body, LGN). Fibers from ipsilateral (temporal) retina terminate in layers *2, 3,* and *5*. Fibers from contralateral (nasal) retina terminate in layers *1, 4,* and *6*. Fibers that originate in neighboring areas of all layers of LGN terminate in same place in striate cortex.

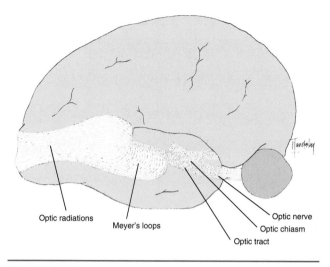

FIGURE 13-18
Location of optic radiations in cerebral hemisphere. Meyer loops pass into temporal lobe before passing into parietal lobe.

Retinotopic representation is present in the striate cortex. Those fibers that are adjacent to one another in the layers of the LGN project to the same area in the visual cortex (see Figure 13-17). That is, corresponding points from the two retinas (*ipsilateral temporal* and *contralateral nasal*) that represent the same target in the visual field will project to neighboring locations in the primary visual cortex. All the cells in a column correspond to a stimulus presented at the same point in the visual field, and cells in an adjacent column correspond to an adjacent point in the visual field.

Clinical Comment: Visual Field Testing

THE VISUAL FIELD is tested monocularly, with the patient looking straight ahead at a fixation point and responding when a target is seen anywhere in the area surrounding that fixation point, usually described to the patient as "seen out of the corner of your eye." The field can be divided into four quadrants by a vertical line and a horizontal line that intersect at the point of fixation. The point of fixation is seen by the fovea and is eccentric because the temporal field is slightly larger than the nasal field. Inversion and reversal of the field are caused by the optical system of the eye. The superior field is imaged on the inferior retina and the inferior field on the superior retina; the nasal field is imaged on the temporal retina and the temporal field on the nasal retina (Figure 13-19). This orientation is maintained in the cortex, where the superior field is projected onto the visual cortex inferior to the calcarine fissure, and where the inferior visual field is projected onto the cortex superior to the calcarine fissure.

the calcarine fissure, and only a small portion is on the posterolateral aspect of the occipital posterior pole.[58]

Fibers from the macular area terminate in the most *posterior* part of the striate cortex, with the superior macular area represented in the cuneus gyrus and the inferior macula represented in the lingual gyrus. The macular projection might extend onto the posterolateral surface of the occipital cortex. The macular area representation occupies a relatively large portion of striate cortex compared with the small macular area in the retina. The macular cells are densely packed, and macular fibers are small caliber. Because macular function involves sharp, detailed vision, the macular representation in the striate cortex is more extensive than the representation of peripheral retinal areas. The most *anterior* part of the striate cortex, the part adjacent to the parietal lobe, represents the periphery of the nasal retina, corresponding to an area of visual field, the **temporal crescent**, that is seen by the contralateral eye only.

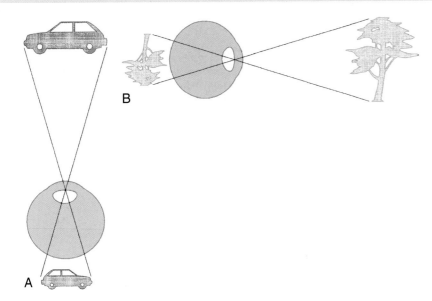

FIGURE 13-19
Orientation of an image on the retina. **A,** Nasal field is imaged on temporal retina. **B,** Superior field is imaged on inferior retina.

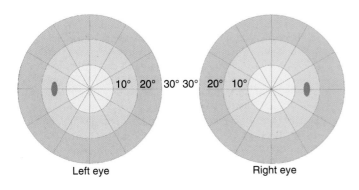

Left eye   Right eye

FIGURE 13-20
Central visual field plots showing scotoma of physiologic blind spot in the temporal field.

The reader is cautioned to be aware of the difference between visual fibers and visual fields. Both can be described as nasal, temporal, superior, and inferior.

*The visual field seen by the right eye is nearly the same as that seen by the left eye. The nasal part of the field for one eye is the same as the temporal part of the field seen by the other eye, with the exception of the far temporal periphery, which is called the **temporal crescent**. The temporal crescent is imaged on the nasal retina of one eye but not on the temporal retina of the other because the depth of the orbit and the prominence of the nose blocks the periphery of the field from the temporal retina. Within each temporal field is an absolute scotoma, the **physiologic blind spot**, a result of the lack of photoreceptors in the optic disc (Figure 13-20).*

*Because the fibers that emanate from nasal retina cross in the chiasm, the postchiasmal pathway carries information from the contralateral temporal field and the ipsilateral nasal field. These combined areas can be described as the **contralateral hemifield** (i.e., the right postchiasmal pathway carries information from the left side of the visual*

field for both eyes). Thus, the left side of the field is "seen" by the right striate cortex, paralleling the involvement of the right hemisphere in the motor and sensory activities of the left side of the body. Similarly, objects in the right side of the field are "seen" by the left striate cortex (see Figure 13-1).

Note that reference to the "left side of the visual field" is not the same as the "visual field of the left eye." Also, some clinicians will refer to the right visual field (meaning the right side of the field) and the left visual field (meaning the left side of the field).

*A defect that affects the nasal field of one eye and the temporal field of the other eye is described as **homonymous**. A defect in the field of just one eye must be caused by a disruption anterior to the chiasm. If there is a defect in the fields of both eyes, there are two lesions, one in each prechiasmal pathway, or there is a single lesion in the chiasm or the postchiasmal pathway, where the fibers for the two eyes are brought together. The pattern of the defect, as well as associated signs or symptoms, might aid in determining the location of the damage.*

Clinical Comment: Characteristic Visual Field Defects

Figure 13-21 depicts examples of various visual field defects.

The regular fiber orientation in each structure of the visual pathway can be correlated with a specific pattern of visual field loss. A lesion of the choroid or outer retina will cause a field defect that is similar in shape to the lesion and is in the corresponding location in the field (e.g., if the lesion is in the superior nasal retina, the defect will be in the inferior temporal field).

*A lesion in the nerve fiber layer will cause a field defect corresponding to the location and configuration of the affected nerve fiber bundle. One of the disease processes that affects the nerve fiber layer is glaucoma. If temporal retinal fibers are affected, an arcuate defect can be produced that curves around the point of fixation from the blind spot to termination at the horizontal nasal meridian (Figure 13-22). This abrupt edge (at the horizontal meridian) is called a **nasal step** and results from the configuration of the fibers at the temporal retinal raphe. Less often, a lesion affects a nasal bundle of nerves, producing a wedge-shaped defect emanating from the physiologic blind spot into the temporal field.*

Injury to the optic nerve is accompanied by a visual field defect, a relative afferent pupillary defect, and atrophy of the affected nerve fibers, which eventually is manifested at the disc. The small-diameter, tightly packed fibers of the macula have the greatest metabolic need and often are affected first in both compressive and ischemic lesions.[12]

*The optic chiasm brings all the visual fibers together; lesions of the chiasm usually will show bitemporal or binasal defects. The most common cause of a **bitemporal field defect** is a pituitary gland tumor, and a visual field defect is often the first clinical sign (Figure 13-23, A). A patient may not recognize the field loss because the nasal field of one eye overlaps the temporal field of the other eye. The crossed fibers seem to be damaged first in compressive lesions such as a tumor.[14] This susceptibility to damage might be attributable to the purported weak blood supply of the median portion of the chiasm. Consequently, the crossed fibers also are more susceptible to ischemia in a vascular event.[41] Involvement of both lateral sides of the chiasm, producing a **binasal defect**, might be caused by an aneurysm of the internal carotid artery that impinges on the chiasm and displaces it against the other internal carotid artery (Figure 13-23, B).*

A single lesion at the optic chiasm and its junction with the optic nerve might be characterized by a central defect in the field of the eye on the same side as the lesion, as well as a superior temporal defect in the field of the opposite eye, because of the inferior nasal fibers that loop into the optic nerve from the contralateral eye. This is known as an anterior junction defect.

*A **homonymous field defect** will be produced by a single lesion in the **postchiasmal** pathway, as the nasal fibers of the contralateral eye join the temporal fibers of the ipsilateral eye; visual acuity usually is not affected because one half the fovea is sufficient for 20/20 Snellen acuity.[14] In this lesion the field loss is present on the side of the field contralateral to the lesion. Other signs or symptoms accompanying a homonymous defect can help the diagnostician determine more exactly the site of the lesion.*

*A lesion involving the optic tract eventually will produce optic nerve atrophy, which usually becomes evident as optic disc pallor. Because the optic tract is relatively small in cross section, a lesion often damages all of the fibers, causing a homonymous field defect that affects the entire half of the field; if a partial hemianopia results, the defects will be incongruent.[59] The defects in a homonymous field are **congruent** if the two defects are similarly shaped and are **incongruent** if the defect shapes are dissimilar. Because crossed fibers outnumber uncrossed fibers, a lesion of the optic tract may be accompanied by a relative afferent pupillary defect of the contralateral eye.[14]*

A lesion in the LGN would affect the contralateral field and eventually also cause optic atrophy; however, there would be no associated pupillary defect. Because of the point-to-point localization in the LGN, lesions here produce moderately to completely congruent field defects.[42]

Damage to the optic radiations or cortex does not normally cause atrophy of the optic nerve because it does not involve the fibers of the retinal ganglion cells. A lesion of the optic radiations causes a contralateral homonymous field defect and, because the fibers are so spread out, the defect often affects only one quadrant. If a lesion of the temporal lobe involves the Meyer loop, a superior quadrant field defect will result; parietal lobe lesions more commonly cause inferior field defects (Figure 13-23, C).[14]

*The characteristic feature of a defect in the occipital lobe is **congruency.** Congruency depends on how closely fibers from corresponding points of each eye (carrying the same visual field information) are positioned to one another at the site of the lesion. As the fibers reach the occipital lobe and finally the striate cortex, the fibers emanating from corresponding points in the field come together to form a point-to-point representation of the field. Therefore, a lesion here will cause a congruent defect (Figure 13-24).*

When visual association areas within the occipital, temporal, and parietal lobes are involved, higher cortical visual processes may be affected. Lesions of the parietal lobe can cause abnormal optokinetic nystagmus and affect visual attention; temporal lobe lesions can cause olfactory hallucinations, formed visual hallucinations, or déjà vu phenomenon; injury involving the occipitotemporal cortex can affect object and facial recognition.[60] Blind sight occurs when there seems to be some sight in a hemifield but there is no conscious awareness of the sight. That is, a motor reflex response can be elicited with presentation of an unexpected stimulus in the affected field, but the patient has no awareness of the vision. It is likely that subcortical visual responses are mediated at the level of the superior colliculus and that the reflex does not initiate from the visual cortex.

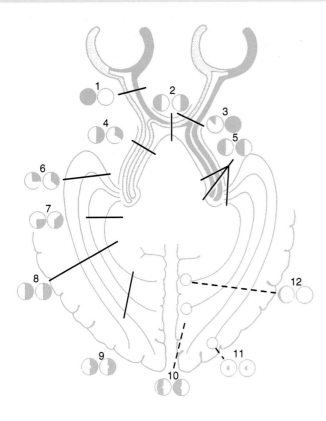

FIGURE 13-21
Visual field defects. Visual pathway is shown, as are sites of interruption of nerve fibers and resulting visual field defects. *1,* Complete interruption of left optic nerve, resulting in complete loss of visual field for left eye. *2,* Interruption in midline of optic chiasm, resulting in bitemporal hemianopia. *3,* Interruption in right optic nerve at junction with chiasm, resulting in complete loss of visual field for right eye and superior temporal loss in field for left eye (due to anterior knees). *4,* Interruption in left optic tract, causing incongruent right homonymous hemianopia. *5,* Complete interruption in right optic tract, lateral geniculate nucleus, or optic radiations, resulting in total left homonymous hemianopia. *6,* Interruption in left optic radiations involving Meyer loop, causing incongruent right homonymous hemianopia. *7,* Interruption in optic radiations in left parietal lobe, causing incongruent right homonymous hemianopia. *8,* Interruption of all left optic radiations, resulting in total right homonymous hemianopia. *9,* Interruption of fibers in left anterior striate cortex, resulting in right homonymous hemianopia with macular sparing. *10,* Interruption of fibers in right striate cortex, resulting in left homonymous hemianopia with macular and temporal crescent sparing. *11,* Interruption of fibers in right posterior striate cortex, resulting in left macular homonymous hemianopia. *12,* Interruption of fibers in right anterior striate cortex, resulting in left temporal crescent loss. (From Hart WM Jr, editor: *Adler's physiology of the eye,* ed 9, St Louis, 1992, Mosby.)

defects with injuries from shrapnel to the occipital lobe. The Holmes map was the most detailed source showing the representation of the visual field in human striate cortex. The macular portion extends from the posterior pole forward, with the periphery of the field represented in the anterior occipital lobe and the uniocular temporal crescent in the most anterior aspect of the striate cortex adjacent to the parietooccipital sulcus. However, detailed mapping of monkey striate cortex using electrophysiologic methods revealed discrepancies between monkey and human data. These findings suggested that either monkey cortex and human cortex were not as alike as believed or the Holmes map required some modification.

Technologies such as MRI have been used to study the human cortex, allowing more direct correlation of a lesion with a field defect. Some investigators suggest revision of the Holmes map[58] similar to Figure 13-25. The primary change concerns the extent of the area depicting macular representation. A much greater area of the visual cortex is thought to be taken up by macular projection,[58] with the central 30 degrees of the visual field represented in approximately 83% of the striate cortex[58] (Figure 13-26). Other imaging studies more closely agree with the Holmes map and show that the central 15 degrees of vision occupies 37% of the surface area of the striate cortex.[62] Some discrepancies may result from the nature of the lesion because an MRI may overestimate the actual area involved when edema is present.[62]

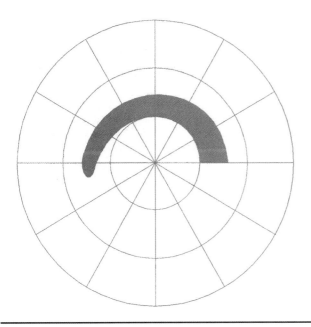

FIGURE 13-22
Automated visual field showing arcuate scotoma and nasal step in field for the left eye.

Striate Cortex Maps

Early study correlating the visual field to striate cortex was done by Holmes and Lister,[61] who studied injured soldiers from World War I and attempted to match visual field

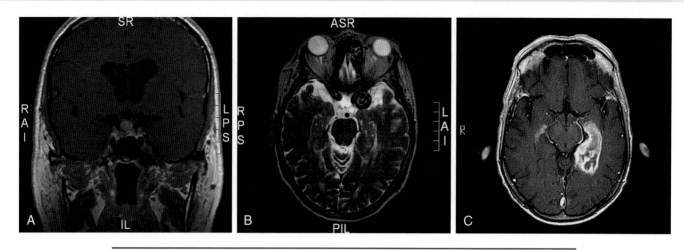

FIGURE 13-23

A, CT scan showing pituitary adenoma causing a bitemporal visual field loss. **B,** CT scan showing aneurysm of left internal carotid artery as it passes through cavernous sinus, resulting in binasal visual field loss, and affecting CN III and CN IV. **C,** MRI showing lesion of left temporal lobe secondary to CVA resulting in right homonymous superior quadrantanopia. (**A-C** courtesy Weon Jun, O.D., Portland VA Medical Center, Portland, Ore.)

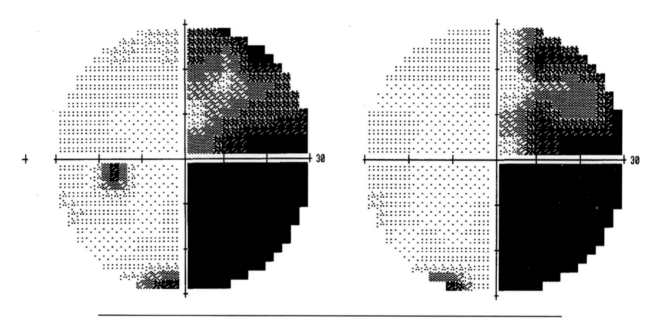

FIGURE 13-24

Automated visual fields showing right congruent homonymous field loss; absolute defect inferior quadrant, relative defect superior quadrant, caused by arteriovenous malformation (AVM in left occipital cortex). AVM successfully obliterated by embolization, visual field loss remained. (Courtesy Edward B. Mallett, O.D., Tillamooh Optometric Clinic, Tillamook, Ore.)

Macular Sparing

Macular sparing occurs when an area of central vision remains within a homonymous field defect. Because fixational eye movements of 1 to 2 degrees do occur during the visual field examination, the area spared within the defect should involve at least 3 degrees in order for macular sparing to be confirmed clinically.[45] Because the macular area often was spared in homonymous defects caused by occipital lobe lesions, it once was supposed that the entire macula was represented in both sides of the striate cortex. We now know that this is not the case. However, even in the presence of an extensive lesion, some of the macular projection area might

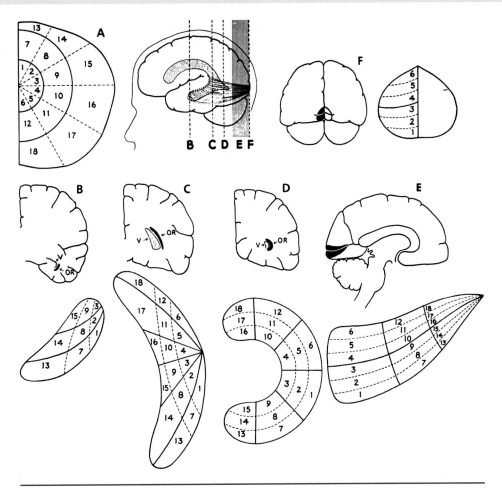

FIGURE 13-25

Schematic representation of architecture of geniculocalcarine pathway with projection of striate cortex and nerve fiber bundles of optic radiation onto visual field. **A,** Right homonymous half field divided into sectors and concentric zones representing projection of various bundles of optic radiations in temporal and parietal lobes and in striate cortex in occipital lobe. **B, C,** and **D,** Coronal sections (seen from in front) through temporal, parietal, and parietooccipital lobes of left cerebral hemisphere showing planes of section, relationship of optic radiations to lateral ventricle, and division of visual fiber bundles in optic radiations into sectors and concentric zones corresponding to their projection onto visual field. Note in plane of section through temporal loop of Meyer **(B)** that only lower half of radiations are represented; in planes **B** and **C,** that section anterior radiations, macular fibers (1 to 6) are laminated on lateral surface of radiations; and in plane **D,** that section's posterior radiations, macular fibers are interposed between and completely separate upper and lower peripheral fibers. **E,** Medial view of left cerebral hemisphere showing striate cortex divided according to its projection on right homonymous half field. **F,** View from behind striate cortex at posterior tip of left occipital pole showing projection of macular portion of right homonymous defect. (From Harrington DO, Drake MV: *The visual fields; text and atlas of clinical perimetry,* ed 6, St Louis, 1990, Mosby.)

remain unaffected, either because the posterior pole of the occipital lobe has such an extensive blood supply or because the macular projection covers a very large area.[14] Macular sparing can also be explained by the size and overlap of the receptive field of the retinal ganglion cells subserving the vertical meridian.[63]

AGING WITHIN THE VISUAL PATHWAY

Neural cell death occurs throughout all structures of the visual pathway, although the extent varies significantly within the population.[64] Age is accompanied

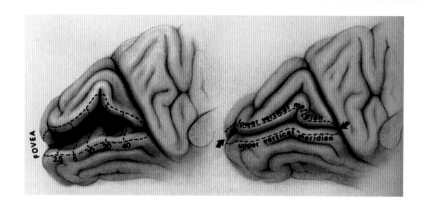

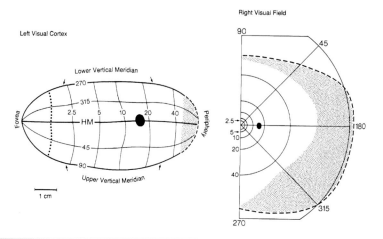

FIGURE 13-26

Revised map of the visual field in the human striate cortex. It is important to emphasize that considerable variation occurs among individuals in the exact size and location of striate cortex. This new map provides the best fit for our data. **A,** View of left occipital lobe with the calcarine fissure opened, exposing the striate cortex. Dashed lines indicate the coordinates of the visual field map. The representation of the horizontal meridian runs approximately along the base of the calcarine fissure. The vertical lines mark the isoeccentricity contours from 2.5 to 40 degrees. The striate cortex wraps around the occipital pole to extend approximately 1cm onto the lateral convexity, where the fovea is represented. **B,** View of the left occipital lobe, showing the striate cortex, which is mostly hidden within the calcarine fissure (*running between arrows*). The boundary (*dashed line*) between the striate cortex (V1) and extrastriate cortex (V2) contains the representation of the vertical meridian, which usually is located along the exposed medial surface of the occipital lobe, as shown, but variation occurs in specimens. **C,** Projection of the right visual hemifield **(D)** on the left visual cortex, depicted by transposing the map illustrated in the top left onto a flat surface. The striate cortex is an ellipse measuring approximately 80 × 40 mm, measuring roughly 2500 square millimeters. The row of dots indicates where the striate cortex folds around the occipital pole: the small region between the dots and the foveal representation is situated on the exposed lateral convexity of the occipital lobe. The black oval marks the region of the striate cortex corresponding to the visual field coordinates of the contralateral eye's blind spot. This region of cortex receives visual input from only the ipislateral eye (HM = horizontal meridian). **D,** Right visual hemifield shows the V4e isopter plotted with a Goldmann perimeter. The stippled region corresponds to the monocular temporal crescent that is mapped within the most anterior 8 to 10% of the striate cortex (see stippled region of map in C). (Reprinted with permission from Horton JC, Hoyt WF: The representation of the visual field in human striate cortex, *Arch Ophthalmol* 109:816, 1991)

by a decrease in the extent of the visual field, caused both by loss of cells and by a decrease in the transparency of the ocular media.[12,65] The ability to perceive accurately the speed of moving objects declines with age, and animal studies have identified an age-related difference in temporal processing speed at the level of the visual cortex.[66] This decline in accurately perceiving the speed of moving objects may contribute to the higher incidence of automobile accidents among the elderly population.

REFERENCES

1. Hoyt WF, Osman L: Visual fiber anatomy in the infrageniculate pathway of the primate, *Arch Ophthalmol* 68:124, 1962.
2. Polyak S: *The vertebrate visual system*, Chicago, 1957, University of Chicago Press.
3. Brouwer B, Zeeman WP: The projection of the retina in the primary optic neuron in monkeys, *Brain* 49, 1926.
4. Boyd JD, Gu Q, Matsubara JA: Overview of the central visual pathways. In Kaufman PL, Alm A, editors: *Adler's physiology of the eye*, ed 10, St Louis, 2003, Elsevier, p 641.
5. Jonas JB, Schmidt AM, Muller-Bergh JA, et al: Human optic nerve fiber count and optic disc size, *Invest Ophthalmol Vis Sci* 33(6):1992, 2012.
6. Sadun AA, Glaser JS: Anatomy of the visual sensory system. In Tasman W, Jaeger EA, editors: *Duane's foundations of clinical ophthalmology*, vol 1, Philadelphia, 1994, Lippincott.
7. Mikelberg FS, Drance SM, Schulzer M, et al: The normal human optic nerve. Axon count and axon diameter distribution, *Ophthalmology* 96:1325, 1989.
8. Warwick R: *Eugene Wolff's anatomy of the eye and orbit*, ed 7, Philadelphia, 1976, Saunders, p 325.
9. Parravano JG, Toledo A, Kucharczyk W: Dimensions of the optic nerves, chiasm, and tracts: MR quantitative comparison between patients with optic atrophy and normals, *J Comput Assist Tomogr* 17(5):688, 1993.
10. Levin LA: Optic nerve. In Kaufman PL, Alm A, editors: *Adler's physiology of the eye*, ed 10, St Louis, 2003, Elsevier, p 603.
11. Unsold R, Hoyt WF: Band atrophy of the optic nerve. The histology of temporal hemianopsia, *Arch Ophthalmol* 98:1637, 1980.
12. Harrington DO: *The visual fields*, ed 5, St Louis, 1981, Mosby.
13. Borchert MS: Vascular anatomy of the visual system, *Ophthalmol Clin North Am* 9(3):327, 1996.
14. Horton JC: The central visual pathways. In Hart WM Jr, editor: *Adler's physiology of the eye*, ed 9, St Louis, 1992, Mosby, p 728.
15. Casagrande VA, Ichida JM: The lateral geniculate nucleus. In Kaufman PL, Alm A, editors: *Adler's physiology of the eye*, ed 10, St Louis, 2003, Elsevier, p 655.
16. Lachica EA, Casagrande VA: The morphology of collicular and retinal axons ending on small relay (W-like) cells of the primate lateral geniculate nucleus, *Vis Neurosci* 10(3):403, 1993.
17. Casagrande VA, Ichida JM: The primary visual cortex. In Kaufman PL, Alm A, editors: *Adler's physiology of the eye*, ed 10, St Louis, 2003, Elsevier, p 669.
18. Krolak-Salmon P, Guenot M, Tiliket C, et al: Anatomy of optic nerve radiations as assessed by static perimetry and MRI after tailored temporal lobectomy, *Br J Ophthalmol* 84(8):884, 2000.
19. Gilbert CD, Kelly JP: The projections of cells in different layers of the cat's visual cortex, *J Comp Neurol* 163:81, 1975.
20. Hubel DH, Wiesel TN: Laminar and columnar distribution of geniculocortical fibers in the macaque monkey, *J Comp Neurol* 146:421, 1972.
21. Horton JC, Dagi LR, McCrane EP, et al: Arrangement of ocular dominance columns in human visual cortex, *Arch Ophthalmol* 108(7):1025, 1990.
22. Zeki S, Watson JD, Lueck CJ, et al: A direct demonstration of functional specialization in human visual cortex, *J Neurosci* 11(3):641, 1991.
23. Livingstone MS, Hubel DH: Segregation of form, color, movement, and depth: anatomy, physiology, and perception, *Science* 240:740, 1988.
24. Hockfield S, Tootell RB, Zaremba S: Molecular differences among neurons reveal an organization of human visual cortex, *Proc Natl Acad Sci U S A* 87(8):3027, 1990.
25. Hubel DH, Livingstone MS: Color and contrast sensitivity in the lateral geniculate body and primary visual cortex in the macaque monkey, *J Neurosci* 10(7):2223, 1990.
26. Silverman SE, Trick GL, Hart WM Jr: Motion perception is abnormal in primary open-angle glaucoma and ocular hypertension, *Invest Ophthalmol Vis Sci* 31(4):722, 1990.
27. Hubel DH, Wiesel TN: Receptive fields and functional architecture of monkey striate cortex, *J Physiol* 195:215, 1968.
28. Hubel DH, Wiesel TN, Stryker MP: Anatomical demonstration of orientation columns in macaque monkey, *J Comp Neurol* 177:361, 1978.
29. Boyd JD, Matsubara JA: Extrastriate cortex. In Kaufman PL, Alm A, editors: *Adler's physiology of the eye*, ed 10, St Louis, 2003, Elsevier, p 686.
30. Catani M, Jones DK, Donato R, et al: Occipito-temporal connections in the human brain, *Brain* 126(pt 9):2093, 2003.
31. Wurtz RH: Vision for the control of movement: the Friedenwald Lecture, *Invest Ophthalmol Vis Sci* 37:2310, 1996.
32. Roland E, Gulyás B, Seitz RJ, et al: Functional anatomy of storage, recall, and recognition of a visual pattern in man, *Neuroreport* 1:53, 1990.
33. Belliveau JW, Kennedy DN Jr, McKinstry RC, et al: Functional mapping of the human visual cortex by magnetic resonance imaging, *Science* 254(5032):716, 1991.
34. Belliveau JW, Kwong KK, Kennedy DN, et al: Magnetic resonance imaging mapping of brain function: human visual cortex, *Invest Radiol* 27(Suppl 2):59, 1992.
35. Kwong KK, Belliveau JW, Chesler DA, et al: Dynamic magnetic resonance imaging of human brain activity during primary sensory stimulation, *Proc Natl Acad Sci U S A* 89(12):5675, 1992.
36. Menon RS, Ogawa S, Kim SG, et al: Functional brain mapping using magnetic resonance imaging: signal changes accompanying visual stimulation, *Invest Radiol* 27(Suppl 2):47, 1992.
37. Le Bihan D, Turner R, Zeffiro TA, et al: Activation of human primary visual cortex during visual recall: a magnetic resonance imaging study, *Proc Natl Acad Sci U S A* 90(24):11802, 1993.
38. Ogawa S, Menon RS, Tank DW, et al: Functional brain mapping by blood oxygenation level-dependent contrast magnetic resonance imaging: a comparison of signal characteristics with a biophysical model, *Biophys J* 64(3):803, 1993.
39. MacKenzie PJ, Cioffi G: Vascular anatomy of the optic nerve head, *Can J Ophthalmol* 43:308–312, 2008.
40. Francoisa J, Neetens A, Collette JM: Vascularization of the optic pathway, *Br J Ophthalmol* 42:80, 1958.
41. Lao Y, Gao H, Zhong Y: Vascular architecture of the human optic chiasma and bitemporal hemianopia, *Chin Med Sci J* 9(1):38, 1994.
42. Ferreira A, Braga FM: Microsurgical anatomy of the anterior choroidal artery, *Arq Neuropsiquiatr* 48(4):448, 1990:(abstract).
43. Margo CE, Hamed KM, McCarty J: Congenital optic tract syndrome, *Arch Ophthalmol* 109(8):1120, 1991.
44. Luco C, Hoppe A, Schweitzer M, et al: Visual field defects in vascular lesions of the lateral geniculate body, *J Neurol Neurosurg Psychiatry* 55(1):12, 1992.
45. McFadzean R, Brosnahan D, Hadley D, et al: Representation of the visual field in the occipital striate cortex, *Br J Ophthalmol* 78(3):185, 1994.
46. Ogden TE: Nerve fiber layer of the macaque retina: retinotopic organization, *Invest Ophthalmol Vis Sci* 24:85, 1983.
47. Hoyt WF, Tudor RC: The course of parapapillary temporal retinal axons through the anterior optic nerve. A NAUTA degeneration study in the primate, *Arch Ophthalmol* 69:503, 1963.
48. Ballantyne AJ: The nerve fiber pattern of the human retina, *Trans Ophthalmol Soc UK* 66:179, 1946.
49. Kupfer C, Chumbley L, Downer J, et al: Quantitative histology of optic nerve, optic tract, and lateral geniculate nucleus of man, *J Anat* 101:393, 1967.
50. Wilbrand HL: Schema des verlaufs der sehnervenfasern durch das chiasma, *Z Augenheilk* 59 135, 1927.

51. Jeffery G: Architecture of the optic chiasm and the mechanisms that sculpt its development, *Physiol Rev* 81(4):1393, 2001.

52. Moore RY: Retinohypothalmic projection in mammals: a comparative study, *Brain Res* 49:403, 1973.

53. Berson M: Phototransduction in ganglion-cell photoreceptors, *Eur J Physiol* 454:849–855, 2007.

54. La Cour M, Ehinger B: The retina. In:Fischbarg J, editor. The biology of the eye. Amsterdam, 2006, Elsevier, p195-252.

55. Kupfer C: The projection of the macula in the lateral geniculate nucleus of man, *Am J Ophthalmol* 54:597, 1962.

56. Hickey TL, Guillery RW: Variability of laminar patterns in the human lateral geniculate body, *J Comp Neurol* 183:221, 1979.

57. Malpeli JG, Baker FH: The representation of the visual fields in the lateral geniculate body of *Macaca mulatta, J Comp Neurol* 161:569, 1975.

58. Horton JC, Hoyt WF: The representation of the visual field in human striate cortex, *Arch Ophthalmol* 109:816, 1991.

59. Reese BE, Cowey A: Fibre organization of the monkey's optic tract. A revision of the classic Holmes map, II. Noncongruent representation of the two half-retinae, *J Comp Neurol* 295(3):401, 1990.

60. Balcer LJ: Anatomic review and topographic diagnosis, *Ophthalmol Clin North Am* 14:1, 2001.

61. Holmes G, Lister WT: Disturbances of vision from cerebral lesions with special reference to the cortical representation of the macula, *Brain* 39:34, 1916.

62. Wong AM, Sharpe JA: Representation of the visual field in the human occipital cortex: a magnetic resonance imaging and perimetric correlation, *Arch Ophthalmol* 117(2):208, 1999.

63. Reinhard J, Trauzettel-Klonsinski S: Nasotemporal overlap of retinal ganglion cells in humans: a functional study, *Invest Ophthalmol Vis Sci* 44(4):1568, 2003.

64. Hirose T, Katsumi O: Functional changes: psychophysical and electrophysiologic measurements. In Albert DM, Jakobiec FA, editors: *Principles and practice of ophthalmology*, Philadelphia, 1994, Saunders, p 728.

65. Trobe JD, Glasser JS: *The visual field manual: a practical guide to testing and interpretation*, Gainesville, Fla, 1983, Triad.

66. Mendelson JR, Wells EF: Age-related changes in the visual cortex, *Vis Res* 42:695, 2002.

Autonomic Innervation of Ocular Structures

The autonomic nervous system innervates smooth muscles, glands, and the heart and consists of (1) the sympathetic system, which when stimulated prepares the body to face an emergency; and (2) the parasympathetic system, which maintains and restores the resting state. Balance is maintained between these two systems and is particularly evident in those structures innervated by both systems. The ocular structures innervated by the autonomic nervous system are the iris muscles, ciliary muscle, smooth muscles of the eyelids, choroidal and conjunctival blood vessels, and the lacrimal gland.

AUTONOMIC PATHWAY

The sympathetic pathway originates in the lateral gray column of the thoracic and upper lumbar segments (T-1 through L-2) of the spinal cord; sympathetic innervation for ocular structures originates in segments T-1 through T-3. The parasympathetic pathway originates in the midbrain, pons, medulla, and sacral spinal cord; parasympathetic innervation of ocular structures originates in the midbrain and pons.

The autonomic efferent pathway consists of two neurons. The cell body of the first, the preganglionic neuron, is located in the brain or spinal cord, whereas the cell body of the second is in a ganglion outside the central nervous system. The preganglionic fiber, which generally is myelinated, terminates in an autonomic ganglion, where a synapse occurs. The postganglionic fiber, which usually is nonmyelinated, exits the ganglion and innervates the target structure. Sympathetic ganglia usually are located near the spinal column, whereas parasympathetic ganglia are located near the target structure.

Ocular structures supplied by the sympathetic system are the iris dilator, ciliary muscle, smooth muscle of the lids, lacrimal gland, and choroidal and conjunctival blood vessels.[1-5] Ocular structures supplied by the parasympathetic system are the iris sphincter, ciliary muscle, lacrimal gland, and blood vessels.

SYMPATHETIC PATHWAY TO OCULAR STRUCTURES

Sympathetic fibers are controlled by the hypothalamus through a pathway that terminates in the lateral column of the cervical spinal cord. The fiber from the preganglionic neuron leaves the spinal cord in one of the first three thoracic nerves via the ventral root and enters the sympathetic ganglion chain located adjacent to the vertebrae (Figure 14-1). These **preganglionic fibers** then ascend in the sympathetic chain to a synapse in the **superior cervical ganglion**, located near the second and third vertebrae.[6,7]

The **postganglionic fibers** leave the ganglion, form the carotid plexus around the internal carotid artery, and enter the skull through the carotid canal. The network of fine sympathetic fibers destined for orbital structures leaves the plexus in the cavernous sinus and takes multiple pathways to the target structures. The fibers most often described in the literature are presented here.

Some of these sympathetic fibers travel with the ophthalmic division of the trigeminal nerve from the cavernous sinus into the orbit.[8] Once in the orbit the sympathetic fibers follow the nasociliary nerve and then travel with the long ciliary nerves to innervate the iris dilator and the ciliary muscle[8-12] (see Figure 14-1).

Other fibers from the carotid plexus follow this same route to the nasociliary nerve and then branch to the ciliary ganglion as the sympathetic root; these fibers pass through the ganglion without synapsing. They enter the globe as the short ciliary nerves to innervate the choroidal blood vessels. Alternately, the sympathetic root to the ciliary ganglion may emanate directly from the internal carotid plexus.[12,13] A sympathetic nerve network accompanies the ophthalmic artery and its branches could have a role in the control of blood flow to ocular structures.[14] The pathway to the conjunctival vasculature may be through either the long or the short ciliary nerves.

Other fibers from the carotid plexus join the oculomotor nerve and travel with it into the orbit to innervate the smooth muscle of the upper eyelid. These fibers follow the same path as the superior division of the

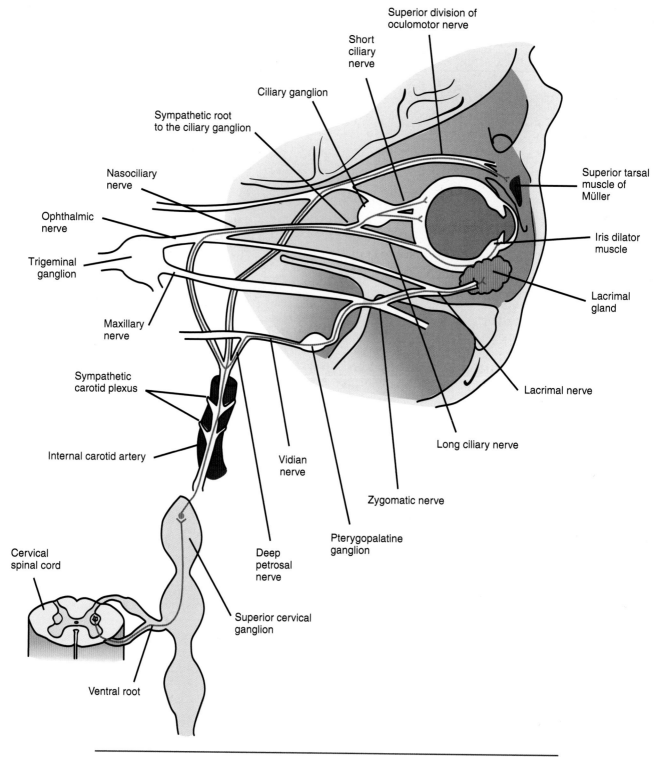

FIGURE 14-1
Sympathetic innervation to iris dilator, Müller muscle, blood vessels, and lacrimal gland.

oculomotor nerve as it supplies the levator muscle[8] (see Figure 14-1). An alternate route to Müller's muscle from the infratrochlear or lacrimal nerve has been suggested.[14]

Sympathetic stimulation activates the iris dilator, causing pupillary dilation and thereby increasing retinal illumination. It also causes vasoconstriction of the choroidal and conjunctival vessels and widening of the palpebral fissure by stimulating the smooth muscle of the eyelids. The sympathetic nerves also exhibit a small inhibitory effect on the ciliary muscle.[1-3,5,15-18]

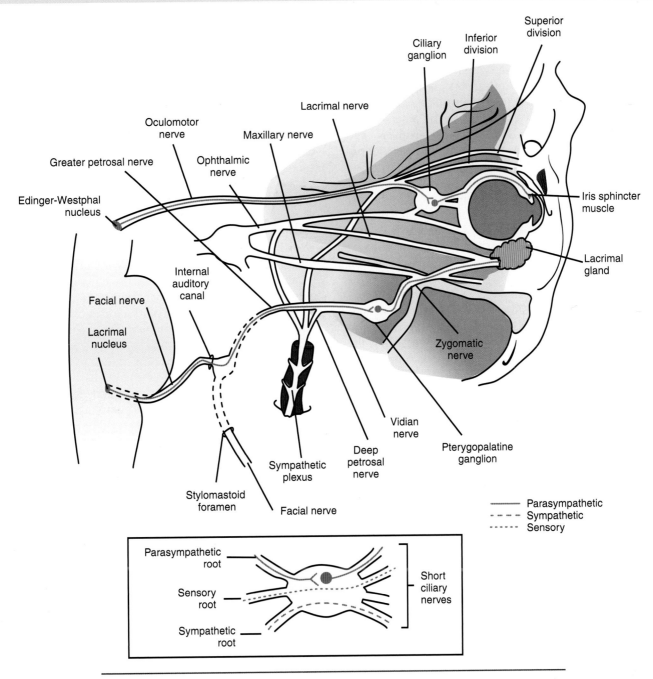

FIGURE 14-2

Parasympathetic innervation to sphincter and ciliary muscles and lacrimal gland. Inset shows sensory, sympathetic, and parasympathetic fibers into ciliary ganglion; only parasympathetic fibers synapse. Each short ciliary nerve carries all three types of fibers.

PARASYMPATHETIC PATHWAY TO OCULAR STRUCTURES

The preganglionic neuron in the parasympathetic pathway to the intrinsic ocular muscles is located in the midbrain in the **parasympathetic accessory third-nerve nucleus,** also called the **Edinger-Westphal nucleus.** The **preganglionic fibers** leave the nucleus with the motor fibers of the oculomotor nerve and follow the inferior division of

that nerve into the orbit.[19] The parasympathetic fibers leave the inferior division and enter the ciliary ganglion as the parasympathetic root[13,20-22] (Figure 14-2).

The **ciliary ganglion** is a small, somewhat flat structure, 2 mm long and 1 mm high, located within the muscle cone between the lateral rectus muscle and the optic nerve, approximately 1 cm anterior to the optic canal.[9,13,23] Three roots are located at the posterior edge of the ganglion: the **parasympathetic root,** mentioned previously; the **sensory root,** which carries sensory fibers from the globe and joins with the nasociliary nerve; and the **sympathetic root,** which supplies the blood vessels. Only the parasympathetic fibers synapse in the ciliary ganglion; the sensory and sympathetic fibers pass through without synapsing (see Figure 14-2).

The short ciliary nerves, located at the anterior edge of the ciliary ganglion, carry sensory, sympathetic, and parasympathetic fibers. The **postganglionic parasympathetic fibers,** which are myelinated,[20] exit the ganglion in the short ciliary nerves, enter the globe, and travel to the anterior segment of the eye to innervate the sphincter and ciliary muscles. Most of the fibers innervate the ciliary body; only approximately 3% supply the iris sphincter.[20,21] The two groups of neurons likely share some characteristics and differ in others, but specifics have not been identified.[24]

Parasympathetic stimulation causes pupillary constriction, thus decreasing retinal illumination and reducing chromatic and spherical aberrations. It also causes contraction of the ciliary muscle, enabling the eye to focus on near objects in accommodation.

Clinical Comment: Iris Equilibrium

The iris contains muscles innervated by both autonomic systems. The parasympathetic system innervates the sphincter, and the sympathetic system innervates the dilator. The parasympathetic and sympathetic nerves are in some state of balance in the normal, healthy, awake individual, and the size of the pupil changes constantly and rhythmically, reflecting this balance. This physiologic pupillary unrest is called hippus and is independent of changes in illumination. During sleep the pupils are small because the sympathetic system shuts down and the parasympathetic system predominates.

Clinical Comment: Inhibition of Ciliary Muscle

Parasympathetic activation causes contraction of the ciliary muscle in accommodation. Many investigators, using pharmacologic,[25,26] electrophysiologic,[27] and anatomic[20,28,29] evidence, have demonstrated the presence of both sympathetic receptors and fibers in animals and humans.[30,31] The sympathetic effect on the ciliary muscle appears to be a small, slow inhibition that is a function of the level of parasympathetic activity.[1-5]

AUTONOMIC INNERVATION TO LACRIMAL GLAND

The efferent autonomic pathway to the lacrimal gland follows a complex route. Fibers controlling the parasympathetic innervation originate in the pons in an area within the nucleus for cranial nerve VII designated as the lacrimal nucleus. These preganglionic fibers exit the

pons with the motor fibers of the facial nerve, enter the internal auditory canal, and pass through the geniculate ganglion of the facial nerve without synapsing. They leave the ganglion as the **greater petrosal nerve,** which exits the petrous portion of the temporal bone.[32] The greater petrosal nerve is joined by the **deep petrosal nerve,** composed of sympathetic postganglionic fibers from the carotid plexus. The greater petrosal and the deep petrosal nerves together form the **vidian nerve** (nerve of the pterygoid canal) (see Figures 14-1 and 14-2).

The vidian nerve enters the **pterygopalatine ganglion,** where the parasympathetic fibers synapse. The pterygopalatine ganglion (also called the **sphenopalatine ganglion**) lies in the upper portion of the pterygopalatine fossa (see Figure 12-5). It is a parasympathetic ganglion because it contains parasympathetic cell bodies and synapses; sympathetic fibers pass through without synapsing.

The autonomic fibers (all of which are now postganglionic) leave the ganglion, join with the maxillary branch of the trigeminal nerve, pass into the zygomatic nerve, and then form a communicating branch to the lacrimal nerve (see Figures 14-1 and 14-2). An alternate pathway bypasses the zygomatic nerve and travels from the ganglion directly to the gland.[33] The parasympathetic fibers that innervate the lacrimal gland are of the secretomotor type and thus cause increased secretion. The sympathetic fibers innervate the blood vessels of the gland and might indirectly cause decreased production of lacrimal gland secretion by restricting blood flow.[14] Parasympathetic stimulation causes increased lacrimation. Figure 14-3 provides a flow chart of the common autonomic nerve pathways to orbital structures. Sympathetic fibers from the zygomatic nerve also branch into the lower eyelid to innervate Müller's muscle of the lower lid.[34]

Parasympathetic innervation to the choroidal blood vessels is believed to emanate directly from the sphenopalatine ganglion through a network of fine nerves, the rami oculares.[35] Parasympathetic activation presumably causes vasodilation, which might raise intraocular pressure.[33,36]

Irritation of any branch of the trigeminal nerve activates a reflex afferent pathway, precipitating increased lacrimation.[7,37]

Clinical Comment: Corneal Reflex

Corneal touch initiates the three-part corneal reflex: lacrimation, miosis, and a protective blink (Figure 14-4). The pain sensation elicited by the touch travels to the trigeminal ganglion and then into the pons as the trigeminal nerve. Communication from the trigeminal nucleus to the Edinger-Westphal nucleus causes activation of the sphincter muscle. Communication to the facial nerve nucleus activates the motor pathway to the orbicularis muscle, causing the blink, and communication to the lacrimal nucleus and the parasympathetic pathway to the lacrimal gland stimulates increased lacrimation.

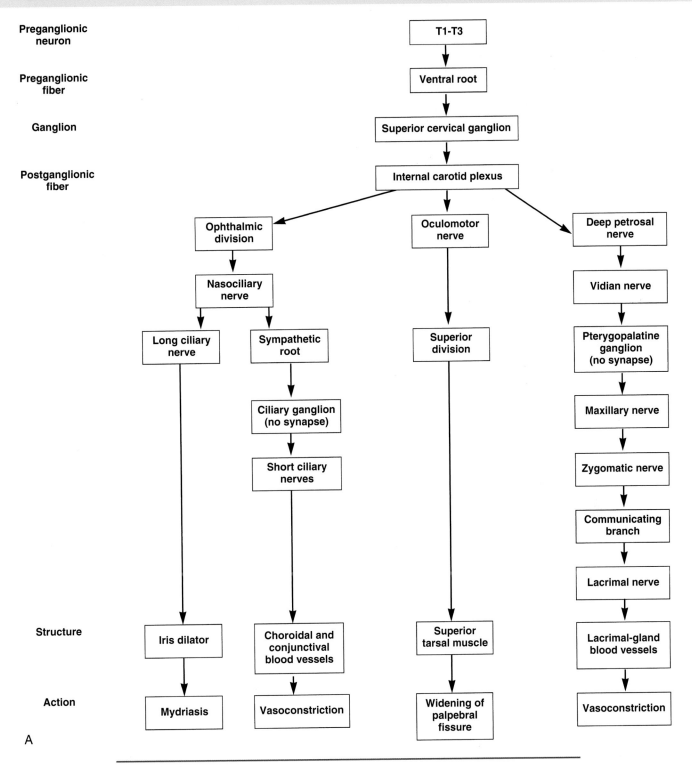

FIGURE 14-3
Flow chart of autonomic nervous system. **A,** Sympathetic innervation.

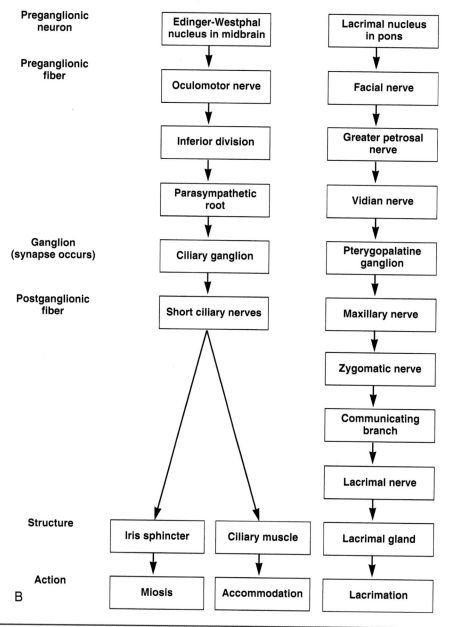

FIGURE 14-3, cont'd
B, Parasympathetic innervation.

PHARMACOLOGIC RESPONSES OF INTRINSIC MUSCLES

Pharmacologic agents can alter autonomic responses. Topical ophthalmic drugs, which readily pass through the cornea, can be used to activate or inhibit the intrinsic ocular muscles.

After a brief discussion of neurotransmitters and drug types relative to iris musculature, this section presents specific drugs that induce mydriasis or miosis, as well as drugs used in the differential diagnosis of certain pupillary abnormalities. The reader is encouraged to review a text on pharmacology for detailed information.

NEUROTRANSMITTERS

When an action potential reaches the terminal end of an axon, a neurotransmitter is released that activates either the next fiber in the pathway or the target structure, the effector. In the sympathetic pathway the

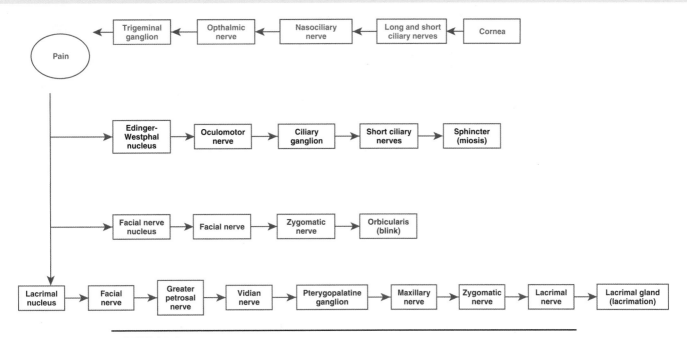

FIGURE 14-4
Corneal touch reflex. Pathways involved when pain from the cornea results in the reflex actions of miosis, blink, and lacrimation.

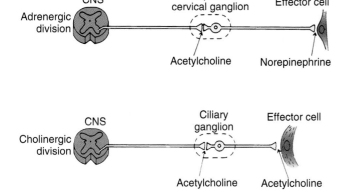

FIGURE 14-5
Autonomic neurotransmitters at their sites of action. *CNS,* Central nervous system. (From Bartlett JD, Jaanus SD: *Clinical ocular pharmacology,* ed 2, Boston, 1989, Butterworth-Heinemann.)

neurotransmitter released by the preganglionic fiber is **acetylcholine,** and the neurotransmitter released by the postganglionic fiber is **norepinephrine.** In the parasympathetic system both preganglionic and postganglionic fibers secrete acetylcholine (Figure 14-5). Fibers that release acetylcholine are called **cholinergic,** and fibers that release norepinephrine are called **adrenergic.**

The neurotransmitter binds to effector sites on the muscle and initiates a contraction. The neurotransmitter

then is released from the muscle and is either inactivated or taken back up by the nerve ending, thus preventing continual muscle spasm; further muscle contraction should occur only with another action potential and release of additional transmitter. At the cholinergic neuromuscular junction, acetylcholinesterase hydrolyzes and inactivates acetylcholine; at the adrenergic neuromuscular junction, norepinephrine is recycled, taken back up by the nerve ending.

DRUGS: AGONISTS AND ANTAGONISTS

A drug that replicates the action of a neurotransmitter is called an **agonist**. A **direct-acting agonist** is usually structurally similar to the transmitter and duplicates the action of the neurotransmitter by acting on the receptor sites of the effector. An **indirect-acting agonist** causes the action to occur either by exciting the nerve fiber, thereby causing release of the transmitter, or by preventing the recycling or reuptake of the transmitter, thus allowing it to continue its activity. **Antagonists** either block the receptor sites or block the release of the neurotransmitter, thus preventing action of the effector.

Ophthalmic Agonist Agents

Epinephrine and *phenylephrine* are **direct-acting adrenergic agonists** that bind to sites on the dilator muscle, causing contraction[38] (Figure 14-6). *Hydroxyamphetamine*

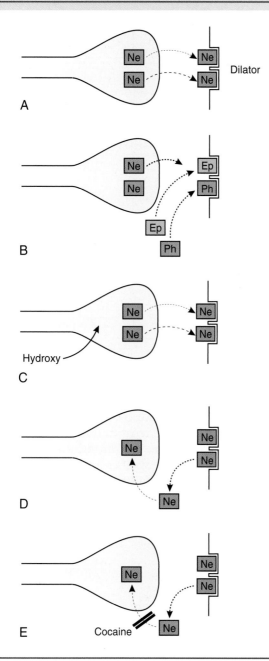

FIGURE 14-6

Adrenergic neuromuscular junction and actions of adrenergic agonists. **A,** Norepinephrine (Ne) is released by axon terminal and binds to sites on iris dilator muscle, causing contraction. **B,** Epinephrine (Ep) and phenylephrine (Ph) are direct-acting adrenergic agonists that bind to those same sites on iris dilator muscle, causing contraction. **C,** Hydroxyamphetamine (Hydroxy) is an indirect-acting adrenergic agonist that acts on nerve fiber, causing release of Ne. **D,** Once released from effector site, Ne is taken back up by nerve ending. **E,** Cocaine, an indirect-acting adrenergic agonist, prevents reuptake of Ne, allowing it to remain in neuromuscular junction and rebind to effector site.

and *cocaine* are **indirect-acting adrenergic agonists.** Hydroxyamphetamine causes the release of norepinephrine from the nerve ending, thus indirectly initiating muscle contraction. Cocaine prevents the reuptake of norepinephrine by the nerve ending; thus norepinephrine remains at the neuromuscular junction and can continue to activate the dilator.[38]

Pilocarpine is a **direct-acting cholinergic agonist** that directly stimulates the sites on the iris sphincter and ciliary muscle, causing contraction[38] (Figure 14-7). *Physostigmine* is an **indirect-acting cholinergic agonist** that inhibits acetylcholinesterase.[38] Therefore, acetylcholine is not broken down but remains in the junction, and the sphincter and ciliary muscle contraction continues in a spasm.

Ophthalmic Antagonist Agents

Dapiprazole is an **adrenergic antagonist** that blocks receptor sites, thereby preventing norepinephrine from activating the dilator muscle. *Atropine, cyclopentolate,* and *tropicamide* are **cholinergic antagonists** that compete with acetylcholine by blocking sphincter and ciliary muscle sites, thereby inhibiting miosis and accommodation[38] (Figure 14-8).

Clinical Comment: Drug-Induced Mydriasis

For maximum pupillary dilation to occur, the dilator muscle should be activated and the sphincter muscle should be inhibited. This end is achieved by the combination of a direct-acting adrenergic agonist and a cholinergic antagonist. A common procedure for a dilated fundus examination involves the use of 2.5% phenylephrine and 1% tropicamide. Phenylephrine-induced mydriasis can be reversed with dapiprazole, which blocks the dilator receptor sites and prevents phenylephrine activity.

ACCOMMODATION-CONVERGENCE REACTION (NEAR-POINT REACTION)

The accommodation-convergence reaction is not a true reflex but rather a synkinesis or an association of three occurrences: convergence, accommodation, and miosis. As an object is brought near along the midline, the medial rectus muscles contract to move the

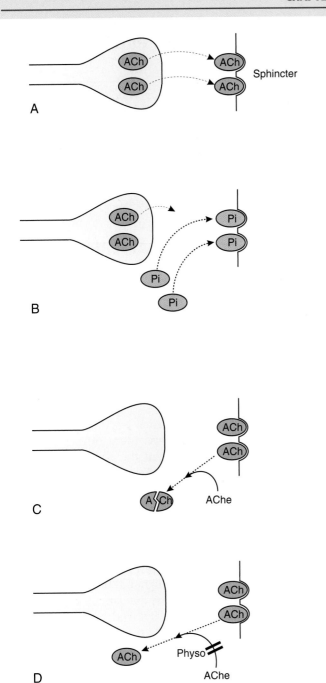

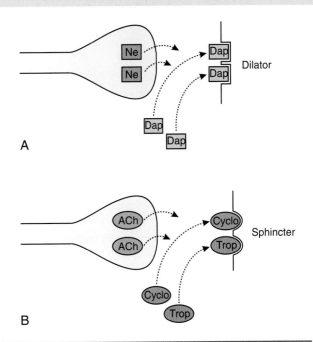

FIGURE 14-8
Actions of adrenergic and cholinergic antagonists at the neuromuscular junction. **A,** Dapiprazole (Dap) is an adrenergic antagonist that blocks receptor sites of iris dilator muscle, preventing norepinephrine (Ne) from binding and causing muscle contraction. **B,** Cyclopentolate (Cyclo) and tropicamide (Trop) are cholinergic antagonists that block receptor sites of iris sphincter muscle, preventing acetylcholine (ACh) from binding and causing muscle contraction.

FIGURE 14-7
Cholinergic neuromuscular junction and actions of cholinergic agonists. **A,** Acetylcholine (ACh) is released by axon terminal and binds to sites on iris sphincter muscle, causing contraction. **B,** Pilocarpine (Pi) is a direct-acting cholinergic agonist that binds to those sites on iris sphincter muscle, causing contraction. **C,** Once released from effector site, ACh is broken down by acetylcholinesterase (AChe), which prevents ACh from rebinding to site. **D,** Physostigmine (Physo) is an indirect-acting cholinergic agonist that inhibits AChe, allowing ACh to remain active in the neuromuscular junction.

image onto each fovea; the ciliary muscle contracts to keep the near object in focus; and the sphincter muscle constricts to decrease the size of the pupil, thereby improving depth of field.

Each of these actions can occur without the others. If plus lenses are placed in front of each eye, pupillary constriction and convergence occur without accommodation. If a base-in prism is placed in front of each eye, pupillary constriction and accommodation occur without convergence.[39]

The afferent pathway for this reaction follows the visual pathway to the striate cortex. From the striate cortex, information is sent to the frontal eye fields, which communicate with the oculomotor nucleus and the Edinger-Westphal nucleus through a pathway that passes through the internal capsule (Figure 14-9). The efferent pathway, via the oculomotor nerve, innervates the medial rectus muscle, and the parasympathetic pathway innervates the ciliary muscle and iris sphincter.

PUPILLARY LIGHT PATHWAY

An understanding of the pupillary light pathway can be an important tool in diagnosing clinical problems with pupillary manifestations. Shining a bright light into an eye normally will initiate pupillary constriction. The afferent fibers that carry this information are called **pupillary fibers,** to distinguish them from visual fibers, which carry visual information. For some time it was unclear whether there were two separate sets of fibers or whether the pupillary fibers were branches of the visual fibers.[39] It now seems that both theories are somewhat correct. One classification model groups retinal ganglion cells as W, X, and Y cells. The W cells project to the pretectum, carrying pupillary afferent information, and project to the colliculi, carrying information for reflexive eye movements. The Y cells send collateral branches to the pretectum and to the colliculi. The X cells primarily carry visual information to the lateral geniculate nucleus, with a few having collateral fibers projecting to the midbrain.[24]

The afferent pupillary light pathway parallels the visual pathway as far as the posterior optic tract, with the nasal fibers crossing in the chiasm. The pupillary fibers exit in the posterior third of the optic tract and travel within the brachium of the superior colliculus to an area of the midbrain known as the **pretectal nucleus,** located near the superior colliculus. Synapse occurs, and the fibers that leave the pretectal region travel to the two Edinger-Westphal nuclei, distributing about equally to both.[39] The fibers that cross to the opposite Edinger-Westphal nucleus travel in the **posterior commissure** (Figure 14-10).

The efferent parasympathetic pathway from the Edinger-Westphal nucleus to the sphincter and ciliary muscles is described earlier under the Parasympathetic Pathway to Ocular Structures section. As the third nerve leaves the midbrain, the pupillomotor fibers generally lie in a *superior* position; but as the nerve leaves the cavernous sinus and enters the orbit, the pupillomotor fibers move into an *inferior* position and travel in the inferior division of the oculomotor nerve.[39]

While the parasympathetic system is activated, an inhibition of the dilator muscle apparently occurs. When light is removed from the eye and the Edinger-Westphal neurons stop firing, the preganglionic sympathetic fibers are no longer inhibited, their firing rate increases, and the dilator muscle increases in tone.[24] The fibers that carry the inhibition message from the retina likely pass through an accessory optic system to the cervical spinal cord. There is similar inhibition of the parasympathetic innervation while the sympathetic nerves cause dilator contraction. These inhibitory fibers course through the midbrain.[24]

Clinical Comment: Pupillary Light Response

> *In assessment of the pupillary light pathway, both the direct response and the consensual response are tested. When a bright light is directed into the eye, both a direct response (constriction of the ipsilateral iris) and a consensual response (constriction of the contralateral iris) occur. The consensual response occurs because of the two crossings of the fibers in the pathway: The nasal retinal fibers cross in the chiasm, and approximately half the fibers from each pretectal nucleus cross in the posterior commissure.*

DISRUPTION IN THE AFFERENT PATHWAY

A disruption in the afferent pathway will affect both direct and consensual responses. For example, in the presence of a disruption in the right afferent pathway, a light directed into the right eye will cause a poor response in both the right and the left eyes, although both responses would be normal if the light were directed into the left eye. If the damage to the afferent pathway is complete (i.e., all the fibers from one eye are affected), there would be no direct and no consensual response when light is directed into the affected eye. More often, only some fibers are damaged, such that the abnormal pupillary responses might be recognized only when compared with the normal pupillary responses; thus the term **relative afferent pupillary defect (RAPD)** is applied.

Disruption can occur anywhere in the afferent pathway: retina, optic nerve, chiasm, optic tract, or superior brachium. The swinging-flashlight test can be used to determine the presence of an RAPD. Damage posterior to the crossing in the chiasm might not be evident with the swinging-flashlight test unless the damage affects a great number of fibers from one eye and significantly fewer fibers from the other eye.[40] There are more crossed (contralateral) fibers in the optic tract than uncrossed (ipsilateral); therefore, with a complete optic tract lesion the pupillary constrictions may be greater with light into the ipsilateral eye than with light into the contralateral eye.

Clinical Comment: Swinging-Flashlight Test

> *The patient is asked to fixate on a distant object, and then the practitioner swings a light from eye to eye, several times rhythmically, taking care to illuminate each pupil for an equal length of time, about 2 or 3 seconds. If both pathways are normal, little or no change in pupil size will be noted; the eye will not recover from the consensual response before it is subjected to the direct light beam. The normal, symmetric response is characterized by equal pupillary*

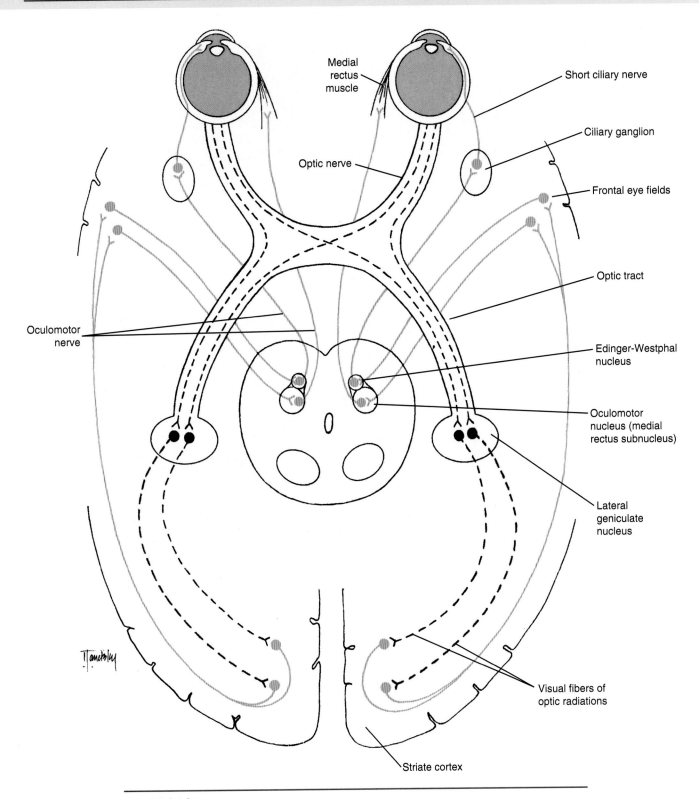

FIGURE 14-9
The near pupillary response. Dotted lines indicate visual pathway fibers carrying visual information from the eye to the visual cortex. Solid lines indicate pathway from the striate cortex to the frontal eye fields, then to the oculomotor nucleus, and from there to the medial rectus, ciliary, and sphincter muscles.

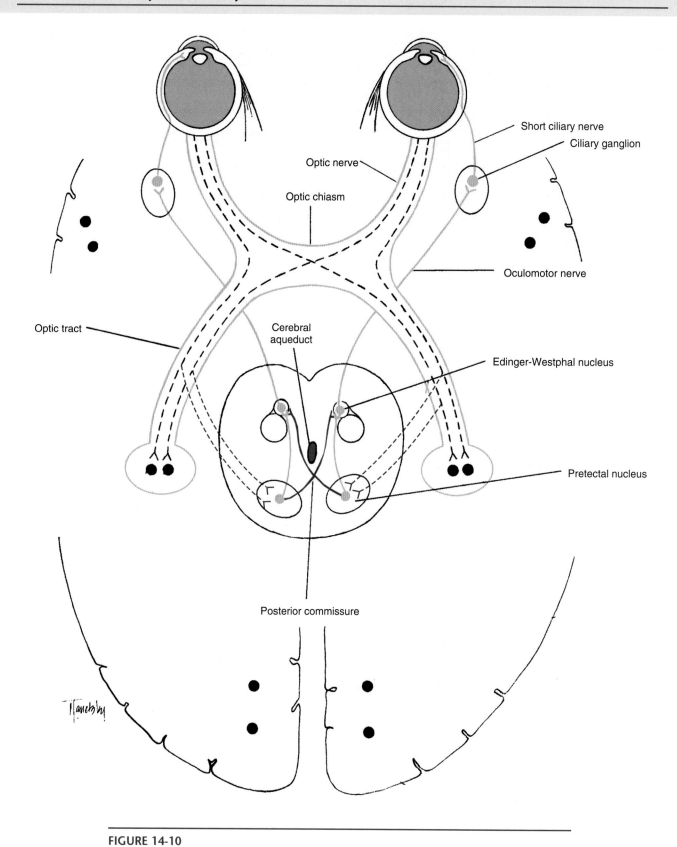

FIGURE 14-10
The pupillary light pathway. Dotted lines indicate the afferent pathway and solid lines the efferent pathway.

constriction in both eyes when the light is presented to either eye. An abnormal response is characterized by larger pupils when the light is directed into the affected eye than when the light is directed into the normal eye (Figure 14-11).

As the intensity of the light increases, stronger constrictions occur when light is presented to a normal eye. There is a threshold, however, beyond which no increase occurs. A very bright light can be used for detecting subtle defects; however, the luminance level should be recorded because a future change in the measured RAPD might reflect only a different light condition.[41,42]

Clinical Comment: Afferent Pupillary Defect in Cataract

It would appear likely that a dense cataract would cause an RAPD because less light penetrates a cataract to stimulate the retina. In a clinical situation, however, a dense cataract has been found to cause an RAPD in the contralateral eye.[43,44] Light scattered back to the retina from the lens opacity probably produces an enhanced pupillary response, which is manifested as an RAPD of the contralateral eye.

Clinical Comment: Optic Neuritis

The most common site of damage in an RAPD is the optic nerve. Ninety percent of patients with optic neuritis exhibit an RAPD during some stage of the disease.[39]

DISRUPTION WITHIN THE CENTRAL NERVOUS SYSTEM

A lesion in the midbrain can involve the pretectal nucleus, the fibers leaving the nucleus, or the parasympathetic Edinger-Westphal nucleus. Damage to the pretectal nucleus might not cause a pupillary defect as fibers from the other pretectal nucleus still supply both parasympathetic nuclei.

Injury to the dorsal tegmentum of the midbrain, that interrupts the fibers from the pretectal nucleus to the parasympathetic third-nerve nucleus, if limited to one side and affecting all fibers into the Edinger-Westphal nucleus, results in a pupil that shows a poor direct and consensual response but does constrict with the near response. This pupillary response is commonly called the **Argyll Robertson pupil** and is said to show a "light-near dissociation.[45]" Since the fibers carrying the message for the near reaction approach the Edinger-Westphal nucleus from a more ventral location, they do not pass through the affected area of the midbrain. Since the pathway from the frontal eye fields is intact and the efferent path is viable, the sphincter and ciliary muscle still will constrict to a near object.[46] In the Argyll Robertson pupil, the retained near response exceeds the best direct-light response (Figure 14-12), and when the patient looks from near to distant, the pupils redilate briskly.

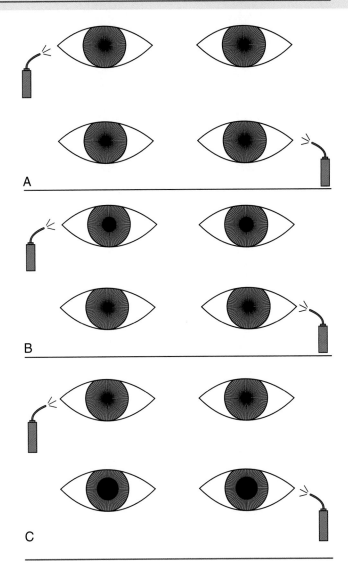

FIGURE 14-11

Swinging-flashlight test. A, Response is equal and symmetric, indicating no relative pupillary defect. **B,** Response is unequal, with both pupils growing larger as light is directed into the right eye, indicating a grade 1+ (relative afferent pupillary defect, right eye (RAPD OD). **C,** Unequal pupillary response in which both pupils enlarge as light is directed into the left eye, indicating a grade 3+ relative afferent pupillary defect, left eye (RAPD OS).

Because the fibers that carry inhibitory feedback to the parasympathetic nucleus also pass through the dorsal midbrain, miosis is a component of the Argyll Robertson syndrome and is evident in darkness, with the affected pupil smaller than would be seen in the normal individual.[24] The Argyll Robertson syndrome is bilateral in approximately 80% to 90% of cases, but the two sides may be affected unequally.[24] Diabetic neuropathy, alcoholic neuropathy, or neurosyphilis is suspected in a complete Argyll Robertson pupil that involves both sides. A near response that exceeds the light response is always a sign of a pathologic pupil.[24]

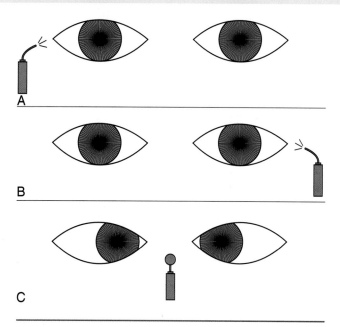

FIGURE 14-12
Argyll Robertson pupil, right eye (OD). A, Poor direct response OD and normal consensual response left eye (OS). **B,** Normal direct response OS and poor consensual response OD. **C,** Normal near response in both eyes.

DISRUPTION IN THE EFFERENT PATHWAY

A lesion in the efferent pathway will cause the eye to show poor direct and consensual pupillary responses and a poor near response. The pupil appears large on clinical presentation, and other ocular structures are involved. Damage in the oculomotor nucleus or nerve could involve the superior rectus, medial rectus, inferior rectus, inferior oblique, or levator muscle, and the patient should be examined for related ocular motility impairment. The parasympathetic fibers in the oculomotor nerve are often spared in ischemic lesions, as from diabetes, but are especially vulnerable to compression because the fibers are superficial as the nerve emerges from the midbrain.[24] Third nerve involvement that includes a dilated pupil is highly suspicious of a compressive intracranial lesion.

Damage to the ciliary ganglion or the short ciliary nerves could be caused by local injury or disease and results in a **tonic pupil,** which is characterized by poor pupillary light response and loss of accommodation. Decreased corneal sensitivity often occurs because some afferent sensory fibers from the cornea pass through the short ciliary nerves and the ganglion.[47] The affected muscle may exhibit *cholinergic denervation supersensitivity,* a physiologic phenomenon resulting from injury to the fibers directly innervating muscles.[48] The near response is retained, but it is delayed and slow, and the pupil redilates sluggishly. One theory postulates that

because the density of the innervation to the ciliary muscle is much greater than the density of innervation to the sphincter, some ciliary muscle nerve fibers remain intact. With near stimulation, these fibers release acetylcholine, which diffuses into the aqueous humor and then causes the supersensitive sphincter to constrict.[49] In late stages of this condition, the pupil becomes tonic and the miotic near reaction difficult to demonstrate, but the accommodative facility appears to recover, perhaps as a result of regeneration of the fibers.[20,50]

Clinical Comment: Adie's Tonic Pupil

If the cause of the tonic pupil is not apparent, the syndrome is called **Adie's tonic pupil.** The typical patient with Adie's pupil is a woman 20 to 40 years of age; 90% of these patients also have diminished tendon reflexes. Because of this systemic manifestation, it is believed that similar degenerative processes are occurring in the ciliary ganglion and in the dorsal column of the spinal cord,[51] but the cause is unknown.[52] If pupillary constriction in early Adie's pupil is examined with the biomicroscope, segmental constriction affecting only a section of the iris may be evident.[53] An Adie's pupil that has been tonic for years eventually becomes smaller and does not dilate well in the dark; thus it is the larger pupil in light and the smaller one in darkness.[50]

In the differential diagnosis of Adie's pupil, a very mild, direct-acting cholinergic agonist can be used because the sphincter muscle is supersensitive.[20,54] A dilute concentration of pilocarpine (0.125%) has minimal effect on a normal sphincter but will cause significant clinical miosis in a supersensitive sphincter. Some investigators believe that a normal pupil can respond to the 0.125% pilocarpine and recommend using a 0.0625% pilocarpine solution.[55] With one drop instilled in each eye, the Adie's pupil should show a much greater constriction than the normal pupil (Figure 14-13). There is indication that a tonic pupil might in some cases be associated with autoimmune disease.[56]

Clinical Comment: Fixed, Dilated Pupil

Recent onset of a fixed, dilated pupil could be caused by accidental drug-induced mydriasis. Investigation of the individual's profession might indicate the handling of drugs (pharmacists, nurses) or chemicals that could exert such an effect (farmers, crop dusters, exterminators). Such a pupil will not respond to 0.125% pilocarpine. Some over-the-counter drops that promise to "get the red out" may also cause a dilated pupil.

DISRUPTION IN THE SYMPATHETIC PATHWAY

An interruption in the sympathetic pathway causes miosis. The usual tone that the dilator muscle normally exerts is not present, and there is no counteracting pull against the sphincter muscle, making the pupil smaller

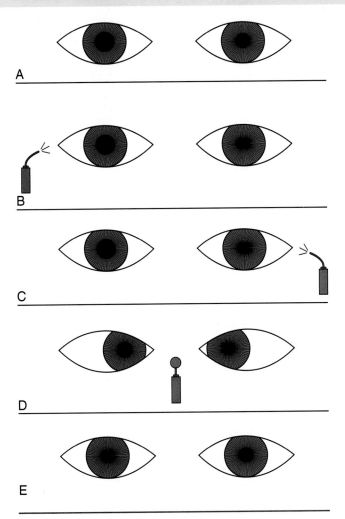

FIGURE 14-13
Adie's pupil OD. A, Presenting anisocoria; right pupil is larger than left pupil. **B,** Poor direct response OD and normal consensual response OS. **C,** Normal direct response OS and poor consensual response OD. **D,** Slow and long-lasting near response. **E,** Pilocarpine 0.125% instilled in both eyes. Miosis OD, no response OS.

than normal. **Anisocoria** (a difference in pupil size) is present under normal room light conditions but is more pronounced in dim light, with the normal eye having the larger pupil. The pupil responds briskly to light, but with slow and incomplete dilation in the dark. If the anisocoria decreases in bright lights and the pupils react normally to a light stimulus, the disruption is likely a sympathetic interruption to the dilator muscle or benign anisocoria.[50]

Clinical Comment: Benign Anisocoria

*Approximately 20% of the population have **benign anisocoria** (also called simple or physiologic anisocoria), which is usually more apparent in dim light than in room light, with the*

difference between pupils usually less than 1 mm.[50] Sometimes the anisocoria may switch sides, but both pupils are round and react well to all stimuli and dilate equally with the lights off. It represents an asymmetric balance between the sympathetic and parasympathetic innervation to the iris. Benign anisocoria may be caused by asymmetric supranuclear inhibition of the Edinger-Westphal nucleus.[50]

Clinical Comment: Horner's Syndrome

CLINICAL FEATURES
*Damage in the sympathetic pathway to the head can cause **Horner's syndrome**, which consists of ptosis, miosis, and facial anhidrosis (absence of sweat secretion). Loss of innervation to the smooth muscle of the upper eyelid causes ptosis, whereas loss of innervation to the lower eyelid causes it to rise slightly such that the palpebral fissure appears narrow, simulating enophthalmos (Figure 14-14).*

The damage can occur anywhere along the sympathetic pathway in the brain, spinal cord, preganglionic path, or postganglionic path. Involvement of the central neuron, which sends its fiber from the hypothalamus through the spinal cord to a synapse with the preganglionic neuron in the cervical dorsal column, can also cause other problems (e.g., vertigo).

The preganglionic fibers leave the dorsal column of the spinal cord, pass into the chest, course over the apex of the lung, and loop around the subclavian artery en route to the superior cervical ganglion (Figure 14-15). These fibers can be damaged in thoracic injury or surgery or in metastatic disease involving the chest.[6]

The postganglionic fibers that enter the skull through the carotid plexus can be damaged by a fracture of the skull base or an injury to the internal carotid artery. Painful Horner's syndrome is a classical symptom of carotid artery dissection and should be treated as an emergent situation.[56] Horner's in combination with a sixth nerve paresis indicates cavernous sinus involvement and a mass in or near the sinus must be ruled out.[56] Damage along the rest of the postganglionic neuron can involve the nasociliary or long ciliary nerves.

IRIS HETEROCHROMIA IN HORNER'S PUPIL
Normal sympathetic innervation is necessary for the development and maintenance of iris melanocyte pigmentation. In congenital Horner's syndrome, normal iris pigmentation fails to develop, and heterochromia is present (Figure 14-16). Heterochromia is rarely seen in acquired Horner syndrome but may develop after long-standing conditions.[24]

DIFFERENTIAL DIAGNOSIS
In addition to the clinical presentation of ptosis and miosis, dilation lag occurs in dim illumination, and this will differentiate Horner's pupil from simple anisocoria. The normal pupil dilates within 5 seconds of lights being off because of the normal sympathetic activity to the dilator and the parasympathetic inactivation of the sphincter. In the Horner's pupil there is no sympathetic activity, and the pupil thus dilates only from inactivation of the sphincter muscle and dilates more slowly, taking

10 to 20 seconds.[50,56] Dilation lag does not occur with physiologic anisocoria.[56]

The location of the disruption of the sympathetic pathway is useful in determining appropriate care. In the differential diagnosis of Horner's syndrome, diagnostic drugs used to determine the site of interruption include cocaine and hydroxyamphetamine, the effects of which are shown in Figures 14-17 and 14-18. If the sympathetic pathway is intact, instillation of one drop of a 5% or 10% ophthalmic cocaine solution, an indirect-acting adrenergic agonist, causes dilation in 30 to 60 minutes.[50,57,58] In contrast, with a disruption anywhere in the pathway, norepinephrine is lacking in the neuromuscular junction, and therefore cocaine has little or no effect, and the pupil dilates poorly.

Hydroxyamphetamine 1% can be administered to determine whether the damage is in the preganglionic or postganglionic pathway.[59-61] A topical administration of this indirect-acting adrenergic agonist acts on the postganglionic fiber, causing release of norepinephrine. If the lesion is in the preganglionic pathway, the postganglionic fiber still is viable and will contain stores of norepinephrine. Instillation of hydroxyamphetamine will cause release of the neurotransmitter, and dilation will occur. If the damage is in the ganglion or the postganglionic fiber, norepinephrine will not be stored in the nerve endings, and therefore no dilation will occur with instillation of hydroxyamphetamine. The instillation should occur 24 to 48 hours after the cocaine test, and dilation may take up to an hour.[50,62]

In the presence of preganglionic and central lesions, the pupil on the affected side usually dilates more than the normal eye with hydroxyamphetamine instillation, either because of enhanced receptor sensitivity or because the adrenergic nerve endings have accumulated more norepinephrine.[62,63] In adults, central Horner's syndrome is often related to stroke, preganglionic Horner's often is associated with neoplasm, and postganglionic Horner's syndrome may have a vascular cause.[50]

An alternative drug might be used in diagnosing postganglionic involvement because the dilator muscle could be supersensitive to a sympathomimetic and a solution of 1% phenylephrine could cause contraction. In the normal pupil, 1% phenylephrine will generally cause

continued on page 271

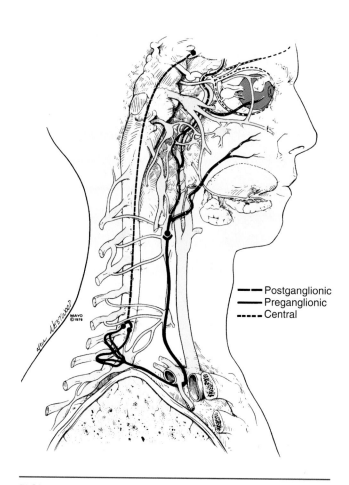

FIGURE 14-15

Sympathetic innervation of the eye. Preganglionic pathway courses from the superior cervical ganglion into the thoracic cavity before entering the skull. (From Maloney WF, Younge BR, Moyer NJ: Evaluation of the causes and accuracy of pharmacologic localization in Horner's syndrome, *Am J Ophthalmol* 90:394, 1980. With permission from the Mayo Foundation.)

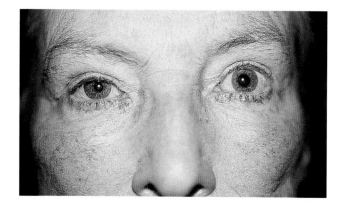

FIGURE 14-14

Ptosis and miosis in Horner's syndrome. (From Kanski JJ, Nischal KK: *Ophthalmology: clinical signs and differential diagnosis*, St Louis, 1999, Mosby.)

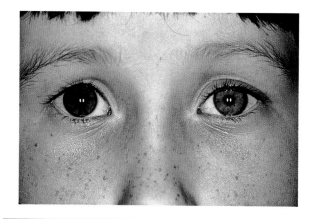

FIGURE 14-16

Iris heterochromia in congenital Horner's syndrome. (From Kanski JJ, Nischal KK: *Ophthalmology: clinical signs and differential diagnosis*, St Louis, 1999, Mosby.)

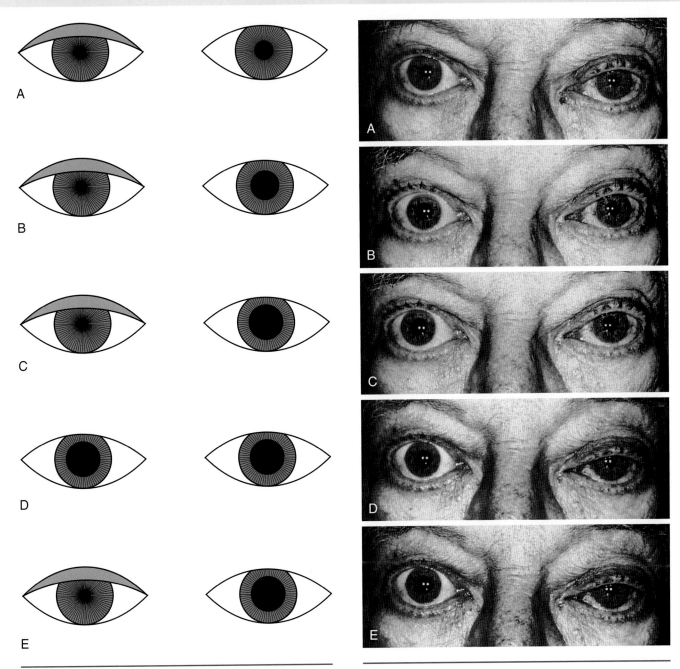

FIGURE 14-17

Horner's syndrome. A, Presenting anisocoria; left pupil is larger than right pupil. Ptosis OD. **B,** Anisocoria greater in dim illumination. **C,** Cocaine 5% instilled in each eye (OU). No response OD, mydriasis OS, interruption in sympathetic pathway OD. **D,** Hydroxyamphetamine 1% instilled OU. Mydriasis OU, interruption in preganglionic pathway OD. **E,** Hydroxyamphetamine 1% instilled OU. No response OD, mydriasis OS, interruption in postganglionic pathway OD. Note also ptosis OD due to involvement of Müller's muscle.

FIGURE 14-18

Dilation lag in 72-year-old man with Horner's syndrome in left eye. **A,** Obvious anisocoria in bright illumination. **B,** Greater anisocoria at 4 to 5 seconds in darkness compared with (**C**) anisocoria at 10 to 12 seconds in darkness. **D,** Cocaine test for Horner's syndrome. After instillation of 10% cocaine OU, there is dilation of normal right pupil but absence of dilation in left Horner's pupil. **E,** Hydroxyamphetamine test in Horner's syndrome. After instillation of 1% hydroxyamphetamine OU, there is dilation of normal right pupil but absence of dilation of left Horner's pupil, indicating a postganglionic lesion. (From Bartlett JD, Jaanus SD: *Clinical ocular pharmacology*, ed 2, Boston, 1989, Butterworth-Heinemann.)

only minimal dilation but in some clinical patients with a postganglionic lesion, the Horner's pupil was found to respond sooner and more vigorously than the unaffected pupil.[64] With a preganglionic lesion, the Horner's pupil would be expected to only dilate minimally although validation with published findings has yet to occur.

In evaluating a patient with anisocoria, if the difference between the pupils is greater in dim light, the smaller pupil is the defective one and the clinician must differentiate between benign anisocoria and Horner's pupil. With benign anisocoria, the pupil will react well to all stimuli and will redilate well in the dark. The Horner's pupil reacts well to all stimuli but redilates poorly in the dark.

If the anisocoria is more evident in bright light, it occurs because the pupil constricts poorly and the larger pupil is the pathologic one. This may be caused by drugs, it may be a tonic pupil, or it may be caused by an efferent defect. Associated symptoms will assist in the diagnosis, and such a pupil abnormality, if accompanied by headache, requires a workup for intracranial involvement.

REFERENCES

1. Olmsted JMD, Morgan MW: The influence of the cervical sympathetic nerve on the lens of the eye, *Am J Physiol* 133:720, 1941.
2. Olmsted JMD: The role of the autonomic nervous system in accommodation for near and far vision, *J Nerv Ment Dis* 99:794, 1944.
3. Morgan MW: The nervous control of accommodation, *Am J Optom* 21:87, 1944.
4. Gilmartin B: A review of the role of sympathetic innervation of the ciliary muscle in ocular accommodation, *Ophthalmic Physiol Opt* 6(1):23, 1986.
5. Rosenfield M, Gilmartin B: Oculomotor consequences of beta-adrenoceptor antagonism during sustained near vision, *Ophthalmic Physiol Opt* 7(2):127, 1987.
6. Maloney WF, Younge BR, Moyer NJ: Evaluation of the causes and accuracy of pharmacologic localization in Horner's syndrome, *Am J Ophthalmol* 90:394, 1980.
7. Doxanas MT, Anderson RL: *Clinical orbital anatomy*, Baltimore, 1984, Williams & Wilkins, pp 93, 131.
8. Pick TP, Howden R, editors: *Gray's anatomy*, ed 15, New York, 1977, Crown, p 799.
9. Warwick R: *Eugene Wolff's anatomy of the eye and orbit*, ed 7, Philadelphia, 1976, Saunders, p 306.
10. Mohney JB, Morgan MW, Olmsted JMD, et al: The pathway of sympathetic nerves to the ciliary muscles in the eye, *Am J Physiol* 135:759, 1942.
11. Ruskell GL: Sympathetic innervation of the ciliary muscle in monkeys, *Exp Eye Res* 16:183, 1973.
12. Natori Y, Rhoton AL: Microsurgical anatomy of the superior orbital fissure, *Neurosurgery* 36:762–775, 1995.
13. Izci Y, Gonul E: The microsurgical anatomy of the ciliary ganglion and its clinical importance in orbital traumas: an anatomic study, *Minim Invasive Neurosurg* 49:156–160, 2006.
14. Thakker MM, Huang J, Possin DE, et al: Human orbital sympathetic nerve pathways, *Ophthal Plast Reconstr Surg* 24:360–366, 2008.
15. Gilmartin B, Hogan RE: The relationship between tonic accommodation and ciliary muscle innervation, *Invest Ophthalmol Vis Sci* 26:1024, 1985.
16. Gilmartin B, Bullimore MA, Rosenfield M, et al: Pharmacological effects on accommodative adaptation, *Optom Vis Sci* 69(4):276, 1992.
17. Winn B, Culhane HM, Gilmartin B, et al: Effect of ß-adrenoceptor antagonists on autonomic control of ciliary smooth muscle, *Ophthalmic Physiol Opt* 22(5):359, 2002.
18. Gilmartin B, Mallen EAH, Wolffsohn JS: Sympathetic control of accommodation: evidence for inter-subject variation, *Ophthalmic Physiol Opt* 22(5):366, 2002.
19. Warwick R: The ocular parasympathetic nerve supply and its mesencephalic sources, *J Anat* 88:71, 1954.
20. Ruskell GL: Accommodation and the nerve pathway to the ciliary muscle: a review, *Ophthalmic Physiol Opt* 10(3):239, 1990.
21. Burde RM: Direct parasympathetic pathway to the eye: revisited, *Brain Res* 463:158, 1988.
22. Reiner A, Erichsen JT, Cabot JB, et al: Neurotransmitter organization of the nucleus of Edinger-Westphal and its projection to the avian ciliary ganglion, *Vis Neurosci* 6(5):451, 1991.
23. Duke-Elder W: *The anatomy of the visual system, vol 2, System of ophthalmology*, St Louis, 1961, Mosby, p 497.
24. Loewenfeld IE: *The pupil: anatomy, physiology, and clinical applications*, Boston, 1999, Butterworth-Heinemann.
25. Tornqvist G: The relative importance of the parasympathetic and sympathetic nervous systems for accommodation in monkeys, *Invest Ophthalmol Vis Sci* 6:612, 1967.
26. Hurwitz BS, Dacidowitz J, Chin NB, et al: The effects of the sympathetic nervous system on accommodation. I. Beta sympathetic nervous system, *Arch Ophthalmol* 87:668, 1972.
27. Tornqvist G: Effect of cervical sympathetic stimulation on accommodation in monkeys. An example of a beta-adrenergic inhibitory effect, *Acta Physiol Scand* 67:363, 1967.
28. Van Alphen GW: The adrenergic receptors of the intraocular muscles of the human eye, *Invest Ophthalmol Vis Sci* 15:502, 1976.
29. Wax MB, Molinoff PB: Distribution and properties of beta-adrenergic receptors in human iris/ciliary body, *Invest Ophthalmol Vis Sci* 25(Suppl):305, 1984:(ARVO abstract).
30. Stephens KG: Effect of the sympathetic nervous system on accommodation, *Am J Optom Physiol Opt* 62(6):402, 1985.
31. Miller RJ, Takahama M: Arousal-related changes in dark focus accommodation and dark vergence, *Invest Ophthalmol Vis Sci* 29(7):1168, 1988.
32. Monkhouse WS: The anatomy of the facial nerve, *Ear Nose Throat J* 69:677, 1990.
33. Ruskell GL: An ocular parasympathetic nerve pathway of facial nerve origin and its influence on intraocular pressure, *Exp Eye Res* 106:323, 1970.
34. Rodriguez-Vazquez JF, Merida-Velasco JR, Jimenez-Collado J: Orbital muscle of Müller: observations on human fetuses measuring 35-150 mm, *Acta Anat (Basel)* 139(4):300, 1990.
35. Ruskell GL: Facial nerve distribution to the eye, *Am J Optom Physiol Opt* 62(11):793, 1985.
36. Stjernschantz J, Bill A: Vasomotor effects of facial nerve stimulation: non-cholinergic vasodilation in the eye, *Acta Physiol Scand* 109:45, 1980.
37. Wobig JL: The lacrimal apparatus. In Reeh MJ, Wobig JL, Wirtschafter JD, editors: *Ophthalmic anatomy*, San Francisco, 1981, American Academy of Ophthalmology, p 55.
38. Jaanus SD, Pagano VT, Bartlett JD: Drugs affecting the autonomic nervous system. In Bartlett JD, Jaanus SD, editors: *Clinical ocular pharmacology*, ed 3, Boston, 1995, Butterworth-Heinemann, p 168.
39. Thompson HS: The pupil. In Hart WM Jr, editor: *Adler's physiology of the eye*, ed 9, St Louis, 1992, Mosby, p 412.
40. Newman SA, Miller NR: The optic tract syndrome. Neuro-ophthalmologic considerations, *Arch Ophthalmol* 101:1241, 1983.
41. Johnson LN: The effect of light intensity on measurement of the relative afferent pupillary defect, *Am J Ophthalmol* 109(4):481, 1990.
42. Lam BL, Thompson HS: Brightness sense and the relative afferent pupillary defect, *Am J Ophthalmol* 108(4):462, 1989.

43. Sadun AA, Bassi CJ, Lessell S: Why cataracts do not produce afferent pupillary defects, *Am J Ophthalmol* 110(6):712, 1990.

44. Lam BL, Thompson HS: A unilateral cataract produces a relative afferent pupillary defect in the contralateral eye, *Ophthalmology* 97(3):334, 1990.

45. Loewenfeld IE: The Argyll Robertson pupil, 1869-1969: a critical survey of the literature, *Surv Ophthalmol* 14:199, 1969.

46. Thompson HS: Light-near dissociation of the pupil, *Ophthalmologica* 189:21, 1984.

47. Purcell JJ, Krachmer JH, Thompson HS: Corneal sensation in Adie's syndrome, *Am J Ophthalmol* 84:496, 1977.

48. Scheie HG: Site of disturbance in Adie's syndrome, *Arch Ophthalmol* 24:225, 1940.

49. Wirtschafter JD, Volk CR, Sawchuk RJ: Transaqueous diffusion of acetylcholine to denervated iris sphincter muscle: a mechanism for the tonic pupil syndrome (Adie syndrome), *Ann Neurol* 4:1, 1978.

50. Kawasaki A, Kardon R: Disorders of the pupil, *Ophthalmol Clin North Am* 14(1):149, 2001.

51. Selhorst JB, Madge G, Ghatak N: The neuropathology of the Holmes-Adie syndrome, *Ann Neurol* 16:138, 1984.

52. Harriman DG, Garland H: The pathology of Adie's syndrome, *Brain* 91:401, 1968.

53. Thompson HS: Segmental palsy of the iris sphincter in Adie's syndrome, *Arch Ophthalmol* 96:1615, 1978.

54. Bourgon P, Pilley FJ, Thompson HS: Cholinergic supersensitivity of the iris sphincter in Adie's tonic pupil, *Am J Ophthalmol* 85:373, 1978.

55. Leavitt JA, Wayman LL, Hodge DO, et al: Pupillary response to four concentrations of pilocarpine in normal subjects: application to testing for Adie tonic pupil, *Am J Ophthalmol* 133:333, 2002.

56. Wilhelm H: The pupil *Curr Opin Neurol* 21:36–42, 2008.

57. Kardon RH, Denison CE, Brown CK, et al: Critical evaluation of the cocaine test in the diagnosis of Horner's syndrome, *Arch Ophthalmol* 108(3):384, 1990.

58. Thompson HS, Mensher JH: Horner's syndrome, *Am J Ophthalmol* 72:472, 1974.

59. Cremer SA, Thompson HS, Digre KB, et al: Hydroxyamphetamine mydriasis in normal subjects, *Am J Ophthalmol* 110(1):66, 1990.

60. Thompson HS, Mensher JH: Adrenergic mydriasis in Horner's syndrome: hydroxyamphetamine test for diagnosis of postganglionic defects, *Am J Ophthalmol* 72:472, 1971.

61. Salvesen R, di-Souza CD, Sjaastad O: Horner's syndrome: sweat gland and pupillary responsiveness in two cases with a probable 3rd neurone dysfunction, *Cephalalgia* 9(1):63, 1989.

62. Patel S, Ilsen PF: Acquired Horner's syndrome: clinical review, *Optometry* 74(4):245, 2003.

63. Cremer SA, Thompson HS, Digre KB, et al: Hydroxyamphetamine mydriasis in Horner's syndrome, *Am J Ophthalmol* 110(1):71, 1990.

64. Danesh-Meyer HV, Savino P, Sergott R: The correlation of phenylephrine 1% with hydroxyamphetamine 1% in Horner's syndrome, *Br J Ophthalmol* 88:592–593, 2004.

Index

Page references followed by "f" indicate figure, by "b" indicate box, and by "t" indicate table.